Date Due

MAR 27 2002			

BRODART, CO.   Cat. No. 23-233-003   Printed in U.S.A.

Atherosclerosis XII

Atherosclerosis XII

Proceedings of the XIIth International Symposium on
Atherosclerosis held in Stockholm on 25–29 June 2000

Editors:

Sten Stemme
Associate Professor
Karolinska Institute
Center for Molecular Medicine
Karolinska Hospital
Stockholm
Sweden

Professor Anders G. Olsson
Department of Medicine and Care
University Hospital
Linköping
Sweden

2000

ELSEVIER

Amsterdam – London – New York – Oxford – Paris – Shannon – Tokyo

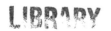
This work is protected under copyright by Elsevier Science, and the following terms and conditions apply to its use:

Photocopying

Single photocopies of single chapters may be made for personal use as allowed by national copyright laws. Permission of the Publisher and payment of a fee is required for all other photocopying, including multiple or systematic copying, copying for advertising or promotional purposes, resale, and all forms of document delivery. Special rates are available for educational institutions that wish to make photocopies for nonprofit educational classroom use.

Permissions may be sought directly from Elsevier Science Global Rights Department, PO Box 800, Oxford OX5 1DX, UK; phone: (+44) 1865 843830, fax: (+44) 1865 853333, e-mail: permissions@elsevier.co.uk. You may also contact Global Rights directly through Elsevier's home page (http://www.elsevier.nl), by selecting 'Obtaining Permissions'.

In the USA, users may clear permissions and make payments through the Copyright Clearance Center, Inc., 222 Rosewood Drive, Danvers, MA 01923, USA; phone: (978) 7508400, fax: (978) 7504744, and in the UK through the Copyright Licensing Agency Rapid Clearance Service (CLARCS), 90 Tottenham Court Road, London W1P 0LP, UK; phone: (+44) 207 631 5555; fax: (+44) 207 631 5500. Other countries may have a local reprographic rights agency for payments.

Derivative Works

Tables of contents may be reproduced for internal circulation, but permission of Elsevier Science is required for external resale or distribution of such material.
Permission of the Publisher is required for all other derivative works, including compilations and translations.

Electronic Storage or Usage

Permission of the Publisher is required to store or use electronically any material contained in this work, including any chapter or part of a chapter.

Except as outlined above, no part of this work may be reproduced, stored in a retrieval system or transmitted in any form or by any means, electronic, mechanical, photocopying, recording or otherwise, without prior written permission of the Publisher.
Address permissions requests to: Elsevier Science Rights & Permissions Department, at the mail, fax and e-mail addresses noted above.

Notice

No responsibility is assumed by the Publisher for any injury and/or damage to persons or property as a matter of products liability, negligence or otherwise, or from any use or operation of any methods, products, instructions or ideas contained in the material herein. Because of rapid advances in the medical sciences, in particular, independent verification of diagnoses and drug dosages should be made.

First edition 2000

Library of Congress Cataloging in Publication Data
A catalog record from the Library of Congress has been applied for.

ISBN: 0-444-50551-2
ISSN: 0531-5131
International Congress Series No. 1215

⊗ The paper used in this publication meets the requirements of ANSI/NISO Z39.48-1992 (Permanence of Paper).

Printed in the Netherlands

Preface

This book, the Proceedings of the XII International Symposium on Athero-sclerosis, differs from previous ISA proceedings in that it is considerably less volu-minous than its predecessors. The Executive Committee decided that it was cru-cial, in these times with rapid research development and fast communication media, to publish highlights very soon after the Symposium. Therefore we decided to limit the proceedings to the most important new findings within the area of atherosclerosis research as presented in Plenary sessions and Workshops.

A different way of composing the scientific programme was used at the XII ISA. Expert scientists were invited as chairpersons according to their expertise in their respective workshop topics. The chairpersons, of whom one was a host chairperson from within Scandinavia and the second from outside Scandinavia, had the freedom to create their own programme. One-half of the speakers were invited by the chairpersons and the remaining presentations were selected from the submitted abstracts. Their selection was supported by a review system where every chairperson was asked to rate 50–100 abstracts. The procedure was very successful and resulted in up-to-date presentations in all workshops. The Execu-tive Committee of the XII ISA is grateful to the workshop chairpersons for their hard and devoted work to make their workshop so exciting.

The XII ISA was attended by 4,240 registered delegates, representing more than 74 countries. The continental distribution was Africa 1%, the Americas 15%, Australasia 17%, and Europe 67%. The number of submitted abstracts were 1,574, of which 925 were presented either orally during a workshop or at a poster session.

The Executive Committee is indebted to the Young Investigator Award Com-mittee, led by Dr Robert Mahley, for its hard and skillful work in selecting 10 awardees out of 377 applicants. The 10 Young Investigator Awards, made possible through a grant from Novartis, were bestowed to:

1st prize: Yadong Huang, U.S.A.
Apolipoprotein E modulates hepatic very low density lipoprotein assembly and secretion

2nd: Marielle Kaplan, Israel
Oxidized LDL binds to macrophage secreted extracellular matrix and is taken up by macrophages

3rd: Rajendra K. Tangirala, U.S.A.
Monocyte chemoattractant protein-1 promotes macrophage oxidation of low density lipoprotein

Honorable mention:
J. Burden, U.K.
Investigation of a novel defect in patients with familial hypercholesterolemia

M.C. Jong, The Netherlands
VLDL receptor deficient mice are protected against diet-induced obesity and insulin resistance

J. Laukkanen, Finland
Secreted macrophage scavenger receptor gene transfer in LDL receptor knock-out mice reduces atherosclerotic lesion area

A. Luttun, Belgium
Paradoxical increase of plaque growth and collagen deposition in atherosclerotic mice lacking plasminogen activator inhibitor-1

U. Schönbeck, U.S.A.
Human vascular smooth muscle cells express an endogenous inhibitor of caspase-1

S. Tsimikas, U.S.A.
Noninvasive imaging and quantitation of atherosclerosis with radiolabeled oxidation-specific antibodies

D.M. Wuttge, Sweden
Cellular immunity in atherosclerosis: T cells specifically recognize oxidatively derived aldehyde adducts

Thanks to a generous support from Dr Alan Howard, Cambridge, UK, all scientists who were present at the first ISA in Athens in 1966 were invited to a celebration in Stockholm. Nineteen colleagues, who attended the 1966 Athens meeting, took the opportunity to meet at this occasion. The first part of this book contains some memorable moments and events in the history of the International Atherosclerosis Society and its Symposia.

The Executive Committee of the XII International Symposium on Atherosclerosis Bo Angelin, Göran K. Hansson, Lars-Åke Pellborn (General Secretary) and Olov Wiklund (Scientific Secretary) and myself would like to thank the sponsors who allowed us to create an attractive atmosphere for the Symposium with regard to exhibition and social programme:

Platinum Medal Sponsors: Bristol-Myers Squibb Company / Sankyo Pharma, Groupe Fournier, Parke Davis, a Division of Warner Lambert, and Pfizer Inc.

Gold Medal Sponsors: AstraZeneca, M.S.D. (Merck Sharp & Dohme), Negma Laboratoires / Kowa Company, Novartis

Silver Medal Sponsor: F. Hoffmann-La Roche Ltd

Sponsors: SAAB, SAS, The City of Stockholm, The Stockholm County Council

It is our hope that this volume will convince you that the XII International Symposium on Atherosclerosis really brought new knowledge to the atherosclerosis scientific community.

Anders G. Olsson
President

International Atherosclerosis Society

Rodolfo Paoletti, President
Antonio M Gotto, Jr, Past President
Heiner Greten, President Elect
Maryvonne Rosseneu, Secretary
Daniel Pometta, Treasurer
Christian Ehnholm, Member-at-Large
Yuji Matsuzawa, Member-at-Large
Gustav Schonfeld, Member-at-Large
Emanuela Folco, Executive Director, Administration, Education and Scientific Affairs
Ann Stephens Jackson, Executive Director, Fellowships, Finance and Legal Affairs

IAS constituent societies

Asian Pacific Society of Atherosclerosis and Vascular Diseases
Australian Atherosclerosis Society
Austrian Atherosclerosis Society
Belgian Atherosclerosis Society
British Atherosclerosis Society
Canadian Atherosclerosis Society
Chinese Atherosclerosis Society
Croatian Atherosclerosis Society
Commonwealth of Independent States (CIS) Atherosclerosis Society
Cuban Atherosclerosis Society
Czech Atherosclerosis Group
Czech Atherosclerosis Society
Dutch Society for Atherosclerosis and Vascular Biology
Egyptian Society of Atherosclerosis
European Atherosclerosis Society
French Atherosclerosis Society
Georgian Atherosclerosis Association
German Society for the Study of Arteriosclerosis
Hellenic Society of Lipidology and Atherosclerosis
Hungarian Atherosclerosis Society
Indian Society for Atherosclerosis Research
Indonesian Council on Atherosclerosis
Iranian Heart Foundation-Council on Atherosclerosis, Nutrition and Lipid Research
Israel Medical Association-Society for Research Prevention and Treatment of Atherosclerosis
Italian Society for the Study of Atherosclerosis
Japan Atherosclerosis Society
Korean Society for Lipidology
Lipid and Atherosclerosis Society of Southern Africa
Mediterranean Society of Atherosclerosis
Mexican Society of Atherosclerosis

New Zealand Atherosclerosis Society
Philippine Lipid Society
Polish Society for Atherosclerosis Research
Portuguese Atherosclerosis Society
Rumanian Association for Atherosclerosis and Lipidology
Scandinavian Society for Atherosclerosis Research
Slovak Atherosclerosis Section of Slovak Medical Association
Sociedad Argentina de Aterosclerosis
Sociedad Iberolatinoamericana de Aterosclerosis
Sociedad Latinoamericana de Aterosclerosis (SOLAT)
Society of Lipids & Atherosclerosis, ROC
Spanish Society of Arteriosclerosis
Swiss Working Group on Lipids and Atherosclerosis
Taiwan Society of Atherosclerosis & Vascular Diseases, ROC
Turkish Cardiology Association, Lipid Working Group
Council on Arteriosclerosis, Thrombosis and Vascular Biology / American Heart Association
Venezuelan Atherosclerosis Association
Yugoslav Atherosclerosis Society

XIIth International Symposium on Atherosclerosis Executive Committee

Anders G Olsson, Chairman
Lars Åke Pellborn, Secretary General
Olov Wiklund, Scientific Secretary
Bo Angelin
Göran K Hansson

Co-opted:
Mats Eriksson
Johannes Hulthe
Mats Rudling
Sten Stemme
Bo Ziedén

Young Investigator Award Committee

Chairman: Robert W Mahley, USA
Members: John Chapman, France
Harald Funke, Germany
Markolf Hanefeld, Germany
Toru Kita, Japan
Marek Naruszewicz, Poland
Michael Oliver, United Kingdom
Daniel Steinberg, USA
Lale Tokgozoglu, Turkey

Contents

Workshop abstracts

Memorable moments in the history of the IAS

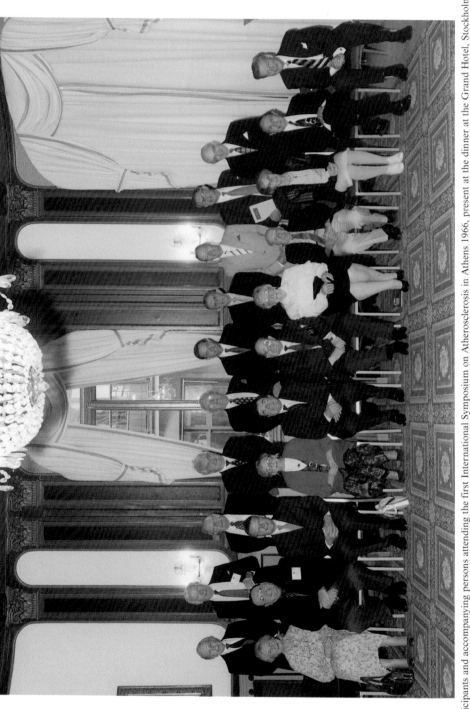

Participants and accompanying persons attending the first International Symposium on Atherosclerosis in Athens 1966, present at the dinner at the Grand Hotel, Stockholm. *Back row:* R Smith (husband of E Smith) M Oliver (London) T Clarkson (Winston-Salem) V Blaton (Bruges) N Sternby (Malmö) J Howard (son of A Howard) Y Stein (Jerusalem) D Bowyer (Cambridge) J Boberg (Uppsala) P Alaupovic (Oklahoma) *Front row:* E Smith (Aberdeen) A L Robertson (Stanford) A Olsson* (Linköping) G Howard (wife of A Howard) A Howard (Cambridge) R Paoletti (Milan) D Haust (London, Ontario) J Stamler (Chicago) O Stein (Jerusalem) A Scanu (Chicago) LA Carlson (Stockholm) *President of XIIth International Symposium as a guest.

©2000 Elsevier Science B.V. All rights reserved.
Atherosclerosis XII.
S. Stemme and A.G. Olsson, editors.

The First International Symposium on Atherosclerosis in Athens, 1966

Alan N. Howard

Downing College, University of Cambridge, Cambridge, CB2 1DQ, UK

A soiree and dinner was held at the Grand Hotel, Stockholm on June 27th 2000 to commemorate the First International Symposium held in Athens in May 1966. Among those present were 18 participants who attended the first Symposium (see photograph) including the general secretary Alan Howard (Cambridge) and the publication secretary Rodolfo Paoletti (Milan), currently the President of the International Atherosclerosis Society (IAS). Honoured guests were Anders G. Olsson (Linköping) President of the XIIth International Symposium and Daniel Pometta (Geneva), the Treasurer of the IAS.

Alan Howard traced the history of the first Symposium from its conception. In late 1963, Rodolfo Paoletti asked him to convene a meeting in Paris to discuss the formation of an Atherosclerosis Group and to liaise with Jean Cottet (Paris) who could provide travel expenses for the steering committee. Nine scientists representing France (2), Germany (2), Greece (1), Italy (2), UK (2) met at the Hopital St Antoine. Included were Gotthard Schettler (Heidelberg), later a President of the IAS, Rodolfo Paoletti and Costas Miras (Athens). It was decided to form a European Atherosclerosis Group (EAG) to promote and support atherosclerosis research in Europe which would be limited in membership, along the lines of the British Atherosclerosis Discussion Group formed in the 1950s. Under the presidency of Anders G. Olsson, in 1988, the EAG changed its name to the European Atherosclerosis Society (EAS). At the next two meetings in Milan, the group expanded and included George Boyd (Edinburgh) and Lars Carlson (Stockholm) among others. At the 4th meeting in Heidelberg on April 28th, 1965, it was decided to hold an international symposium in Athens with Costas Miras as local secretary and Alan Howard as the general scientific secretary. The latter would liaise with Robert Wissler (Chicago) and O.J. Pollak (Dover, Delaware) of the Arteriosclerosis Council of the American Heart Association who wished to arrange for a substantial North American delegation to attend.

The first International Symposium was intentionally small and consisted of only about 100 scientists from 22 countries (as detailed by Daria Haust, London, Ontario, below) and included some distinguished scientists of the day such as Paul Dudley White, physician to President Eisenhower, G. Biörck, physician to the King of Sweden and Ancel Keys who organised the famous seven countries study in the 1950s. The 4-day Symposium consisted of only one session at which oral communications were presented. At that time, poster presentations were not at all common. This contrasts with over 4,000 scientists who attended the XIIth International Symposium with six simultaneous sessions and more than 1,000 presentations.

An important part of the meeting were the excursions to historic sites in the surrounding countryside including a business meeting of the EAG in Delphi, cocktail parties at the Athens Yacht Club and Acropolis. and a dinner-dance at Asteria Beach (costing only $8). At 3 pm one afternoon the scientific sessions were discontinued and all the participants were transported by bus to Cape Sounion for a swim. Everyone was expected to join in the social events which were considered as important as the scientific sessions. They helped establish international contacts which led to further international meetings especially the second Symposium organised by Robert Wissler in Chicago.

During the after-dinner speeches at the Grand Hôtel commemorate reunion, the original participants emphasised the great importance of this first meeting in the development of International Atherosclerosis research for the rest of the century. Participants were specifically asked to give what they considered the most significant advances since the first Symposium. The following topics were mentioned: The discovery of the LDL receptor concept. The development of new effective drugs for lowering plasma cholesterol, especially the statins. Drugs to lower blood pressure. Definitive confirmation of the cholesterol hypothesis. Understanding the underlying cellular process in atherosclerosis and broadening of the concepts in acknowledging that many blood contents and arterial components participate in the inception and progression of the disease. Role of inflammatory and immune mechanisms in athero-thrombosis. The oxidation hypothesis. Vascular oxidation stresses and gene regulation. New concepts on plaque instability and rupture. Chemistry and metabolism of lipoproteins. Discovery of apoprotein(a) and its significance. Recognition of risk factors other than lipoproteins. Homocysteine as a risk factor. Development of surgical procedures for temporary relief of complications. Thrombolysis. Emphasis on nutritional intervention and changes in lifestyle. The cardiovascular benefits of soy phyto-oestrogens and fish oils. The reductions of atherogenesis by oestrogen treatment. The global concept of treatment of risk factors in secondary and primary CHD prevention. Macro-vascular control in diabetes. Control of the X syndrome. Introduction of transgenic animals to atherosclerosis research. The rapid and promising advances in gene therapy.

What were the reasons for establishing the first Symposium on atherosclerosis at that time? Many of the International Society meetings such as those for Biochemistry, Pathology, and Physiology were extremely large and too diversified. Scientists were becoming more interested in a multidisciplinary approach to research on a disease. Another factor was the availability of cheaper air transportation but probably more important, finance for travel expenses was made available by a growing pharmaceutical industry interested in the development of new drugs.

All those present at the Grand Hôtel soiree expressed the view that the establishment of an international symposium on atherosclerosis in 1966 was very timely, and they personally were proud to be associated with and to have attended the very first Symposium.

The meeting was sponsored by the Howard Foundation, Cambridge, UK.

Jean Cottet and the origin of the fibrates

Michael F. Oliver

Keepier Wharf, 12 Narrow St, London E14 8DH, UK

In 1953, Jean Cottet — a physician in Clermont-Ferrand (France) — noticed that many farm workers and farmers were being admitted to the principal hospital with nausea, vomiting and recent weight loss. He speculated that these features might be related to exposure to a new insecticide developed by Imperial Chemical Industries (ICI) of Britain. For reasons lost with time, Cottet also measured the plasma cholesterol of these men and found that most had concentrations less than 150 mg/dl. Cottet guessed that this was a specific effect of the insecticide.

ICI withdrew the insecticide which was alpha-phenyl-butyric acid and explored alternative derivatives. One developed by Jeff Thorp, a chemist in the pharmaceutical division of ICI, was chloro-phenoxy-isobutyrate (CPIB). Thorp came to the Edinburgh group (George Boyd and Michael Oliver), since at that time we were the only laboratory team in the UK measuring cholesterol and lipoproteins. He asked us to determine the cholesterol-lowering capability of this new compound, first in rats and later in man. We had no idea of the dose that might be effective and, having shown that CPIB did indeed lower beta (LDL) lipoproteins in rats without adverse effects, we began by testing a very low dose (50 mg) in hypercholesterolaemic men. This was before ethics committees and the rules of human experimentation had been established and nowadays direct transfer of animal-derived data to man would be much harder to achieve. After 2 more years, we established that an effective dose was 1–1.5 g daily. We reported this finding in the Lancet in 1961. The compound was first given the name of Atromid-S, then Atromid but later it was called Clofibrate — the first fibrate [1].

Jean Cottet, meanwhile, became more and more interested in cholesterol metabolism and suggested that some group might be formed to meet regularly to discuss its relevance to disease. From this arose the European Atherosclerosis Group and later the Society. Jean Cottet was a prime mover in its foundation but did not attend the first Symposium. Jeff Thorp was an outstanding eccentric and charming chemist who drank very heavily without any evident ill effects and finally constructed a rocket in order to blow his ashes 100 metres over Manchester! He did participate in the Athens meeting presenting a paper on Atromid-S. George Boyd also attended.

These early findings led to the establishment in 1965 of the first major trial to determine whether cholesterol lowering would influence the incidence of coronary heart disease (CHD). Clofibrate 1 g morning and night was compared with an identical placebo (1 g olive oil). The trial was initiated in Edinburgh in an exploratory manner, since at that time there were no established guidelines about the design and conduct of clinical trials. Blood donors were recruited and those with hypercholesterolaemia were randomised to Clofibrate or placebo. Eventually, 15,000 men were included and the trial was extended to Budapest (George Lamm) and Prague (Jiri Widimsky). The World Health Organisation (Zdenek Fejfar) helped with communications, funding and travel in Hungary and Czechoslovakia which were both under Russian domination. The MRC Statistics Unit (Austin Heady and Jerry Morris) was the co-ordinating centre.

The WHO Cooperative Trial of Clofibrate reported first in 1976 and demonstrated a significant reduction in CHD rates but an increase also in noncoronary deaths, mostly cancer [2]. The WHO trial was the first to demonstrate the benefit of cholesterol reduction but because of the adverse effect, also shown later in the Helsinki Heart Study using gemfibrozil, world opinion was cautious about promoting cholesterol lowering. Indeed, this remained the case until the results of the statin trials became available in the early 1990s.

References

1. Oliver MF. Further observations on the effects of Atromid and ethylchlorophenoxyisobutyrate on serum lipid levels. J Atheroscler Res 1963;3:427–444.
2. Report from the Committee of the Principal Investigators (WHO trial). A cooperative trial in the primary prevention of ischaemic heart disease using clofibrate. Br Heart J 1978;40: 1069–1118.

The significance and importance of the Athens symposium

M. Daria Haust
Department of Pathology, the University of Western Ontario, London, Ontario, N6A 5C1 Canada

It is of note that with the passing of time the first Symposium assumes an increasing importance. At first it appeared only important that we met face-to-face with investigators in our own respective fields, whose publications we quoted in our own writing.

Looking back, additional facets of significance of this first Symposium emerge:
   1. In reviewing the Athens program one realises that for the very first time a Symposium not only brought together investigators from 22 countries (and of four continents) (see Table 1), but that the topics covered a wide spectrum of the multifaceted atherosclerotic disease, i.e., the role of various arterial components; plasma lipoproteins and defects in their metabolism; platelets; coagulation factors and thrombosis; hormones; and the role of oxidative and lipolytic enzymes; the use of tissue culture and experimental animals (both primates and nonprimates) in the study of atherogenesis; risk factors; prevention and treatment of the disease by diets and pharmacological agents, and epidemiological studies. This wide spectrum is of note, because in the past, a conference or a Symposium, organised with the participation of a few international authorities in Europe or in North America, was limited usually to a narrow aspect of atherosclerosis, e.g., that in 1962 organised by the Chicago Heart Association was focused on "The Atherosclerotic Plaque".

Table 1. Number of presentations by countries at the Athens Symposium, 1966.

	Country	No. of presentations		Country	No. of presentations
1	USA	33	12	Switzerland	3
2	England	12	13	Belgium	2
3	Argentina	6	14	Czechoslovakia	2
4	Canada	4	15	Finland	2
5	Germany	4	16	Poland	2
6	India	4	17	USSR	2
7	Italy	4	18	Denmark	1
8	Greece	3	19	France	1
9	Israel	3	20	Hungary	1
10	Scotland	3	21	Japan	1
11	Sweden	3	22	Netherlands	1

2. The other and most significant role of the Athens Symposium lies in the recognition that such international, multidisciplinary exchanges must not remain sporadic if progress were to be made in the field of atherosclerosis. Rather, encounters of similar nature and depth are required at a well-determined time intervals and on a geographically rotating basis. This conclusion was reached at the closing of a general meeting, and Robert Wissler and Robert Furman invited the participants for the next gathering to the USA. The International Symposia on Atherosclerosis were born and firmly established with the second Symposium in 1969 in Chicago; Robert Wissler who unfortunately could not be present in Stockholm deserves much credit for carrying that banner in organising that second Symposium with the support of Jerry Stamler and the late Louis Katz.

3. Of personal interest is the fact that of the approximately 100 participants at the Athens Symposium only four were female scientists, i.e., Ruth Pick of the USA, Elspeth Smith of the UK, Olga Stein of Israel and myself from Canada. On the other hand over one-third of the participants of this the XIIth International Symposium on Atherosclerosis are female scientists.

4. I wish to acknowledge that the permanent record of the Athens Symposium, the proceedings [1], exists through the efforts of Rodolfo Paoletti and to pay tribute to the "heroes" of the Symposium. Alan Howard was one of the scientists of the day who conceived the idea of the first Symposium and, serving as secretary, was largely responsible for contacting the potential participants and devising the programme. The other is Costas Miras who was the host in Athens. His warm hospitality and unforgettable congeniality (created with his charming wife Zizika) provided an atmosphere in which many lifelong friendships blossomed.

Reference

1. International Symposium on Recent Advances in Atherosclerosis, Athens 1966. In: Miras CJ, Howard AN, Paoletti R (eds) Progress in Biochemical Pharmacology 4. Basel, Switzerland: Karger, 1967.

Plenary session

Genetics of atherosclerosis: studies in humans and mice

Jan L. Breslow

The Rockefeller University, Laboratory of Biochemical Genetics and Metabolism, New York, USA

Abstract. Atherosclerotic cardiovascular disease is a complex genetic disorder with many genes involved and significant gene-environment interactions. Extensive study of candidate genes in pathways relevant to atherosclerotic cardiovascular disease risk factors has had limited success in explaining population susceptibility to this disease. With the advent of the Genome Program, it is now becoming possible to use positional cloning techniques to identify new atherosclerosis susceptibility genes. With this goal in mind, several laboratories at Rockefeller University are engaged in a comprehensive epidemiological and genetic study on the Pacific Island of Kosrae, one of the four states that make up the Federated States of Micronesia, to map genes involved in dyslipidemia, hypertension, diabetes and obesity. In our own laboratory, we are also using apo E knockout mice to identify atherosclerosis modifier genes in a cross between a susceptible strain, C57Bl/6J E0, and a resistant strain, FVB/N E0. These projects should lead to the identification of new genes and pathways predisposing to atherosclerosis that might improve the early diagnosis of susceptible individuals in the population and suggest new and improved mechanism-based treatments.

Keywords: apo E knockout mice, gene mapping, Pacific islanders, positional cloning.

Atherosclerotic cardiovascular disease is the major cause of morbidity and mortality in much of the world [1]. Susceptibility to atherosclerosis is not inherited in a simple Mendelian fashion, but rather has multiple genetic and environmental determinants with significant gene-environment interactions [2]. Genes that control risk factors for atherosclerotic cardiovascular disease, such as lipoprotein levels, blood pressure, glucose levels and obesity, are involved, as are presumably genes involved in blood vessel wall function, the clotting system and the immune system, especially macrophage function. Environmental factors such as cigarette smoking, nutrition and physical exercise are also important, as are the body's responses to these environmental factors.

Extensive study of candidate genes involved in lipoprotein metabolism has revealed some variation in the general population influencing lipoprotein levels and coronary heart disease susceptibility. The three allelic forms of apo E [3] have different metabolic fates and account for 5–10% of the population variance in cholesterol levels [4] and affect the relative risk of coronary heart disease [5]. Variants at the apo A-I/CIII/A-IV locus predict hypertriglyceridemia [6,7], probably by influencing the level of expression of the apo CIII gene [8]. Variants of

Address for correspondence: Dr Jan L. Breslow, Rockefeller University, 1230 York Avenue, New York, NY 10021, USA. Tel.: +1-212-327-7704. Fax: +1-212-327-7165.
E-mail: Breslow@rockvax.rockefeller.edu

the LPL and HL genes influence HDL cholesterol levels [9—11]. Sib pair analysis has implicated the apo AI/CIII/AIV and hepatic lipase loci in the control of HDL cholesterol levels [12], whereas in another study linkage analysis in families implicated the apo A-II and CETP loci [13]. Sib pair analysis has shown the Cyp7 locus controls LDL cholesterol levels [14]. Linkage analysis with candidate genes has suggested the involvement of the apo AI/CIII/AIV, LCAT/CETP, and MnSOD loci in the Familial Combined Hyperlipidemia (FCHL) phenotype [15—17]. Candidate gene studies have been useful but clearly the full range of genetic variation underlying lipoprotein levels and coronary heart disease susceptibility has not yet been described.

Another approach to human atherosclerotic cardiovascular disease genes involves positional cloning. Human populations around the world are now being gathered and assessed for coronary heart disease or its risk factors. With the aid of the tools being developed by the Human Genome Project, genome scans are being undertaken to identify new genes involved in atherosclerosis susceptibility. For example, in a recent study linkage analysis in Finnish FCHL families revealed a locus for the lipoprotein phenotype on human 1q21—23, distinct from the apo A-II locus [18]. At Rockefeller, the Friedman, Stoffel, Ott and Breslow laboratories have initiated a comprehensive epidemiologic and genetic study on the Pacific Island of Kosrae, one of the four states in the Federated States of Micronesia, to positionally clone genes involved in several of the main risk factors for atherosclerosis, dyslipidemia, hypertension, diabetes and obesity.

Kosrae is located 2,500 miles north east of Australia. Kosrae was originally settled by a small number of founders (estimated to be 50), originating from Polynesia around 50 AD. Kosrae was first sighted by Westerners in 1804 and first visited in 1824. During the 19th century the combined effects of a typhoon (in 1835) and exposure of the native population to Western communicable diseases reduced the indigenous population from 3,000 to about 300 individuals by 1888. Historical and genealogical records indicate that these 300 survivors were the result of extensive admixture between native Kosraen females and male Caucasian whalers from New England and Europe who visited the island in mid to late 19th century. As late as 1945 Kosraens consumed a diet consisting mostly of fish and fruits and vegetables and the average individual was noted to be lean. After WWII Kosrae was designated a US Protectorate and this led to drastic lifestyle change, with islanders becoming much more sedentary and consuming large quantities of high fat foods, such as spam, turkey tails, hamburgers and ice cream, supplied through US aid. Since 1945 there has been a large increase in the Kosraen population and this has been accompanied by a dramatically increased prevalence of obesity, an outcome similar to that of other indigenous populations, such as the Pima Indians of Arizona and the Nahruans. In 1994, concern over the epidemic of obesity led to screening of all adult Kosraens for obesity, dyslipidemia, diabetes and hypertension. In addition, blood was obtained for DNA analysis and an extensive family tree was constructed for the entire Island.

In the current study, markers in or near seven candidate genes previously implicated in lipoprotein abnormalities, apo E, apo CIII, apo AII, hepatic lipase, cholesteryl ester transfer protein (CETP), microsomal triglyceride transfer protein (MTP) and cholesterol 7α-hydroxylase (cyp7), were tested in a family-based association study for contributing to lipid and lipoprotein variation on Kosrae. The findings suggested a codominant apo CIII allele for triglycerides and a recessive apo CIII allele for cholesterol and apo B, a recessive apo A-II allele for increased triglycerides and decreased apo A-I, and recessive CETP and cyp7 alleles for apo A-I. Compared to the E3 allele, the E4 allele was associated with increased triglycerides, cholesterol, apo B and decreased apo A-I, whereas the E2 allele was associated with decreased cholesterol and apo B levels. Compared to general population association studies, the family-based association study described here is more likely to reveal true associations because it is less prone to false-positive associations from population stratification and the subjects are living in a more homogenous environment.

In addition to positional cloning in human genetic studies, parallel approaches are being undertaken to identify atherosclerosis susceptibility genes in animal models. The most ideal mammal for such studies is the laboratory mouse [19]. Mice are small (25 to 40 g), have short generation times (9—10 weeks) and large litter sizes (five to ten offspring), and there are many inbred strains available. Early attempts to use the mouse to positionally clone atherosclerosis susceptibility genes confronted the difficulty that mice are quite resistant to atherosclerosis and do not naturally develop lesions. To circumvent this problem dietary approaches were tried. In the 1980s, Paigen used a diet containing 15% fat, 1.25% cholesterol, and 0.5% cholic acid to study ten inbred mouse strains and found differences in atherosclerosis susceptibility that did not correlate well with plasma cholesterol levels [20]. In a series of studies, using the diet-induced mouse atherosclerosis model in a number of crosses, Paigen mapped 8 atherosclerosis susceptibility loci (designated Ath-1 through Ath-8) [21—27]. Ath-1, Ath-3 and Ath-6 were mapped to chromosomes 1, 7 and 12, respectively, and the other Ath genes were not mapped. None of the Ath loci have progressed to gene identification, although a putative antioxidant gene in the region of Ath-1 (Aop2) has been identified [28]. One of the main difficulties in using the diet-induced mouse model to identify atherosclerosis susceptibility genes is, even in the susceptible mouse strains, the lesions are quite small and variable making it appear that the atherosclerosis trait is incompletely penetrant [27].

In recent years, Lusis has done considerable work to place atherosclerosis candidate genes on the mouse genomic map [29]. He has also done considerable QTL mapping of atherosclerosis risk factors using crosses between several inbred mouse strains. He has mapped a locus controlling HDL levels on a chow diet to chromosome 1, and three other loci that control the decrease in HDL levels in response to the Paigen diet to chromosomes 3, 5, and 11 [30], a locus for combined hyperlipidemia to chromosome 3 [31], loci controlling body fat, lipoprotein levels and insulin levels to chromosomes 2 and 9, a locus controlling leptin levels to chromosome 4 [32], and in an autoimmune model loci controlling lipoprotein levels to chromosomes 5, 8, 15 and 19 [33]. None of the lipoprotein QTLs described above have progressed to gene identification, with the possible exception of the locus on chromosome 1 controlling HDL levels on a chow diet most likely being apo A-II [34,35].

In our laboratory Hayes Dansky, Jonathan Smith and I have been using the more recently developed apo E knockout (E0) mouse to map atherosclerosis susceptibility genes [36]. In this mouse atherosclerosis model, even on a chow diet, lesions are much larger and the atherosclerosis trait is fully penetrant. In initial studies we bred the E0 trait onto different backgrounds to assess whether genetic background influences atherosclerotic lesion area in this model. The E0 trait was originally created in 129 ter/SV embryonic stem cells and a line established by crossing chimeras with C57BL/6J mice. Outbred mice were then backcrossed using classical techniques onto the C57BL/6J and FVB/N backgrounds. Utilizing these mice, mean aortic root atherosclerotic lesion area was 7 (males) to 9 (females) times higher in chow fed C57Bl/6J E0 mice compared to FVB/N E0 mice at 16 weeks of age. Lesion area in F1 mice was intermediate in size compared to parental values and lesion area in F2 mice spanned the range of lesion areas in both parental strains. In the F2 mice there were no correlations between lesion area and total cholesterol, non-HDL cholesterol, HDL cholesterol, apo A-I, apo A-II, apo J, or anticardiolipin antibodies [37]. This study established that genetic background influences atherosclerosis susceptibility in E0 mice and also suggested that the genes responsible did not act through influencing lipoprotein levels. This study also suggested that a genomic approach might succeed in identifying genes responsible for the strain differences in atherosclerosis susceptibility that act independently of the measured plasma parameters.

In preliminary experiments, now almost completed, we have used bone marrow transplantation to determine whether the atherosclerosis susceptibility phenotype can be partially or entirely transmitted through bone marrow-derived cells. In these experiments recipient 6-week-old male mice are irradiated and donor 12-week-old male mice bone marrow cells transplanted. Transplanted animals are sacrificed at 20 weeks of age to assess atherosclerotic lesion area. To insure that bone marrow transplantation did not disrupt the atherosclerosis susceptibility difference between the strains, C57Bl/6J E0 bone marrow was transplanted to irradiated C57Bl/6J E0 mice and FVB/N E0 bone marrow to irradiated FVB/N E0 mice. A highly significant 9-fold difference in atherosclerotic lesion area was still observed between the strains. We next tested whether non-bone-marrow-derived host factors influenced atherosclerosis susceptibility by transplanting bone marrow from F1 (C57Bl/6J E0 x FVB/N E0) mice into C57Bl/6J E0 and FVB/N E0 recipients. Utilizing F1 marrow allows the immune system of the host to be replaced by a graft that recognizes as self both C57Bl/6J and FVB/N antigens, preventing the complications of graft-versus-host disease. Transplanting F1 E0 marrow to C57Bl/6J E0 mice resulted in animals with significantly more atherosclerosis than when such marrow was transplanted to FVB/N mice. This result shows that in this cross non-bone-marrow host factors play a role in atherosclerosis susceptibility. We also tested whether bone-marrow-derived factors play a role by transplanting F1 E0 and C57Bl/6J E0 marrow into C57Bl/6J E0 recipients and F1 E0 and FVB/N E0 marrow into FVB/N E0 recipients. In the former case the F1 E0 marrow resulted in less atherosclerosis and in the latter case more atherosclerosis. Based on these bone marrow transplantation studies, we have concluded that both bone-marrow-derived factors and non-bone-marrow host factors are responsible for the atherosclerosis susceptibility difference between C57Bl/6J E0 and FVB/N E0 mice.

In collaboration with scientists at the Millenium Pharmaceutical Company, our laboratory has now done two independent crosses to search for genes that could explain the atherosclerosis susceptibility difference between C57Bl/6J E0 and FVB/N E0 mice. The initial cross described by Dansky was extended to 364 F2 mice and a second cross was done in which 197 F2 mice were generated. There were two differences between the crosses. In cross 1 the animals were fed a chow diet (4.5% fat), whereas in cross 2 the mice were fed a breeder chow diet (9% fat). In addition, cross #1 was started before fully inbred E0 mouse strains were available and, based on a genome scan of 145 markers, the parental C57Bl/6J E0 mice carried only 92% of their genetic material from C57BL/6J and the parental FVB/N E0 mice carried only 91% of their genetic material from FVB/N. Cross 2 was started later and begun with fully backcrossed C57Bl/6J and FVB/N E0 mice. The parental strains used to generate crosses 1 and 2 had very similar lipoprotein levels and atherosclerotic lesion areas. A preliminary analysis for loci influencing atherosclerosis susceptibility has been carried out on 200 F2 mice from cross 1 and on 197 F2 mice from cross 2 for which there is both phenotypic and genotypic data. The QTL analysis, based on a 10 cM genome scan carried out with 187 markers that differ between C57Bl/6J and FVB/N mice, was done using the MAPMANAGER QT Program [38]. Atherosclerosis susceptibility loci were identified on chromosomes 10, 14 and 19, and a strong lipoprotein level locus on chromosome 1. We are now creating secondary congenics for each of the atherosclerosis susceptibility loci as the next step in gene isolation.

References

1. Murray CJ, Lopez AD. Alternative projections of mortality and disability by cause 1990—2020: global burden of disease study. Lancet 1997;349:1498—1504.
2. Lusis A, Weinreb A, Drake TA. Genetics of atherosclerosis. In: Topol EJ (ed) Textbook of Cardiovascular Medicine. Philadelphia: Lipincott-Raven Publishers, 1997;2389—2413.
3. Zannis VI, Just PW, Breslow JL. Human apolipoprotein E isoprotein subclasses are genetically determined. Am J Hum Genet 1981;33:11—24.
4. Davignon J, Gregg RE, Sing CF. Apolipoprotein E polymorphism and atherosclerosis. Arteriosclerosis 1988;8:1—21.
5. Wilson PW, Schaefer EJ, Larson MG, Ordovas JM. Apolipoprotein E alleles and risk of coronary disease. A meta-analysis. Arterioscl Thromb Vasc Biol 1996;16:1250—1255.

6. Dammerman MM, Sandkuijl LA, Halaas JL, Chung W, Breslow JL. An apolipoprotein CIII haplotype protective against hypertriglyceridemia is specified by promoter and 3' untranslated region polymorphisms. Proc Natl Acad Sci USA 1993;90:4562–4566.

7. Surguchov AP, Page GP, Smith L, Patsch W, Boerwinkle E. Polymorphic markers in apolipoprotein C-III gene flanking regions and hypertriglyceridemia. Arterioscler Thromb Vasc Biol 1996;16:941–947.

8. Li WW, Dammerman MM, Smith JD, Metzger S, Breslow JL, Leff T. Common genetic variation in the promoter of the human apo CIII gene abolishes regulation by insulin and may contribute to hypertriglyceridemia. J Clin Invest 1995;96:2601–2605.

9. Fisher RM, Humphries SE, Talmud PJ. Common variation in the lipoprotein lipase gene: effects on plasma lipids and risk of atherosclerosis. Atherosclerosis 1997;135:145–159.

10. Murtomaki SE, Tahvanainen E, Antikainen M, Tiret L, Nicaud V, Jansen H, Ehnholm C. Hepatic lipase gene polymorphisms influence plasma HDL levels. Results from Finnish EARS participants. European atherosclerosis research study. Arterioscl Thromb Vasc Biol 1997;17:1879–1884.

11. Zambon A, Deeb SS, Hokanson JE, Brown BG, Brunzell JD. Common variants in the promoter of the hepatic lipase gene are associated with lower levels of hepatic lipase activity, buoyant LDL, and higher HDL2 cholesterol. Arterioscl Thromb Vasc Biol 1998;18:1723–1729.

12. Cohen JC, Wang Z, Grundy SM, Stoesz MR, Guerra R. Variation at the hepatic lipase and apolipoprotein AI/CIII/AIV loci is a major cause of genetically determined variation in plasma HDL cholesterol levels. J Clin Invest 1994;94:2377–2384.

13. Bu X, Warden CH, Xia YR, De Meester C, Puppione DL, Truya S, Lokensgard B, Daneshmand S, Brown J, Gray RJ et al. Linkage analysis of the genetic determinants of high density lipoprotein concentrations and composition: evidence for involvement of the apolipoprotein A-II and cholesteryl ester transfer protein loci. Hum Genet 1994;93:639–648.

14. Wang J, Freeman DJ, Grundy SM, Levine M, Guerra R, Cohen JC. Linkage between cholesterol 7alpha-hydroxylase and high plasma low-density lipoprotein cholesterol concentrations. J Clin Invest 1998;101:1283–1291.

15. Wojciechowski AP, Farrall M, Cullen P, Wilson TM, Bayliss JD, Farren B, Griffin BA, Caslake MJ, Packard CJ, Shepherd J et al. Familial combined hyperlipidaemia linked to the apolipoprotein AI-CII- AIV gene cluster on chromosome 11q23-q24. Nature 1991;349:161–164.

16. Dallinga-Thie GM, van Linde-Sibenius Trip M, Rotter JI, Cantor RM, Bu X, Lusis AJ, de Bruin TW. Complex genetic contribution of the apo AI-CIII-AIV gene cluster to familial combined hyperlipidemia. Identification of different susceptibility haplotypes. J Clin Invest 1997;99:953–961.

17. Allayee H, Aouizerat BE, Cantor RM, Dallinga-Thie GM, Krauss RM, Lannin CD, Rotter JI, Lusis AJ, de Bruin TW. Families with familial combined hyperlipidemia and families enriched for coronary artery disease share genetic determinants for the atherogenic lipoprotein phenotype. Am J Hum Genet 1998;63:577–585.

18. Pajukanta P, Nuotio I, Terwilliger JD, Porkka KV, Ylitalo K, Pihlajamaki J, Suomalainen AJ, Syvanen AC, Lehtimaki T, Viikari JS, Laakso M, Taskinen MR, Ehnholm C, Peltonen L. Linkage of familial combined hyperlipidaemia to chromosome 1q21-q23. Nat Genet 1998;18:369–373.

19. Silver LM. Mouse Genetics. New York, Oxford: Oxford University Press, 1995.

20. Paigen B, Morrow A, Brandon C, Mitchell D, Holmes P. Variation in susceptibility to atherosclerosis among inbred strains of mice. Atherosclerosis 1985;57:65–73.

21. Paigen B, Mitchell D, Reue K, Morrow A, Lusis AJ, LeBoeuf RC. Ath-1, a gene determining atherosclerosis susceptibility and high density lipoprotein levels in mice. Proc Natl Acad Sci USA 1987;84:3763–3767.

22. Paigen B, Albee D, Holmes PA, Mitchell D. Genetic analysis of murine strains C57BL/6J and C3H/HeJ to confirm the map position of Ath-1, a gene determining atherosclerosis susceptibility. Biochem Genet 1987;25:501–511.

23. Paigen B, Nesbitt MN, Mitchell D, Albee D, LeBoeuf RC. Ath-2, a second gene determining atherosclerosis susceptibility and high density lipoprotein levels in mice. Genetics 1989;122: 163—168.

24. Stewart-Phillips JL, Lough J, Skamene E. ATH-3, a new gene for atherosclerosis in the mouse. Clin Invest Med 1989;12:121—126.

25. Paigen B. Genetics of responsiveness to high-fat and high-cholesterol diets in the mouse. Am J Clin Nutr 1995;62:458S—462S.

26. Mu JL, Naggert JK, Svenson KL, Collin GB, Kim JH, McFarland C, Nishina PM, Levine DM, Williams KJ, Paigen B. Quantitative trait loci analysis for the differences in susceptibility to atherosclerosis and diabetes between inbred mouse strains C57BL/6J and C57BLKS/J. J Lipid Res 1999;40:1328—1335.

27. Pitman WA, Hunt MH, McFarland C, Paigen B. Genetic analysis of the difference in diet-induced atherosclerosis between the inbred mouse strains SM/J and NZB/BINJ. Arterioscler Thromb Vasc Biol 1998;18:615—620.

28. Phelan SA, Johnson KA, Beier DR, Paigen B. Characterization of the murine gene encoding Aop2 (antioxidant protein 2) and identification of two highly related genes. Genomics 1998; 54:132—139.

29. Welch CL, Xia YR, Shechter I, Farese R, Mehrabian M, Mehdizadeh S, Warden CH, Lusis AJ. Genetic regulation of cholesterol homeostasis: chromosomal organization of candidate genes [published erratum appears in J Lipid Res 1996;37(10):2269]. J Lipid Res 1996;37:1406—1421.

30. Machleder D, Ivandic B, Welch C, Castellani L, Reue K, Lusis AJ. Complex genetic control of HDL levels in mice in response to an atherogenic diet. Coordinate regulation of HDL levels and bile acid metabolism. J Clin Invest 1997;99:1406—1419.

31. Castellani LW, Weinreb A, Bodnar J, Goto AM, Doolittle M, Mehrabian M, Demant P, Lusis AJ. Mapping a gene for combined hyperlipidaemia in a mutant mouse strain. Nat Genet 1998; 18:374—377.

32. Mehrabian M, Wen PZ, Fisler J, Davis RC, Lusis AJ. Genetic loci controlling body fat, lipoprotein metabolism, and insulin levels in a multifactorial mouse model. J Clin Invest 1998;101: 2485—2496.

33. Gu L, Johnson MW, Lusis AJ. Quantitative trait locus analysis of plasma lipoprotein levels in an autoimmune mouse model: interactions between lipoprotein metabolism, autoimmune disease, and atherogenesis. Arterioscl Thromb Vasc Biol 1999;19:442—453.

34. Doolittle MH, LeBoeuf RC, Warden CH, Bee LM, Lusis AJ. A polymorphism affecting apolipoprotein A-II translational efficiency determines high density lipoprotein size and composition. J Biol Chem 1990;265:16380—16388.

35. Mehrabian M, Qiao JH, Hyman R, Ruddle D, Laughton C, Lusis AJ. Influence of the apoA-II gene locus on HDL levels and fatty streak development in mice [published erratum appears in Arterioscl Thromb 1993 Mar;13(3):466]. Arterioscl Thromb 1993;13:1—10.

36. Smith JD, Breslow JL. The emergence of mouse models of atherosclerosis and their relevance to clinical research. J Intern Med 1997;242:99—109.

37. Dansky H, Charlton SA, Sikes JL, Heath SC, Simantov R, Levin LF, Shu P, Moore KJ, Breslow JL, Smith JD. Genetic Background Determines the Extent of Atherosclerosis in ApoE-Deficient Mice. Arterioscl Thromb Vasc Biol 1999;19:1960—1968.

38. Manly KF, Olson JM. Overview of QTL mapping software and introduction to map manager QT. Mamm Genome 1999;10:327—334.

X-ceptors, nuclear receptors for metabolism

Johan Auwerx[1] and David Mangelsdorf[2]

[1]*Institut de Génétique et de Biologie Moléculaire et Cellulaire, CNRS/INSERM/ULP, Illkirch, France;*
and [2]*Howard Hughes Medical Institute, Southwestern Medical Center, University of Texas, Dallas,*
Texas, USA

Abstract. We designate permissive RXR heterodimer partners as X-ceptors. These X-ceptors
include nuclear receptors such as the peroxisome proliferator-activated receptors (PPAR), the liver
X receptors (LXR), the pregnane X receptor or steroid and xenobiotic receptor (PXR/SXR), and
the farnesol X receptor (FXR; also termed bile acid receptor or BAR). The ligands for these X-ceptors are found in excess (Xs) in humans in an industrialized westernized society and include compounds of dietary origin, such as fatty acids (PPARs) and sterols (LXRs), compounds induced by a
western-style diet, such as bile acids (FXR), and drugs and xenobiotics (SXR, PXR). X-ceptors
can therefore be considered as receptors for excess, or thrifty receptors, and they are thought to
play an important role in many common disorders, such as obesity, insulin resistance, type 2 diabetes, hyperlipidemia, gallbladder disease, etc., often commonly referred to as "syndrome X". The
central role of X-ceptors in common disorders makes them also excellent drug targets. The above
points are illustrated by reviewing the biology of PPARγ a master controller of adipogenesis, lipid
and glucose homeostasis and of LXR and FXR, which together control cholesterol and bile acid
homeostasis.

Keywords: atherosclerosis, cholesterol, FXR, gene expression, LRH-1, LXR, nuclear receptors,
oxysterols, PPARγ, RXR, SREBP.

X-ceptors, a new subclass of nuclear receptors controlling affluence

Alterations in nutrient intake and composition alter gene expression, ultimately
resulting in metabolic adaptation. The interest in understanding the mechanisms
by which nutrients change gene expression is driven by the association of alterations in nutrient intake and the development of metabolic diseases. Indeed, diets
rich in lipids and carbohydrates predispose to diseases such as obesity, non-insu-
lin-dependent diabetes mellitus, hyperlipidemia and atherosclerosis. Recently it
has become clear that a subset of the nuclear hormone receptor superfamily are
key signaling factors in translating nutritional events in changes in gene expression.

Nuclear hormone receptors are ligand-activated transcription factors that
mediate the transcriptional activity of small lipophilic-signaling molecules such
as steroids, retinoids and thyroid hormones. In order to bind efficiently to
response elements in DNA, most nuclear receptors form dimers with other

Address for correspondence: Johan Auwerx, Institut de Génétique et de Biologie Moléculaire et Cellulaire (IGBMC), 1 rue Laurent Fries, F-67404 Illkirch, France. E-mail: auwerx@igbmc.u-strasbg.fr

22

nuclear receptors. The classical steroid hormone receptors all form homodimers, as is the case for the glucocorticoid (GR) and estrogen receptors (ER) for example. An important number of receptors, including the retinoid acid receptor (RAR), thyroid hormone receptor (TR), the vitamin D receptor (VDR), the various peroxisome proliferator-activated receptors (PPAR), the liver X receptors (LXR), the pregnane X receptor or steroid and xenobiotic receptor (PXR/SXR), and the farnesol X receptor (FXR also termed bile acid receptor), form heterodimers with the retinoid X receptor (RXR). The RXR heterodimers can be further subdivided in two subgroups, based on the activation properties of the heterodimer. Nonpermissive heterodimers such as RXR/RAR, RXR/TR or RXR/VDR cannot be activated solely by the RXR ligand, but only by the ligand of the partner, i.e., RAR, TR, or VDR. In contrast, permissive RXR heterodimers can be both activated by ligands for RXR and the respective partner. We designate this group of permissive RXR heterodimer partners as X-ceptors (Fig. 1). This terminology was chosen as it not only reflects that most of them carry the letter X, but also because, as discussed in the sections below, the natural ligands for these X-ceptors are compounds which are found in excess (Xs) in people living in an industrialized westernized society. These ligands include compounds of dietary origin, such as fatty acids (PPARs) and sterols (LXRs), compounds induced by a western-style diet, such as bile acids (FXR), and drugs and xenobiotics (SXR, PXR) (Fig. 1). One can therefore consider that X-ceptors are receptors for excess or thrifty receptors.

X-ceptors seem to play a predominant role in many common disorders in our industrialized societies, such as obesity, insulin resistance, type 2 diabetes, hyperlipidemia, gallbladder disease, etc., often commonly referred to as "syndrome X". This central role of several of these X-ceptors in common disorders also

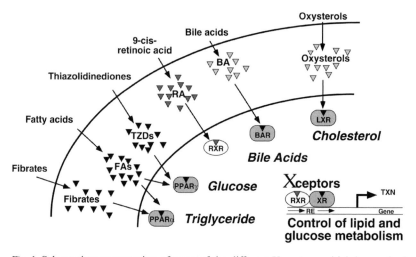

Fig. 1. Schematic representation of some of the different X-ceptors, which have roles in metabolism, and the pathways they control. Natural ligands for the various X-ceptors are depicted.

makes these receptors excellent drug targets. The activity of X-ceptor/RXR heterodimers can pharmacologically be modulated either by specific X-ceptor ligands or by ligands for RXR. This double activation mechanism therefore allows not only the development of highly specific drugs, affecting only selective metabolic pathways (for example PPAR-controlled pathways), but also the development of "broad-spectrum" metabolic modulators, which affect numerous X-ceptor signaling pathways.

Below we will illustrate the above principles by exploring the biology of PPARγ, an X-ceptor involved in the control of fat formation, and lipid and glucose homeostasis and by discussing the emerging role of two other X-ceptors, i.e., LXR and FXR, in the control of cholesterol and bile acid homeostasis.

PPARγ, the thrifty receptor

PPARγ (NR1C3), a coordinator of adipocyte differentiation and energy conservation

The human PPARγ gene translates into two proteins, these being PPARγ1, which is ubiquitously expressed, and PPARγ2, which contains 28 additional amino acids at its NH_2-terminus, and which is only expressed to a significant extent in adipose tissue, where it makes up about 20% of total PPARγ mRNA [1,2]. PPARγ is bound and activated by 15-deoxy-$\Delta^{12,14}$-prostaglandin J_2 [3,4], 9- and 13-hydroxyoctadecadienoic acids [5], thiazolidinedione (TZD) [6] and L-tyrosine-based [7,8] antidiabetic compounds, and a number of nonsteroidal anti-inflammatory drugs (NSAIDs) [9]. The high level of expression of PPARγ in general and the restriction of PPARγ2 expression to adipose tissue points to an important role of this transcription factor in adipocyte differentiation.

Adipogenesis, as well as the maintenance of the fully differentiated adipocyte phenotype, requires an interplay between the PPARγ/RXR heterodimer and two other groups of transcription factors: the CCAATT enhancer-binding proteins (C/EBP) and the helix-loop-helix transcription factor Adipocyte Differentiation and Determination factor-1 (ADD-1)/Sterol regulatory element binding protein 1 (SREBP-1) [10,11]. Although all of these transcription factors can independently induce adipocyte differentiation in vitro, they act synergistically in vivo. During the initial phases of adipogenesis C/EBPβ and δ are induced in response to adipogenic hormones such as insulin or glucocorticoids [12—14]. Both C/EBPs then induce the transcription the PPARγ2 promoter [14—17]. PPARγ2 in its turn then stimulates the expression of PPARγ1 [17]. ADD-1/SREBP-1 [18,19], which is involved in cholesterol homeostasis, enhances PPARγ activity early during adipogenesis on the one hand by inducing PPARγ transcription [20] and on the other hand by controlling the generation of fatty acid-like PPARγ ligands [21—24]. Furthermore, terminal adipocyte differentiation requires the concerted action of PPARγ and C/EBPα [16,25,26], which appears only relatively late in the differentiation process. PPARγ controls not only the expression of C/EBPα, but this last factor in its turn also induces PPARγ gene expression [16,17,27]. Finally, RXR, the obligate heterodimeric partner of PPARγ, is also of importance during adipocyte differentiation [28]. On DR-1 response elements, RXR is a nonpermissive inactive partner when heterodimerized with RAR, whereas it is permissive in the context of the PPARγ/RXR heterodimer. The decrease in RAR expression in the wake of a significant increase in PPARγ levels will drive RXR to switch from RAR to PPARγ as dimerization partner [28,29] and change RXR activity from a nonpermissive to a permissive X-ceptor state, ultimately translating in an alteration of the transcriptional activity of the downstream target genes [28].

The enhanced adipocyte differentiation, which ensues from PPARγ activation, translates in the induction of the expression of adipocyte-specific genes, such as aP2 [30], phosphoenol pyruvate carboxykinase (PEPCK) [31], acyl CoA synthase (ACS) [32,33], fatty acid translocase/CD36 (FAT/CD36) [34], fatty acid transport protein-1 (FATP-1) [35,36], and lipoprotein lipase (LPL) [37]. A number of these genes are involved in the generation and/or cellular uptake of fatty acid ligands of PPARγ, supporting the hypothesis that PPARγ in conjunction with its target genes, enhances adipocyte conversion and maintenance through a positive feedback "thrifty" regulatory loop [10,38,39].

Two cytokines produced by the adipocytes, leptin and TNFα, also appear to be functioning in this adipocyte-sustaining positive regulatory loop. The expression of leptin, a protein that controls body weight and energy expenditure [40], is regulated in an opposite fashion by PPARγ and C/EBPα, the first one reducing [41–43], whereas the second induces its expression [44–46]. Lower leptin levels will trigger food intake, increasing energy delivery to the adipocyte and facilitating energy storage. TNFα is a potent inhibitor of adipocyte differentiation [47,48], an effect based in part on the down-regulation of the expression of adipogenic factors such as C/EBPα [49,50] and PPARγ [51–53]. Interestingly, obesity characterized by increased adipose tissue mass is associated with increased TNFα expression in adipose tissue. Although the exact role of high TNFα levels in obesity is unclear, it might constitute a regulatory mechanism to limit further increase in adipose tissue mass. This increase in TNFα levels in obesity also interferes with the insulin-signaling pathways [54,55] contributing to the insulin resistance characteristic of the obese state [56,57]. Interestingly, PPARγ activation will reduce TNFα expression, thereby again stimulating fat accumulation [58,59].

The drawback to insulin sensitization by PPARγ is the induction of obesity

It is interesting that even mechanisms underlying the insulin-sensitizing actions of PPARγ agonists are part of a "thrifty response". Although other adipose-independent mechanisms can contribute to the insulin-sensitizing effects of PPARγ agonists, since these compounds retain activity in transgenic mice that lack adipose tissue [60], it is currently thought that adipose tissue is their main site of action. Treatment with PPARγ agonists is invariably associated with an increase in adipose tissue mass, which seems at first illogical since obesity is associated with insulin resistance. Lack of adipose tissue, such as seen in subjects [61] and animals with lipoatrophy [62,63] is, however, associated with extreme insulin resistance. Storage of energy in the adipocytes therefore seems to favor insulin sensitivity, suggesting that the important adipogenic activity of PPARγ contributes to the insulin sensitization. PPARγ activation induces in fact a "fatty acid steal" by "trapping" the fatty acids in adipose tissue [64,65]. This results in a decreased systemic availability and a diminished fatty acid uptake by the muscle, improving insulin sensitivity according to Randle [66]. The local decrease in adipocyte TNFα production [58,59] and the decrease in circulating leptin levels [41−43] consequent to PPARγ activation, which also improves insulin signaling, will further enhance fat accumulation. Although all the data above suggest that trapping of energy in adipose tissue will ameliorate insulin sensitivity, this comes at a cost. Whereas in the short-term storage of excess energy by pharmacological PPARγ activation might be beneficial, the resulting accumulation of fat, which ultimately will lead to obesity, will be associated with insulin resistance. Therefore, we expect that long term stimulation of PPARγ activity will lead to a state of resistance to its beneficial actions once a critical adipose mass threshold has been surpassed.

Genetic evidence in support of PPARγ being a thrifty transcription factor

Genetic studies of the PPARγ gene support its role as adipogenic factor [67−71]. A rare Pro115Gln mutation in the NH_2-terminal ligand-independent activation domain of PPARγ was found in four very obese subjects [68]. This mutation, which results in a more active PPARγ, led to increased adipocyte differentiation capacity in vitro [68]. In contrast, a much more common Pro12Ala substitution in the PPARγ2-specific exon B (frequency ± 0.12 in Caucasians and ± 0.02), was associated with a lower body mass index (BMI), improved insulin sensitivity, and higher plasma HDL cholesterol levels [70]. The association with insulin sensitivity disappeared when corrected for BMI, indicating that the primary effect of this mutation was on body weight. The PPARγ Pro12Ala allele exhibited a reduced ability to transactivate responsive promoters, pointing to the importance of the PPARγ2 specific B exon in determining the activity of PPARγ more particularly in adipocytes, the only tissue known to express significant amounts of PPARγ2. Support of the role of the NH_2-terminus of PPARγ in transcriptional activity not only comes from the presence of a ligand-independent AF-1 domain in this part of the molecule [72] but also from its allosteric effects on ligand-dependent transcriptional activity through interdomain communication [73].

These human genetic studies were validated by the analysis of heterozygous PPARγ KO mice, eliminating the potential confounding effect of gene-environment interactions in human studies. Whereas homozygous PPARγ −/− mice are not viable [74,75], mainly due to defects in placentation, heterozygous PPARγ −/+ mice are characterized by a decrease in adipose tissue mass and, contrary to expectations, by a marked insulin sensitization [75,76]. These data from the

PPARγ $-/+$ mice demonstrate that the prime activity of PPARγ is to stimulate adipocyte differentiation and that its effect on insulin sensitivity is secondary to these changes in adipose tissue [75,76]. Whereas these animal data might seem conflicting with our current knowledge on PPARγ, which is mainly derived from pharmacological studies, they are fully in line with the genetic studies, supporting a role of PPARγ in the control of adipogenesis in vivo, such that a more active PPARγ (Pro115Gln) results in an increased BMI and insulin resistance [68], whereas the opposite is seen with a less active PPARγ (Pro12Ala) [70]. Hence, like humans with the Pro12Ala mutation, heterozygous PPARγ $-/+$ mice have a deficiency in the PPARγ system resulting in a decreased capacity to generate adipose tissue with a subsequent improvement in insulin sensitivity.

PPARγ and atherogenesis and inflammation another tale of maladaptation

Just as the functions of PPARγ in adipose tissue can be viewed as an adaptive "thrifty response", other PPARγ-controlled activities might also be part of a similar adaptive response, which carried some benefits under certain environmental conditions. A good example is PPARγ's role in the macrophage differentiation. Macrophages are a crucial component of the innate immune system. Since PPARγ is barely present in undifferentiated resting monocytes [34,77,78], whereas its expression increases strongly during macrophage differentiation [34,78], it was suggested that PPARγ was important for this differentiation process. This was supported by the observation that activation of the PPARγ/RXR heterodimer furthermore enhances macrophage differentiation [34]. Interestingly, exposure of monocytes to oxidized LDL (oxLDL), but not regular LDL, induces PPARγ expression [34,78], which in turn stimulates the transcription of the oxLDL receptor, FAT/CD36, thus establishing a positive feedback loop enhancing macrophage differentiation into foam cells [34]. Exposure of monocyte/ macrophages to oxLDL not only induces PPARγ expression, but provides the cells also with two new PPARγ ligands, i.e., 9- and 13-hydroxyoctadecadienoic acids, both oxidative metabolites of linoleic acid present in oxLDL [5]. This role of PPARγ in macrophage differentiation suggests potential contributions to the development of atherosclerosis. In fact, high amounts of PPARγ were observed in human [78,79] and mouse [34] atherosclerotic lesions, where PPARγ colocalized with oxLDL [78,79]. The strong expression of PPARγ in macrophage foam cells and atherosclerotic lesions, as well as the important amounts of 9- and 13-hydroxyoctadecadienoic acids present in oxLDL, suggest that PPARγ might have a predominantly pro-atherogenic activity when the appropriate dietary conditions are met. Although this pro-atherogenic activity might be counterbalanced or neutralized by other effects of PPARγ on vascular smooth muscle cells [80] or other organ systems, further in vivo studies are clearly necessary to define the exact role of PPARγ in atherosclerosis.

Based on the general antagonism between PPARγ and TNFα, PPARγ activation could also limit inflammatory responses in macrophages. In fact, in both adipocytes and macrophages, PPARγ agonists seem to limit the production of proinflammatory cytokines [81,82]. This is mediated by interference with the transcription factors NF-kB, AP-1, and STAT, all of which regulate cytokine gene expression [81,82]. It is therefore tempting to hypothesize that some of the beneficial effects of nonsteroidal anti-inflammatory drugs (NSAIDs) might be due to a PPARγ-mediated suppression of cytokine synthesis. Consistent with this is the fact that the effective doses of nonsteroidal anti-inflammatory drugs (NSAIDs) are in the micromolar range, and exceed those required inhibition of cyclooxygenases, but are in the range of those required to activate PPARγ.

PPARγ and obesity: parallels with insulin signaling and dauer formation

So far, experimental evidence seems to support the hypothesis that PPARγ is a master controller of the "thrifty response". During most of evolution, such a response was selected by genetic pressure. In fact, a "thrifty response", associated with efficient energy storage was highly beneficial in stressful episodes and allowed the individual to survive episodes of famine and food shortage. Like efficient energy conservation used to be beneficial, a solid innate immune response was clearly of interest to combat infection, inflammation and neoplasia. This "thrifty response" carries strong resemblance with some aspects of the insulin signaling system. How PPARγ interfaces with the insulin signaling, another key hormonal axis involved in energy storage, is unknown. However, the fact that PPARγ agonists are insulin sensitizers suggests a significant overlap of both signaling pathways. Insulin has been associated with the physiological response to food intake throughout the animal kingdom. For instance, in the primitive worm *Caenorhabditis elegans*, animals with mutations in the insulin signaling pathway (Daf-2/Daf-16) are growth arrested, store energy under the form of fat in a condition resembling dauer, and significantly extend their life-span [83]. Wild-type animals can also enter diapause or dauer under unfavorable conditions, such as in the absence of adequate nutrition and/or crowding, making this situation similar to a "thrifty response". Similarly, Drosophila interference with insulin signaling, as occurs in chico mutants that lack the Drosophila homolog of the insulin receptor substrate, is characterized by fat accumulation [84]. It is likely that PPARγ acts on a similar energy-saving pathway in higher mammals and enhances fat accumulation and a "thrifty response".

The nuclear receptors LXR and FXR: feedback regulation of cholesterol metabolism

Liver X receptor (LXR), the sterol X-ceptor

LXRα is an X-ceptor originally isolated from liver [85]. Two different LXR genes exist, termed LXRα (RLD-1 or NR1H3) [85,86] and LXRβ (NER, UR, OR-1 or NR1H2) [87–89]. LXRα, the best-characterized form, is expressed to a high extent in liver and macrophages, with lower levels being present in kidney, intestine, spleen and adipose tissue [2,86]. In contrast to LXRα, LXRβ is more ubiquitously expressed. Despite its more ubiquitous expression pattern, relatively little is known about the function of LXRβ. Therefore, the subsequent discussion is mainly focussed on LXRα.

LXR binds as a heterodimer with RXR (NR2B1) to a LXR response element (LXRE), preferentially consisting of a direct repeat of the hormone receptor response element half site spaced by four nucleotides (DR-4) [85,86,88,89]. Consistent with the definition of X-ceptors, the LXR/RXR heterodimer can be activated on the one hand by oxysterol intermediates of the cholesterol synthesis pathways and on the other hand by RXR ligands [90,91]. This suggests that the presence of RXR ligands is capable of inducing a conformational change in the LXR AF-2 domain, necessary for the transcriptional activation of the RXR/LXR heterodimer. If both RXR and LXR ligands are present, a synergistic activity is obtained.

The finding that LXR is activated by cholesterol metabolites is not too surprising since most ligands for nuclear receptors are lipophilic derivatives of acetyl CoA and several of them are cholesterol metabolites (i.e., the steroid hormones and vitamin D_3). Interestingly, only a very confined group of metabolites of the sterol synthesis pathways are powerful activators [92—95] and ligands [96]. Structure activity studies have in fact demonstrated that position-specific monooxidation of the sterol side chain is a requisite for LXR binding and activation [96]. 24, 25(S)-epoxycholesterol, which is produced from squalene and builds up in the liver after cholesterol feeding, is the most effective activator. In contrast to other oxysterols, 24, 25(S)-epoxycholesterol is derived from a shunt in the classical cholesterol biosynthesis pathway. Another equally potent but less effective activator is 22(R)-hydroxycholesterol. This compound is synthesized mainly in the gonads, the adrenal glands and the placenta and might play an important role in developmental signalling by LXR. A third molecule that elicits an LXR response at a concentration that is within the physiological range, is 20(S)-OH-cholesterol. Finally, a fourth compound capable of significantly activating LXR is 24(S)-hydroxycholesterol or cerebrosterol, which is produced to a great extent in the development of the brain. The constitutive activity of LXRα led Forman et al. to examine whether this was dependent on endogenous lipid metabolism [95]. Inhibition of de novo cholesterol synthesis by HMG-CoA reductase inhibitors, led to a significantly repressed LXRα activity, which could be restored by addition of mevalonic acid or any of the above-mentioned oxysterols [95]. Furthermore, the amount of these cholesterol-derived signaling molecules present in tissues which express LXRα and LXRβ is in a concentration range of their dissociation constant for the receptors (0.1-1 μM), lending credibility to the hypothesis that these compounds could act as putative natural ligands. In addition to these natural agonists, some synthetic LXR ligands were recently described with some improved characteristics, relative to the natural ligands. Sterols with a 24-oxo group, which act as hydrogen bond acceptors, have enhanced capacity to bind and activate LXR [96]. Furthermore, introduction of an oxygen on the sterol B-ring results in ligands with a slight LXRα selectivity [96].

Oxysterols are clearly not the only compounds capable of modulating LXR activity, since it has been reported that transactivation by ligand-activated LXRs may be further modulated through other signal transduction pathways involving phosphorylation by protein kinases, such as PKA and PKC [97]. Consistent with this last observation, Tamura et al. recently demonstrated that LXR plays a critical role in inducing both renin and c-Myc transcription after activation of the cAMP signal transduction cascade [98]. In addition, these authors demonstrated that LXRα binds both the classical DR-4 and a newly identified LXR response element corresponding to the binding sequence of the cAMP-inducible transcription activator (CNRE), thereby mediating cAMP responsiveness of a subset of target genes [98].

Unequivocal evidence for a specific role in cholesterol homeostasis has been provided by studies in LXRα-deficient mice, which demonstrated that LXRα is involved in oxysterol-induced excretion of cholesterol [94]. When LXRα −/− mice are fed a high-cholesterol diet, they develop hepatomegaly due to excessive hepatic cholesterol accumulation. More elaborate expression studies of genes involved in cholesterol synthesis and removal revealed that LXR mutant mice are not able to upregulate the 7α-hydroxylase (CYP 7A1) gene after cholesterol feeding [94]. In wild-type animals, induction of CYP 7A1 by excessive amounts of cholesterol results in excretion of the excess of cholesterol in the bile. The incapacity to upregulate the initial and rate-limiting enzyme of the bile acid synthesis pathway would explain the development of hepatomegaly observed in LXRα deficient mice. Interestingly, the mouse CYP 7A1 gene was previously shown to contain a DR-4 LXR response element in its promoter (Fig. 2) [92,93]. The recent identification of a series of new target genes for LXR, further underscores the role of this X-ceptor in almost every aspect of cholesterol homeostasis. First, LXRα controls ATP cassette-binding protein (ABC)-mediated reverse cholesterol transport from the peripheral tissues to the liver [99] (Repa et al., unpublished observations). By regulating the expression of the cholesterol ester transfer protein (CETP), LXRα furthermore favors transfer of cholesterol to the liver [100]. In the liver LXR controls cholesterol catabolism through its regulatory effects on CYP 7A1 [94]. Finally, in the gut, activation of LXRα has been recently shown to decrease intestinal cholesterol absorption, through its effects on intestinal ABC expression (Repa et al., unpublished observations). All of these actions of LXRα activation seem to favor cholesterol catabolism and excretion and hence contribute to lowering total body cholesterol content.

One last recent publication worth mentioning related to LXRα's role in lipid homeostasis is the observation that the expression of the LXRα gene is induced by fatty acids via a PPAR-driven mechanism. This observation hints to a potential cross-talk between fatty acid and cholesterol metabolism and suggests that such cross-regulatory circuits might underlie the body's capacity to handle lipids ingested through the diet.

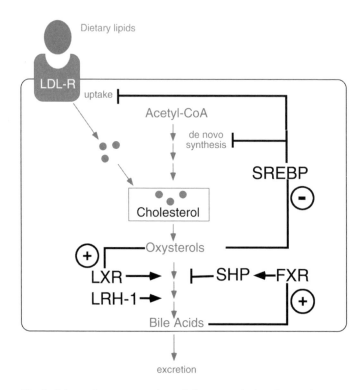

Fig. 2. Schematic representation of the transcription factors involved in the feedforward (LXRα, FXR/BAR, LRH-1, SHP) and feedback (SREBP) regulation of cholesterol metabolism.

Farnesol X receptor (FXR or NR1H4) or bile acid receptor (BAR)

Rat FXR [101] and its mouse ortholog RIP-14 [102] are X-ceptors that were isolated independently by different approaches and that show most homology with the Drosophila ecdysone receptor (EcR or NR1H1). Analogous to the known dimerization of EcR and Ultraspiracle (Usp or NR2B4) and consistent with it being an X-ceptor, FXR forms a permissive heterodimer with RXR, the mammalian ortholog of Usp, and binds to DNA sequences consisting of an inverted repeat spaced by one nucleotide (IR-1) [103]. FXR is most highly expressed in liver, gut, kidney and adrenal cortexes.

FXR was originally identified as an X-ceptor whose transcriptional activity was modulated by a large variety of endogenous isoprenoids, including farnesol [101]. In addition, FXR was also shown to be activated by all-trans-retinoic acid and synthetic retinoids such as TTNPB [104]. Although the compounds discussed above could induce moderately the activity of FXR, none of them were shown to be direct ligands for FXR. A lot of excitement was generated recently when FXR was shown to be bound and activated by a number of bile acids, including chenodeoxycholic acid (CDCA), litocholic acid (LCA) and deoxycholic acid (DCA) [105–107]. Due to this fact, FXR earned the name of nuclear Bile Acid Receptor (BAR). Bile acids are mostly conjugated to glycine or taurine, a derivative of cysteine. Unlike the nonconjugated bile acids CDCA, LCA, and DCA, their conjugated forms were only capable of activating FXR if the intestinal bile acid transporter (IBAT) was cotransfected in the cells, enabling their access to the cell [105,107]. This control of ligand entry in the cell restricts receptor activation to cells expressing the transporter protein.

Interestingly, FXR was also shown to control a number of proteins involved in bile acid homeostasis. Most notably, FXR stimulated the expression of the cytosolic intestinal bile acid-binding protein (IBABP), which acts as a carrier protein facilitating the re-uptake of bile acids from the gut [106,108]. This regulation explains in part the efficacy of the enterohepatic recirculation of bile acids, which is crucial to maintain the bile acid pool. Furthermore FXR was involved in the reduction of de novo bile acid synthesis by down-regulating the transcription of the rate-limiting enzyme in bile acid synthesis, CYP 7A1 [105,106]. This down-regulation of CYP 7A1 was, however, not due to a direct negative regulation of FXR on the CYP 7A1 promoter, but rather was secondary to the FXR-mediated transcriptional induction of the short heterodimeric partner (SHP or NR0B2), an atypical orphan nuclear receptor, which like the related receptor DAX-1 lacks a DNA-binding domain (Fig. 2). Similar to DAX-1, SHP has been shown to decrease the transcriptional activity of several nuclear receptors, by several mechanisms including recruitment of corepressors and completion of coactivator binding to the receptor [109–112]. The FXR-mediated induction of SHP by bile acids attenuated the positive effects of another nuclear receptor, the liver receptor homolog-1 (LRH-1 or NR5A2) on CYP 7A1 production and hence will lead to a decrease in CYP7A1 levels (Lu et al., unpublished data and Fig. 2). Furthermore, a recent paper demonstrated that FXR regulates the expression of the human phospholipid transfer protein (PLTP), a protein that catalyzes the transfer of phospholipids and cholesterol from triglyceride-rich lipoproteins to high-density lipoproteins [113]. These authors also identified potential FXR binding sites in the carnitine palmitoyltransferase II and phenylethanolamine N-methyltransferase, although data demonstrating that these last two genes are regulated by FXR in vivo are as of yet lacking [113].

Conclusions and future perspectives

We speculate that X-ceptors arose early during evolution in order to help organisms adapt to changes in nutrient composition and supply, which were often important evolutionary bottlenecks. In order to get a maximal profit from the presence of nutrients, it would clearly be beneficial if organisms would possess an efficient autoregulatory mechanism stimulating in a feedback fashion use and metabolism of these nutrients. Such a regulation could be achieved if the nutrient would also have a signaling function triggering this regulatory circuit. The observation that nutrient-derived fatty acids are not only important energy sources but also potent signaling molecules, activating the PPAR subfamily of X-ceptors, suggests that such a mechanism might in fact be active. The PPARs can therefore be considered as important sensors and effectors in such a feedback regulatory loop governing the use of fatty acids. Hence PPARs would condition the use of fatty acids either as direct substrates for β-oxidation, in a process controlled by PPARα, or as building blocks for triglyceride synthesis in the adipocyte, under the impetus of a PPARγ. The importance of these regulatory circuits is underscored by diseases, such as morbid obesity, associated with genetic defects in certain PPAR-controlled homeostatic processes [68].

The situation for cholesterol is somewhat different. Cholesterol is an important building block for membrane synthesis and organisms definitely need a constant cholesterol supply. High cholesterol concentrations are, however, toxic and hence an intricate transcriptional control circuit limits exposure to excess cholesterol both at a cellular and whole body level. Variations in intracellular sterol concentrations can affect the activity of transcription factors via two completely distinct control mechanisms, i.e., by modulating proteolytic cleavage of the SREBP family of helix-loop-helix factors [114], or by direct binding and activation of LXR (Fig. 2). These redundant control mechanisms underscore the importance of cholesterol homeostasis and suggest that even moderate changes in cholesterol levels beyond an optimal range could have an important impact on developmental and homeostatic processes. Good examples demonstrating the impact of aberrant regulation of cholesterol homeostasis are provided by the severe malformations associated with decreased cholesterol synthesis in early development [115–118] and the negative impact of elevated cholesterol levels in subjects with familial hypercholesterolemia on atherosclerotic vascular disease.

Nutrients, such as meat, a rich source in fatty acids and cholesterol, were rather limited in supply during much of evolution. It is certainly to make optimal use of such nutrients that organisms developed these nutrient-sensitive transcription factors, allowing metabolic adaptation and survival by stimulating a "thrifty response". Such a "thrifty response", which used to be necessary for survival for the hunter-gatherer, became unfortunately completely maladapted in our affluent societies today, and we speculate that "overstimulation" of the transcription factors underlying such a "thrifty response" underlies in part the recent rise in prevalence of common diseases, such as obesity, atherosclerosis, or chronic inflammation. In fact, "overstimulation" of PPARγ, by excess dietary-derived PPARγ agonists, could underlie the current epidemic of obesity and associated disorders. Likewise our high intake of cholesterol-rich nutrition could perturb the fine-tuned transcriptional regulation of cholesterol and bile acid homeostasis, contributing to the increased frequency of hypercholesterolemia and gallbladder disease. More detailed understanding of the function of these X-ceptors in whole body homeostasis will therefore be indispensable before chronic therapeutic use of X-ceptor modulators can be advocated in the treatment of some of these common disorders. For instance, based upon the evidence discussed above, we speculate that PPARγ antagonists or partial agonists could in fact hold more promise then very efficacious and potent agonists for some chronic conditions such as obesity, insulin resistance, and chronic inflammatory disorders. Likewise, we speculate that the understanding of the novel feedback regulatory pathways of cholesterol homeostasis will lead to alternative lipid-lowering strategies based on stimulation of LXR and/or inhibition of FXR signaling, and will emerge as valid additions to therapeutic inhibition of de novo cholesterol synthesis.

Acknowledgements

Helpful discussions with members of the Auwerx lab are acknowledged. Work in the laboratories of the authors is supported by grants of CNRS, INSERM, ULP, Hopital Universitaire de Strasbourg, HHMI, and HFSP (RG0041/1999-M). J. Auwerx is a research director with CNRS, and K. Schoonjans is a research assistant with INSERM.

References

1. Fajas L, Fruchart JC, Auwerx J. PPARγ3 mRNA: a distinct PPARγ mRNA subtype transcribed from an independent promoter. FEBS Lett 1998;438:55−60.
2. Auboeuf D, Rieusset J, Fajas L, Vallier P, Frering V, Riou JP, Laville M, Staels B, Auwerx J, Vidal H. Tissue distribution and quantification of the expression of PPARs and LXRα in humans: no alterations in adipose tissue of obese and NIDDM patients. Diabetes 1997;48:1319−1327.
3. Kliewer SA, Lenhar JM, Willson TM, Patel I, Morris DC, Lehman JM. A prostaglandin J2 metabolite binds peroxisome proliferator-activated receptor γ and promotes adipocyte differentiation. Cell 1995;83:813−819.
4. Forman BM, Tontonoz P, Chen J, Brun RP, Spiegelman BM, Evans RM. 15-Deoxy-Δ12,14 prostaglandin J2 is a ligand for the adipocyte determination factor PPARγ. Cell 1995;83:803−812.
5. Nagy L, Tontonez P, Alvarez JG, Chen H, Evans RM. Oxidized LDL regulates macrophage gene expression through ligand activation of PPARγ. Cell 1998;93:229−240.
6. Lehmann JM, Moore LB, Smith-Oliver TA, Wilkison WO, Willson TM, Kliewer SA. An antidiabetic thiazolidinedione is a high affinity ligand for Peroxisome Proliferator-Activated Receptor γ (PPARγ). J Biol Chem 1995;270:12953−12956.
7. Cobb JE, Blanchard SG, Boswell EG, Brown KK, Charifson PS, Cooper JP, Collins JL, Dezube M, Henke BR, Hull-Ryde EA, Lake DH, Lenhard JM, Oliver W Jr, Oplinger J, Pentti M, Parks DJ, Plunket KD, Tong WQ. N-(2-Benzoylphenyl)-L-tyrosine PPARgamma agonists. 3. Structure-activity relationship and optimization of the N-aryl substituent. J Med Chem 1998;41: 5055−5069.
8. Collins JL, Blanchard SG, Boswell GE, Charifson PS, Cobb JE, Henke BR, Hull-Ryde EA, Kazmierski WM, Lake DH, Leesnitzer LM, Lehmann J, Lenhard JM, Orband-Miller LA, Gray-Nunez Y, Parks DJ, Plunkett KD, Tong WQ. N-(2-Benzoylphenyl)-L-tyrosine PPARgamma agonists. 2. Structure-activity relationship and optimization of the phenyl alkyl ether moiety. J Med Chem 1998;41:5037−5054.
9. Lehmann JM, Lenhard JM, Oliver BB, Ringold GM, Kliewer SA. Peroxisome proliferator-activated receptors α and γ are activated by indomethacin and other non-steroidal anti-inflammatory drugs. J Biol Chem 1997;272:3406−3410.
10. Fajas L, Fruchart JC, Auwerx J. Transcriptional control of adipogenesis. Curr Opin Cell Biol 1998;10:165−173.
11. Rosen ED, Walkey CJ, Puigserver P, Spiegelman BM. Transcriptional regulation of adipogenesis (In Process Citation). Genes Dev 2000;14:1293−1307.

12. Yeh WC, Cao Z, Classon M, McKnight S. Cascade regulation of terminal adipocyte differentiation by three members of the C/EBP family of leucine zipper proteins. Genes Devel 1995;9: 168–181.

13. Wu Z, Xie Y, Bucher NLR, Farmer SR. Conditional ectopic expression of C/EBPβ in NIH-3T3 cells induces PPARγ and stimulates adipogenesis. Genes Devel 1995;9:2350–2363.

14. Wu Z, Bucher NLR, Farmer SR. Induction of peroxisome proliferator-activated receptor γ during the conversion of 3T3 fibroblasts into adipocytes is mediated by C/EBPβ, C/EBPδ, and glucocorticoids. Molec Cell Biol 1996;16:4128–4136.

15. Fajas L, Auboeuf D, Raspe E, Schoonjans K, Lefebvre AM, Saladin R, Najib J, Laville M, Fruchart JC, Deeb S, Vidal-Puig A, Flier J, Briggs MR, Staels B, Vidal H, Auwerx J. Organization, promoter analysis and expression of the human PPARγ gene. J Biol Chem 1997;272:18779–18789.

16. Wu Z, Rosen ED, Brun R, Hauser S, Hauser G, Hauser A, Troy AE, McKeon C, Darlington GJ, Spiegelman BM. Cross-regulation of C/EBPα and PPARγ controls the transcriptional pathway of adipogenesis and insulin sensitivity. Molec Cell 1999;3:143–150.

17. Saladin R, Fajas L, Dana S, Halvorsen YD, Auwerx J, Briggs M. Differential regulation of peroxisome proliferator activated receptor γ1 (PPARγ1) and PPARγ2 mRNA expession in early stages of adipogenesis. Cell Growth Differ 1999;10:43–48.

18. Tontonoz P, Kim JB, Graves RA, Spiegelman BM. ADD1: a novel helix-loop-helix transcription factor associated with adipocyte determination and differentiation. Molec Cell Biol 1993;13: 4753–4759.

19. Kim JB, Spiegelman BM. ADD1/SREBP1 promotes adipocyte differentiation and gene expression linked to fatty acid metabolism. Genes Devel 1996;10:1096–1107.

20. Fajas L, Schoonjans K, Gelman L, Kim JB, Najib J, Martin G, Fruchart JC, Briggs M, Spiegelman BM, Auwerx J. Regulation of PPARγ expression by ADD-1/SREBP-1: implications for adipocyte differentiation and metabolism. Molec Cell Biol 1999;19:5495–5503.

21. Shimano H, Horton JD, Hammer RE, Shimomura I, Brown MS, Goldstein JL. Overproduction of cholesterol and fatty acids causes massive liver enlargement in transgenic mice expressing truncated SREBP-1a. J Clin Invest 1996;98:1575–1584.

22. Lopez JM, Bennett MK, Sanchez HB, Rosenfeld JM, Osborne TF. Sterol regulation of acetyl coenzyme A carboxylase: a mechanism for coordinate control of cellular lipid. Proc Natl Acad Sci USA 1996;93:1049–1053.

23. Bennet MK, Lopez JM, Sanchez HB, Osborne TF. Sterol regulation of fatty acid synthase promoter; coordinate feedback regulation of two major lipid pathways. J Biol Chem 1995;270: 25578–25583.

24. Kim JB, Wright HM, Wright M, Spiegelman BM. ADD1/SREBP1 activates PPARγ through the production of endogenous ligand. Proc Natl Acad Sci USA 1998;95:4333–4337.

25. Tontonoz P, Hu E, Spiegelman BM. Stimulation of adipogenesis in fibroblasts by PPARγ2, a lipid-activated transcription factor. Cell 1994;79:1147–1156.

26. Hu E, Tontonoz P, Spiegelman BM. Transdifferentiation of myoblasts by the adipogenic transcription factors PPARγ and C/EBPα. Proc Natl Acad Sci USA 1995;92:9856–9860.

27. Zhu Y, Qi C, Korenberg JR, Chen X-N, Noya D, Rao MS, Reddy JK. Structural organization of mouse peroxisome proliferator activated receptor γ (mPPARγ) gene: alternative promoter use and different splicing yield two mPPARγ isoforms. Proc Natl Acad Sci USA 1995;92:7921–7925.

28. DiRenzo J, Soderstrom M, Kurokawa R, Ogliastro MH, Ricote M, Ingrey S, Horlein A, Rosenfeld MG, Glass CK. Peroxisome proliferator-activated receptors and retinoic acid receptors differentially control the interactions of retinoid X receptor heterodimers with ligands, coactivators and corepressors. Molec Cell Biol 1997;17:2166–2176.

29. Xue JC, Schwarz EJ, Chawla A, Lazar MA. Distinct stages in adipogenesis revealed by retinoid inhibition of differentiation after induction of PPARγ. Molec Cell Biol 1996;16:1567–1575.

30. Tontonoz P, Hu E, Graves RA, Budavari AI, Spiegelman BM. mPPARγ2: tissue-specific regula-

tor of an adipocyte enhancer. Genes Devel 1994;8:1224–1234.

31. Tontonoz P, Hu E, Devine J, Beale EG, Spiegelman BM. PPARγ2 regulates adipose expression of the phosphoenolpyruvate carboxykinase gene. Molec Cell Biol 1995;15:351–357.

32. Schoonjans K, Staels B, Grimaldi P, Auwerx J. Acyl-CoA synthetase mRNA expression is controlled by fibric-acid derivatives, feeding and liver proliferation. Eur J Biochem 1993;216:615–622.

33. Schoonjans K, Watanabe M, Suzuki H, Mahfoudi A, Krey G, Wahli W, Grimaldi P, Staels B, Yamamoto T, Auwerx J. Induction of the Acyl-Coenzyme A synthetase gene by fibrates and fatty acids is mediated by a peroxisome proliferator response element in the C promoter. J Biol Chem 1995;270:19269–19276.

34. Tontonoz P, Nagy L, Alvarez JG, Thomazy VA, Evans RM. PPARγ promotes monocyte/macrophage differentiation and uptake of oxidized LDL. Cell 1998;93:241–252.

35. Martin G, Schoonjans K, Lefebvre A, Staels B, Auwerx J. Coordinate regulation of the expression of the fatty acid transport protein (FATP) and acyl CoA synthetase genes by PPARα and PPARγ activators. J Biol Chem 1997;272:28210–28217.

36. Hui TY, Frohnert BI, Smith AJ, Schaffer JE, Bernlohr DA. Characterization of the murine fatty acid transport protein gene and its insulin response sequence. J Biol Chem 1998;273:27420–27429.

37. Schoonjans K, Peinado-Onsurbe J, Lefebvre AM, Heyman R, Briggs M, Deeb S, Staels B, Auwerx J. PPARα and PPARγ activators direct a tissue-specific transcriptional response via a PPRE in the lipoprotein lipase gene. EMBO J 1996;15:5336–5348.

38. Schoonjans K, Martin G, Staels B, Auwerx J. Peroxisome proliferator-activated receptors, orphans with ligands and functions. Curr Opin Lipid 1997;8:159–166.

39. Spiegelman BM, Flier JS. Adipogenesis and obesity: rounding out the big picture. Cell 1996;87:377–389.

40. Auwerx J, Staels B. Leptin. Lancet 1998;351:737–742.

41. De Vos P, Lefebvre AM, Miller SG, Guerre-Millo M, Wong K, Saladin R, Hamann L, Staels B, Briggs MR, Auwerx J. Thiazolidinediones repress ob gene expression via activation of PPARγ. J Clin Invest 1996;98:1004–1009.

42. Zhang B, Graziano MP, Doebber TW, Leibowitz MD, White-Carrington S, Szalkowski DM, Hey PT, Wu M, Cullinan CA, Bailey P, Lollmann B, Frederich R, Flier JS, Strader CD, Smith RG. Down-regulation of the expression of the obese gene by antidiabetic thiazolidinedione in Zucker diabetic fatty rats and db/db mice. J Biol Chem 1996;271:9455–9459.

43. Kallen CB, Lazar MA. Antidiabetic thiazolidinediones inhibit leptin (ob) gene expression in 3T3-L1 adipocytes. Proc Natl Acad Sci USA 1996;93:5793–5796.

44. Miller SG, De Vos P, Guerre-Millo M, Wong K, Hermann T, Staels B, Briggs MR, Auwerx J. The adipocyte specific transcription factor, C/EBPα modulates human ob gene expression. Proc Natl Acad Sci USA 1996;93:5507–5511.

45. He Y, Chen H, Quon MJ, Reitman M. The mouse obese gene. Genomic organization, promoter activity, and activation by CCAAT/enhancer-binding protein alpha. J Biol Chem 1995;270:28887–28891.

46. Hollenberg AN, Susulic VS, Madura JP, Zhang B, Moller DE, Tontonoz P, Sarraf P, Spiegelman BM, Lowell BB. Functional antagonism between CCAAT/enhancer binding protein-α and peroxisome proliferator-activated receptor-γ on the leptin promoter. J Biol Chem 1997;272:5283–5290.

47. Torti FM, Dieckman B, Beutler B, Cerami A, Ringold GM. A macrophage factor inhibits adipocyte gene expression; an in vitro model for cachexia. Science 1985;229:867–869.

48. Beutler B, Cerami A. Cachectin (tumor necrosis factor): a macrophage hormone governing cellular metabolism and inflammatory response. Endocrine Rev 1988;9:57–66.

49. Williams PM, Chang DJ, Danesch U, Ringold GM, Heller RA. CCAAT/enhancer binding protein expression is rapidly extinguished in TA1 adipocyte cells treated with tumor necrosis factor. Molec Endocrinol 1992;6:1135–1141.

50. Ron D, Brasier AR, McGehee REJ, Habener JF. Tumor necrosis factor-induced reversal of adipocytic phenotype of 3T3-L1 cells is preceded by a loss of nuclear CCAAT/enhancer binding protein (C/EBP). J Clin Invest 1992;89:223–233.

51. Peraldi P, Xu M, Spiegelman BM. Thiazolidinediones block tumor necrosis factor-α-induced inhibition of insulin signalling. J Clin Invest 1997;100:1863–1869.

52. Xing H, Northrop JP, Grove JR, Kilpatrick KE, Su JL, Ringold GM. TNFα-mediated inhibition and reversal of adipocyte differentiation is accompanied by suppressed expression of PPARγ without effects on Pref-1 expression. Endocrinology 1997;138:2776–2783.

53. Hill M, Young M, McCurdy C, Gimble J. Decreased expression of murine PPARγ in adipose tissue during endotoxinemia. Endocrinology 1997;138:3073–3076.

54. Hotamisligil GS, Shargill NS, Spiegelman BM. Adipose tissue expression of tumor necrosis factor-α: direct role in obesity-linked insulin resistance. Science 1993;259:87–91.

55. Hotamisligil GS, Arner P, Caro JF, Atkinson RL, Spiegelman BM. Increased adipose tissue expression of tumor necrosis factor-α in human obesity and insulin resistance. J Clin Invest 1995;95:2409–2415.

56. Hotamisligil GS, Peraldi P, Budavari A, Ellis R, White MF, Spiegelman BM. IRS-1-mediated inhibition of insulin receptor tyrosine kinase activity in TNF-α- and obesity induced insulin resistance. Science 1996;271:665–668.

57. Hotamisligil GS, Murray DL, Choy LN, Spiegelman BM. Tumor necrosis factor α inhibits signaling from the insulin receptor. Proc Natl Acad Sci USA 1994;91:4854–4858.

58. Hofmann C, Lorenz K, Braithwaite SS, Colca JR, Palazuk BJ, Hotamisligil GS, Spiegelman BM. Altered gene expression for tumor necrosis factor-α and its receptor during drug and dietary modulation of insulin resistance. Endocrinology 1994;134:264–270.

59. Okuno A, Tamemoto H, Tobe K, Ueki K, Mori Y, Iwamoto K, Umesono K, Akanuma Y, Fujiwara T, Horikoshi H, Yazaki Y, Kadowaki T. Troglitazone increases the number of small adipocytes without the change of white adipose tissue mass in obese Zucker rats. J Clin Invest 1998; 101:1354–1361.

60. Burant CF, Sreenan S, Hirano K-I, Tai T-AC, Lohmiller J, Lukens J, Davidson NO, Ross S, Graves RA. Troglitazone action is independent of adipose tissue. J Clin Invest 1997;100:2900–2908.

61. Moller DE, Flier JS. Insulin resistance-mechanisms, syndromes, and implications. N Engl J Med 1991;325:938–948.

62. Shimomura I, Hammer RE, Richardson JA, Ikemoto S, Bashmakov Y, Bashmakov JL, Bashmakov G, Brown MS. Insulin resistance and diabetes mellitus in transgenic mice expressing nuclear SREBP-1c in adipose tissue: a model for congenital generalized lipodystrophy. Genes Devel 1998;12:3182–3194.

63. Moitra J, Mason MM, Olive M, Krylov D, Gavrilova O, Marcus-Samuels B, Feigenbaum L, Lee E, Aoyama T, Eckhaus M, Reitman ML, Vinson C. Life without fat: a transgenic mouse. Genes Devel 1998;12:3168–3181.

64. Martin G, Schoonjans K, Staels B, Auwerx J. PPARγ activators improve glucose homeostasis by stimulating fatty acid uptake in the adipocytes. Atherosclerosis 1998;137:75–80.

65. Oakes ND, Camilleri S, Furler SM, Chisholm DJ, Kraege EW. The insulin sensitizer, BRL 49653, reduces systemic fatty acid supply and utilization and tissue availability in the rat. Metabolism 1997;46:935–942.

66. Randle PJ, Garland PB, Hales CN, Newsholme EA. The glucose-fatty acid cycle: its role in insulin sensitivity and metabolic disturbances of diabetes mellitus. Lancet 1961;1:785–789.

67. Vigouroux C, Fajas L, Khallouf E, Meier M, Gyapay G, Auwerx J, Weissenbach J, Capeau, Magre J. Human peroxisome proliferator-activated receptor gamma 2: genetic mapping, identification of a variant in the coding sequence, and exclusion as the gene responsible for lipoatrophic diabetes. Diabetes 1998;47:490–492.

68. Ristow M, Muller-Wieland D, Pfeiffer A, Krone W, Kahn CR. Obesity associated with a mutation in a genetic regulator of adipocyte differentiation. N Engl J Med 1998;339:953–959.

69. Yen CJ, Beamer BA, Negri C, Silver K, Brown KA, Yarnall DP, Burns DK, Roth J, Shuldiner AR. Molecular scanning of the human peroxisome proliferator activated receptor gamma gene in diabetic Caucasians: identification of a Pro12Ala PPARgamma 2 missense mutation. Biochem Biophys Res Commun 1997;241:270—274.

70. Deeb S, Fajas L, Nemoto M, Laakso M, Fujimoto W, Auwerx J. A Pro 12 Ala substitution in the human peroxisome proliferator-activated receptor gamma2 is associated with decreased receptor activity, improved insulin sensitivity, and lowered body mass index. Nature Genet 1998;20: 284—287.

71. Beamer BA, Yen CJ, Andersen RE, Muller D, Elahi D, Cheskin LJ, Andres R, Roth J, Shuldiner AR. Association of the Pro12Ala variant in peroxisome proliferator-activated receptor gamma2 gene with obesity in two Caucasian populations. Diabetes 1998;47:1806—1808.

72. Werman A, Hollenberg A, Solanes G, Bjorbaek C, Vidal-Puig A, Flier JS. Ligand-independent activation domain in the N terminus of peroxisome proliferator-activated receptor γ (PPARγ). J Biol Chem 1997;272:20230—20235.

73. Shao D, Rangwala SM, Bailey ST, Krakow SL, Reginato MJ, Lazar MA. Interdomain communication regulating ligand binding by PPAR gamma. Nature 1998;396:377—380.

74. Barak Y, Nelson MC, Ong ES, Jones YZ, Ruiz-Lozano P, Chien KR, Koder A, Evans RM. PPARgamma is required for placental, cardiac, and adipose tissue development. Molec Cell 1999;4:585—595.

75. Kubota N, Terauchi Y, Miki H, Tamemoto H, Yamauchi T, Komeda K, Satoh S, Nakano R, Ishii C, Sugiyama T, Eto K, Tsubamoto Y, Okuno A, Murakami K, Sekihara H, Hasegawa G, Naito M, Toyoshima Y, Tanaka S, Shiota K, Kitamura T, Fujita T, Ezaki O, Aizawa S, Nagai R, Tobe K, Kimura S, Kadowaki T. PPARg mediates high-fat diet-induced adipocyte hypertrophy and insulin resistance. Molec Cell 1999;4:597—609.

76. Miles PD, Barak Y, He W, Evans RM, Olefsky JM. Improved insulin-sensitivity in mice heterozygous for PPAR-gamma deficiency. J Clin Invest 2000;105:287—292.

77. Greene ME, Blumberg B, McBride OW, Yi HF, Kronquist K, Kwan K, Hsieh L, Greene G, Nimer SD. Isolation of the human peroxisome proliferator activated receptor gamma cDNA: expression in hematopoietic cells and chromosomal mapping. Gene Expression 1995;4:281—299.

78. Ricote M, Huang J, Fajas L, Li A, Welch J, Najib J, Witztum JL, Auwerx J, Palinski W, Glass CK. Expression of the peroxisome proliferator-activated receptor γ (PPARγ) in human atherosclerosis and regulation in macrophages by colony stimulating factors and oxidized low density lipoprotein. Proc Natl Acad Sci USA 1998;95:7614—7619.

79. Marx N, Sukhova G, Murphy C, Libby P, Plutzky J. Macrophages in human atheroma contain PPARgamma: differentiation-dependent PPARgamma expression and reduction of MMP-9 activity through PPARgamma activation in mononuclear phagocytes in vitro. Am J Pathol 1998;153:17—23.

80. Marx N, Schoenbeck U, Lazar MA, Libby P, Plutzky J. Peroxisome proliferator-activated receptor gamma activators inhibit gene expression and migration in human vascular smooth muscle cells. Circ Res 1998;83:1097—1103.

81. Jiang C, Ting AT, Seed B. PPARγ agonists inhibit production of monocyte inflammatory cytokines. Nature 1998;391:82—86.

82. Ricote M, Li AC, Willson TM, Kelly CJ, Glass CK. The peroxisome proliferator-activated receptor γ is a negative regulator of macrophage activation. Nature 1998;391:79—82.

83. Kimura KD, Tissenbaum HA, Liu Y, Ruvkun G. Daf-2, an insulin receptor-like gene that regulates longevity and diapause in Caenorhabditis elegans. Science 1997;277:942—946.

84. Bohni R, Riesgo-Escovar J, Oldham S, Brogiolo W, Stocker H, Andruss BF, Beckingham K, Hafen E. Autonomous control of cell and organ size by CHICO, a drosophila homolog of vertebrate IRS1-4. Cell 1999;97:865—875.

85. Apfel R, Benbrook D, Lernhardt E, Ortiz MA, Salbert G, Pfahl M. A novel orphan receptor specific for a subset of thyroid hormone-responsive elements and its interaction with the reti-

38

noid/thyroid hormone receptor subfamily. Molec Cell Biol 1994;14:7025−7035.

86. Willy PJ, Umesono K, Ong ES, Evans RM, Heyman RA, Mangelsdorf DJ. LXR, a nuclear receptor that defines a distinct retinoid response pathway. Genes Devel 1995;9:1033−1045.

87. Shinar DM, Endo N, Rutledge SJ, Vogel R, Rodan GA, Schmidt A. NER, a new member of the gene family encoding the human steroid hormone nuclear receptor. Gene 1994;147:273−276.

88. Song C, Kokontis JM, Hiipakka RA, Liao S. Ubiquitous receptor: a receptor that modulates gene activation by retinoic acid and thyroid hormone receptors. Proc Natl Acad Sci USA 1994; 91:10809−10813.

89. Teboul M, Enmark E, Li Q, Wikström AC, Pelto-Huikko M, Gustafsson J-A. OR-1, a member of the nuclear receptor superfamily that interacts with the 9-cis-retinoic acid receptor. Proc Natl Acad Sci USA 1995;92:2096−2100.

90. Willy PJ, Mangelsdorf DJ. Unique requirements for retinoid-dependent transcriptional activation by the orphan receptor LXR. Genes Devel 1996;12:289−298.

91. Wiebel FF, Gustafsson J-A. Heterodimeric interaction between retinoid X receptor a and orphan receptor OR-1 reveals dimerization induced activation as a novel mechanism of nuclear receptor activation. Molec Cell Biol 1997;17:3977−3986.

92. Janowski BA, Willy PJ, Devi TR, Falck JR, Mangelsdorf DJ. An oxysterol signalling pathway mediated by the nuclear receptor LXRα. Nature 1996;383:728−731.

93. Lehmann JM, Kliewer SA, Moore LB, Smith-Oliver TA, Oliver BB, Su JL, Sundseth SS, Winegar DA, Blanchard DE, Spencer TA, Willson TM. Activation of the nuclear receptor LXR by oxysterols defines a new hormone response pathway. J Biol Chem 1997;272:3137−3140.

94. Peet DJ, Turley SD, Ma W, Janowski BA, Lobaccaro JM, Hammer RE, Mangelsdorf DJ. Cholesterol and bile acid metabolism are impaired in mice lacking the nuclear oxysterol receptor LXR alpha. Cell 1998;93:693−704.

95. Forman BM, Ruan B, Chen J, Schroepfer GJ, Evans RM. The orphan nuclear receptor LXRalpha is positively and negatively regulated by distinct products of mevalonate metabolism. Proc Natl Acad Sci USA 1997;94:10588−10593.

96. Janowski BA, Grogan MJ, Jones SA, Wisely GB, Kliewer SA, Corey EJ, Mangelsdorf DJ. Structural requirements of ligands for the oxysterol liver X receptors LXRα and LXRβ. Proc Natl Acad Sci USA 1999;96:266−271.

97. Huang CJ, Feltkamp D, Nilsson S, Gustafsson JA. Synergistic activation of RLD-1 by agents triggering PKA and PKC dependent signaling. Biochem Biophys Res Commun 1998;243: 657−663.

98. Tamura K, Chen YE, Horiuchi M, Chen Q, Daviet L, Yang Z, Lopez-Ilasaca M, Mu H, Pratt RE, Dzau VJ. A novel function of LXRa as a cAMP-responsive transcriptional regulator of gene expression. Proc Natl Acad Sci USA 2000 (in press).

99. Venkateswaran A, Repa JJ, Lobaccaro JM, Bronson A, Mangelsdorf DJ, Edwards PA. Human White/Murine ABC8 mRNA levels are highly induced in lipid-loaded macrophages. A transcriptional role for specific oxysterols (in process citation). J Biol Chem 2000;275:14700−14707.

100. Luo Y, Tall AR. Sterol upregulation of human CETP expression in vitro and in transgenic mice by an LXR element. J Clin Invest 2000;105:513−520.

101. Forman BM, Goode E, Chen J, Oro AE, Bradley DJ, Perlmann T, Nooman DJ, Burka LT, McMorris T, Lamph WW, Evans RM, Weinberger C. Identification of a nuclear receptor that is activated by Farnesol metabolites. Cell 1995;81:687−693.

102. Seol W, Choi HS, Moore DD. Isolation of proteins that interact specifically with retinoid X receptor: two novel orphan receptors. Molec Endocrinol 1995;9:72−85.

103. Laffitte BA, Kast HR, Nguyen CM, Zavacki AM, Moore DD, Edwards PA. Identification of the DNA binding specificity and potential target genes for the farnesoid X-activated receptor. J Biol Chem 2000;275:10638−10647.

104. Zavacki AM, Lehmann JM, Seol W, Willson TM, Kliewer SA, Moore DD. Activation of the orphan receptor RIP-14 by retinoids. Proc Natl Acad Sci USA 1997;94:7909−7914.

105. Wang H, Chen J, Hollister K, Sowers LC, Forman BM. Endogenous bile acids are ligands for

the nuclear receptor FXR/BAR. Molec Cell 1999;3:543—553.

106. Makishima M, Okamoto AY, Repa JJ, Tu H, Learned RM, Luk A, Hull MV, Lustig KD, Mangelsdorf DJ, Shan B. Identification of nuclear receptors for bile acids. Science 1999;284: 1362—1365.

107. Parks DJ, Blanchard SG, Bledsoe RK, Chandra G, Consler TG, Kliewer SA, Stimmel JB, Willson TM, Zavacki AM, Moore DD, Lehman JM. Bile acids: natural ligands for orphan nuclear receptors. Science 1999;284:1365—1368.

108. Graham DL, Oram JF. Identification and characterization of a high density lipoprotein-binding protein in cell membranes by ligand-blotting. J Biol Chem 1987;262:7439—7442.

109. Johansson L, Thomsen JS, Damdimopoulos AE, Spyrou G, Gustafsson JA, Treuter E. The orphan nuclear receptor SHP inhibits agonist-dependent transcriptional activity of estrogen receptors ERα and ERβ. J Biol Chem 1999;274:345—353.

110. Crawford PA, Dorn C, Sadovsky Y, Milbrandt J. Nuclear receptor DAX-1 recruits nuclear receptor corepressor N-CoR to steroidogenic factor 1. Molec Cell Biol 1998;18:2949—2956.

111. Nachtigal MW, Hirokawa Y, Enyeart-VanHouten DL, Flanagan JN, Hammer GD, Ingraham HA. Wilms' tumor and Dax-1 modulate the orphan nuclear receptor SF-1 in sex-specific gene expression. Cell 1998;93:445—454.

112. Lee YK, Dell H, Dowhan DH, Hadzopoulou-Cladaras M, Moore DD. The orphan nuclear receptor SHP inhibits hepatocyte nuclear factor 4 and retinoid X receptor transactivation: two mechanisms for repression. Molec Cell Biol 2000;20:187—195.

113. Hammer GD, Ingraham HA. Steroidogenic factor-1: its role in endocrine organ development and differentiation. Front Neuroendocrinol 1999;20:199—223.

114. Brown MS, Goldstein JL. The SREBP pathway: regulation of cholesterol metabolism by proteolysis of a membrane-bound transcription factor. Cell 1997;89:331—340.

115. Roux C, Horvath C, Dupuis R. Teratogenic action and embryo lethality of AY 9944R. Prevention by a hypercholesterolemia-provoking diet. Teratology 1979;19:35—38.

116. Roux C, Dupuis R, Horvath C, Giroud A. Interpretation of isolated agenesis of the pituitary. Teratology 1979;19:39—43.

117. Xu G, Salen G, Shefer S, Ness GC, Chen TS, Zhao Z, Salen L, Tint GS. Treatment of cholesterol biosynthetic defect in Smith-Lemli-Opitz syndrome reproduced in rats with BM 15.766. Gastroenterology 1995;109:1301—1307.

118. Tint GS, Irons M, Elias ER, Batta AK, Frieden R, Chen TS, Salen G. Defective cholesterol biosynthesis associated with the Smith-Lemli-Opitz syndrome. N Engl J Med 1994;330:107—113.

Atherosclerosis XII.
S. Stemme and A.G. Olsson, editors.

41

The role of the extracellular matrix on atherogenesis

Germán Camejo[1,2], Eva Hurt-Camejo[1,2], Urban Olsson[1], Olov Wiklund[1] and Göran Bondjers[1]

[1] Wallenberg Laboratory for Cardiovascular Research, Sahlgrenska University Hospital, Göteborg; and [2] AstraZeneca, Research and Development, Mölndal, Sweden

Abstract. The intima extracellular matrix is where most events leading to atherogenesis take place. This large compartment is made of complex fibrillar macromolecules like collagens, proteoglycans (PGs), hyaluronate, and extracellular multidomain proteins. Proteoglycans rich in sulfated glycosaminoglycan (GAGs) chains appear to be responsible for the retention of apoB-containing lipoproteins, like LDL, IDL and Lp (a) in the arterial intima. This takes place by specific interaction of lysine, arginine-rich segments of the apoB-100. Such associations cause structural modifications of the lipid and protein moieties of the lipoproteins that appear to potentiate their susceptibility to proteases, phospholipases and free radical-mediated processes. The reversible and irreversible association of apoB-lipoproteins with intima PGs increase their uptake by macrophages and smooth muscle cells leading to "foam cell" formation. The secreted PGs of proliferating cells and activated macrophages have a tendency to interact with apoB-lipoproteins, a phenomenon that may explain the preferred deposition of apoB-lipoproteins at sites of smooth muscle cell proliferation and macrophage accretion. Proteoglycans of the arterial intima have a higher affinity for small, dense subfractions of LDL possibly because the small particles expose more of the lysine, arginine-rich GAG-binding sites in its surface. The affinity of LDL for arterial PGs in vitro correlates with the presence of atherosclerotic cardiovascular disease. This suggests that atherosclerosis progress may be modulated by the extent of the association of apoB-lipoproteins with the intima extracellular matrix and the tissue response to lipoprotein modifications that follows this entrapment.

Keywords: apoB lipoproteins, atherosclerosis, extracellular matrix, proteoglycans.

Introduction

One of the most contended views on the hypotheses about atherogenesis is the relative importance of apoB-lipoproteins deposition in the arterial intima and that of a pre-existent cellular inflammatory alteration that conditions such accumulations. The last review article of our late friend Russell Ross exemplifies the cellular viewpoint [1]. The evidence for a chronic inflammatory process in atherosclerosis is strong; however, atherosclerosis cannot be induced in animal models without concurrent induction of abnormalities of the apoB-lipoproteins. Therefore, lipoprotein entrapment in the extracellular matrix of the arterial intima may be a key and very early cause of plaque development. Evidence for such a concept has been extensively reviewed by Williams and Tabas as part of the "Response-to-Retention" hypothesis [2,3]. We will discuss evidence indicating

Address for correspondence: Germán Camejo, AstraZeneca, Mölndal, S-431 83, Sweden. Tel.: +46-31-776-1686. Fax: +46-31-776-3737. E-mail: german.camejo@astrazeneca.com

that retention of apoB-lipoproteins in the intima extracellular matrix goes beyond being a phenomenon that contributes to their accumulation.

Retention of LDL by intima proteoglycans

The extracellular matrix of the arterial intima is a relatively large compartment made of fibrous proteins like the collagens, proteoglycans, hyaluronate, elastin and multidomain proteins like fibronectin, laminin and tenascin. The intima extracellular space extends from the basement membrane of endothelial cells to the internal elastic lamina and forms a continuous space in contact with the pericellular region of smooth muscle cells and macrophages, if they are present in the intima [4]. The proteoglycans of the extracellular intima are highly sulfated proteoglycans such as versican and decorin that are made of core protein and glycosaminoglycan (GAGs) chains of chondroitin sulfate (CS) and dermatan sulfate (DS), and they are truly extracellular. Others like syndecan and perlecan, rich in heparan sulfate (HS) glycosaminoglycan, are anchored in the membrane of endothelial cells and smooth muscle cells. The polycarboxyalted and polysulfated GAGs are the most negatively charged molecules of living tissue. This property favors their reversible and irreversible associations with many growth factors, cytokines, coagulation factors and apolipoproteins with Ca^{++} and Mg^{++} segments in their surface. In addition, via hydrogen bonds, they immobilize large amounts of water providing most of the viscoelastic properties of the intima [4].

ApoB-100- and apoE-containing particles associate with the negatively charged sulfated glycosaminoglycans of intima PGs, mainly by means of at least two arginine, lysine-rich segments of the apolipoprotein. They are 3145-3157 with five positive charges, and 3359-3367, also with five positive charges:

Ser-Val-**Lys**-Ala-Gln-Trp-**Lys**-**Lys**-Asn-**Lys**-His-**Arg**-His-

-**Arg**-Leu-Thr-**Arg**-**Lys**-**Arg**-Gly-Leu-**Lys**-

These segments are more surface exposed in LDL than in VLDL and, within the LDL class, the small, dense LDL (sdLDL) particles seem also to expose better in such segments, due to their lower content of phospholipids, [5,6]. Once the primary sequence of the apoB-100 was established, several peptide segments obtained by controlled proteolysis were identified as regions binding to heparin [7]. We searched with computer modeling for apoB-100 segments that could interact with the human arterial CS-rich versican. Regions with a high probability of residing in the LDL surface and with a high density of positively charged amino acids were selected and synthesized, together with other silent sequences, and their affinity for versican and GAGs evaluated by competition experiments and frontal elution chromatography [8—11]. The two peptides with the highest affinity for isolated arterial versican also completed the association of LDL with rabbit aortic segments. Therefore, they seem to be responsible, at least partially, for the interaction with the intact intima [12].

Additional proof of the affinity for CS-GAG of the most active apoB-100 segment identified (3356—3364) was obtained after anchoring the peptide on the surface of neutral liposomes. The liposomes, initially having had no affinity for PGs or CS, gained high affinity binding after acquiring copies of the peptide 1015 [Olsson, 1993]. It should be pointed out that these segments are part of the proposed receptor-binding region of the apoB-100 [13]. An heterodimer of the above peptides was synthesized and joined by three glycines in order to test the hypothesis that positive segments separated linearly for about 200 amino acids could be efficient contributors to the LDL binding to PGs and GAGs, if brought together by structural constraints in the particle surface. The segments that individually bind GAGs may be close to each other at the LDL surface because a disulfide bridge exists between Cys (3167) and Cys (3296) and this may force a U-turn in this region [13]. The synthetic heterodimer was more effective than the separated peptides in completing the binding of LDL to chondroitin sulfate and to the LDL receptor in fibroblasts [6].

The association of apoB-100 particles with proteoglycans can also be modulated by the secondary and tertiary structures of the protein at the particle surface [14]. The apoB-100 seems to wrap around the lipid spherical particle as a broad belt, with the first part located roughly in one hemisphere and the second half continuing into the other hemisphere. The apoB-100 is anchored in the lipid surface as both α-helices and β-strands have an amphipatic distribution with the nonpolar amino acid side chain interacting with the lipid surface monolayer and the polar amino acids interacting with the external solvent. The hemisphere containing the last half of the apoB-100 has the two more important GAGs binding sites and the receptor-binding domain. This hemisphere contains also a bow structure formed by the segment with the last 500 amino acids crossing over the region that contains the putative receptor-binding region and the GAG-binding segments. The disulfide bridge between Cys (3117) and Cys (3296) may introduce a U-turn. The crossing of the α-helix$_3$ segment over the region containing the proposed GAG- and receptor-binding sequences suggests an additional mechanism for the control of the association with the LDL receptor and also for the association with GAGs [15,16]. Changes in the packing at the particle surface may alter the exposure of the GAG- and receptor-binding regions. Olsson et al. [11] found that the affinity for chondroitin sulfate increases with a decreasing size of VLDL subclasses. We speculate that in large VLDL, and in large LDL, the surface lipids compress the apoB-100, and this may sterically hinder the contact with the GAGs. In small, dense LDL with more area for the apoB-100, the region containing the GAG-binding segments may be more exposed.

Recently, Borén et al. [17] reported on the critical contribution that the association of LDL and PG via the apoB-100 segment 3359-3367 has in lesion progression. Transgenic mice were developed expressing normal human apoB-100 and others with mutations in this region in which a positive arginine was changed to a neutral serine. The animals with mutated apoB-100 that binds little to PGs developed lesions at much slower rate than mice with the normal human apoB-100, in spite of having similar plasma cholesterol level. Lp (a) is another apoB-100 containing a complex that is considered atherogenic and that interacts with the extracellular intima and accumulates there in progressing lesions [18]. In vitro experiments indicate that, once bound to the extracellular matrix, PG secreted by smooth muscle cells Lp (a) increases the subsequent retention of LDL by the matrix. We interpreted these results as evidence of the matrix PG contributing to formation of coaggregates of Lp (a) and LDL [19].

Changes of LDL structure caused by the association with PGs

Studies on LDL-PG complexes and on LDL that has being associated with arterial PG and dissociated from them document some of the structural alterations induced by the association. Low angle X-ray diffraction, differential-scanning calorimetry, nuclear magnetic resonance and differential spectroscopy showed that both the core and surface monolayer organization of LDL is markedly decreased [20−22]. This leads to an increased exposure of arginine, lysine-rich segments that include those responsible for the binding to sulfated GAG [22]. Probably because the association causes increased exposure of polar segments in the particle surface, proteases that act in these peptide bonds degrade the protein of PG-treated LDL faster [22]. The phospholipids of the surface monolayer of LDL can be also enzymatically hydrolyzed, especially by secretory nonpancreatic phospholipase A$_2$ (snpPLA$_2$). This could be the major enzyme acting on the phospholipids of LDL immobilized in the intima because it is also bound by the extracellular GAGs that bind LDL [23]. This enzyme, when bound to PG, acts more rapidly on LDL when the particle is also associated to PGs and GAGs [24]. Furthermore, the actions of snPLA$_2$ on LDL phospholipids potentiate the conversion LDL sphyngomyelin to ceramides [25].

Although the above effects were documented in vitro, they suggest that a similar situation in vivo may contribute to focal generation of lipid products that, like the lysophospholipids and ceramides, have potent cellular actions, many of them proposed as proinflammatory and atherogenic [23,25]. Phospholipid depletion and protein fragmentation characterize lipoproteins isolated from human lesions. Such two effects should contribute to aggregation and fusion of particles in the intima that may be the leading cause of the extracellular lipid deposits that characterize advanced lesions [26,27].

LDL size and the association with extracellular matrix proteoglycans

Studies about the correlation between composition and structure of LDL subclasses and their affinity for PGs were performed by Hurt-Camejo et al. [5]. LDL was fractionated into four subclasses by sequential precipitation with increasing amounts of human versican (decreasing affinity). LDL fraction 1 has the highest affinity for versican and LDL 4 the lowest. The LDL fraction with the highest affinity for versican was associated with smaller particles that were more positive (high isoelectric point). Analysis of the lipid composition of the four fractions showed interesting correlation between the surface and core dimensions of the

LDL subclasses and their reactivity for versican. Table 1 shows the calculated structural parameters of these subclasses [28]. The fraction with higher affinity for the PG has a smaller amount of total lipids, with a higher percent content of cholesterol esters. The most interesting, however, is that the calculated area occupied by the polar lipids, i.e., phospholipids and cholesterol, is inversely related to the affinity. Thus, the particles with higher affinity should have 20–30% more area accessible to accommodate the other surface component, the apoB-100. The four LDL fractions isolated by differential affinity for PG correspond closely in composition and PG-affinity to those obtained by equilibrium density fractions between 1.019–1.030, 1.030–1.040, 1.040–1.050 and 1.050–1.060 g/ml [5]. McNamara et al. reported the calculated volume and area parameters of eight well characterized subfractions of LDL obtained by sequential ultracentrifugation from 66 subjects [29]. With the use of similar calculations to those reported by Hurt-Camejo et al. [5], these authors concluded that with decreasing size and increasing density the LDL particles have less of the nonpolar core covered with the surface monolayer made of phospholipids and cholesterol. They propose also that the apoB-100 was more extended for the small and dense LDL and that this may alter the exposure of binding epitopes of the particle.

Cellular responses to proteoglycan-caused LDL modifications

Two types of complex between LDL and PGs can be induced in vitro depending on the amount of Ca^{++} and the pH used. Irreversible complexes are obtained with more than 10 µM Ca^{++}. However, at conditions similar to those in the extracellular environment, complexes that can be dissociated by raising the ionic strength can be obtained. We used LDL that was dissociated from arterial versican or GAGs and then dissolved in cell culture media in experiments with cells. These preparations are not aggregated but are structurally altered as discussed. The PG-modified LDL, when incubated with human macrophages, is internalized more efficiently than native LDL and leads to formation of lipid-filled cells, probably because the receptors involved are not down-regulated [30,31]. A similar finding is obtained with insoluble complexes of LDL and arterial PGs

Table 1. Volume and area parameters for LDL subclasses of decreasing reactivity for human arterial proteoglycans.

LDL class	Diameter of total lipids (nm)	Diameter of nonpolar core (nm)	Area of polar lipids ($nm^2 \times 10^{-2}$)	% area occupied by polar lipids	% area accessible to protein
LDL1	16.2	15.0	2.5	35.6	64.4
LDL2	17.0	15.4	3.2	42.0	58.0
LDL3	17.4	15.5	4.0	53.1	46.9
LDL4	17.6	15.0	4.7	63.3	36.7
LDL total	17.5	15.6	4.2	55.2	44.8

[32,33]. In smooth muscle cells PG-treated LDL is also more efficiently taken up than native LDL [34]. These effects are probably caused by the irreversible changes in the surface monolayer of the lipoprotein produced by the association with PG. Another interesting alteration induced by the PG effects on LDL structure is a remarkable increase of its susceptibility to oxidation caused by transition metals, hemin, peroxidases and cells [35,36]. This effect increases the uptake of LDL by human macrophages via receptors that are not down-regulated [37].

Pre-existing alterations of the extracellular matrix that may potentiate the entrapment of apoB-lipoproteins

In early studies about the interaction of GAGs with lipoproteins, it was found that the nature of the disaccharide units and the extent of sulfation were important parameters controlling the formation of insoluble complexes between these structures [38—42]. Today we know that there is a large diversity of proteoglycans in the arterial intima. They have different core proteins that are products of multiple genes, form families and contain at least four general classes of GAG chains. Molecular models of the LDL-GAG association point to the importance of the sulfate and carboxylic groups in the GAGs for binding to the arginine-, lysine-rich peptides. Therefore, one molecule of versican with up to 20 chondroitin sulfate chains and 30—80 disaccharide units per chain can bind several LDL molecules. Thus, the capacity and the affinity for entrapping LDL particles in the extracellular environment can vary with the matrix composition.

The amount of PGs, the length of their GAG chains and probably their extent of sulfation may change depending on whether the smooth muscle cells that assemble these molecules are resting or proliferating [43—46]. It is possible then that at sites of intimal thickening, which is mostly induced by matrix accumulation, more and different proteoglycans and other matrix products accumulate [4]. In a rabbit model of atherosclerosis Alavi et al. [47] showed that the CS-PGs from lesions bind more LDL ex vivo than those from normal arteries. In humans, Cardoso et al. [48] documented that LDL bind with higher affinity to the chondroitin sulfate chains isolated from lesion-prone regions of the arterial tree than to those from regions that rarely develop lesions. The authors ascribed the difference to the longer GAG chains of the lesion-prone sites. These results indicate that PGs with higher affinity for apoB-100 lipoproteins may precede the onset of atherosclerotic lesion. Results obtained with pigeons susceptible or not to atherosclerosis also show that the susceptibility is associated with arterial proteoglycans with high affinity for LDL [49]. We found that the versican secreted by proliferating human arterial smooth muscle cells has 3—5 times higher affinity for LDL, at physiological ionic conditions, than the versican of quiescent cells. This property was attributed to the longer chondroitin sulfate chains [50]. The studies discussed suggest that at lesion-prone sites increased production of proteoglycans with longer GAG chains, which can bond more frequently and firmly with LDL, may contribute to its accumulation. If smooth muscle cells and macrophages that invade the intima during atherogenesis produce more of these PGs, the conditions for generating a self-supporting pathogenic cycle may be reached [51].

One of the main results of the action of secretory phospholipases and other lipases on lipids of apoB-lipoproteins entrapped in the intima should be the release of nonesterified fatty acids (NEFA). In dyslipidemias associated with insulin resistance and type 2 diabetes, conditions in which the prevalence of arterial disease is high, the vasculature is exposed to a permanently high influx of albumin-bound NEFA originating from the hydrolysis of postprandial lipoproteins and from increased lipolysis of adipose tissue triglycerides. Cell culture studies with endothelial cell monolayers show that high levels of albumin-NEFA cause an increase of the permeability of their basement membrane. This effect is associated with a reduction of the synthesis of heparan PGs of the extracellular matrix and an increase in the synthesis of chondroitin sulfate PG [52]. The authors suggested that an analogous situation in vivo might contribute to increase permeability of the arterial and capillary endothelium. Olsson et al. [53] found recently that human arterial smooth muscle cells exposed for 48 h to high physiological levels of albumin-bound NEFA (300 μm) show a substantial increase in the expression of the genes for the core proteins of the proteoglycans syndecan, versican and decorin. This increase is associated to elevations of the immuno-detectable gene products. More remarkable, the matrix produced by cells exposed to high NEFA bond more efficiently to LDL. Interestingly, the effect of NEFA on expression of decorin is dose-dependently inhibited by the PPARγ agonist darglitazone [53]. Hypothetically, a similar effect of chronic exposure to high levels of NEFA could lead to increased production by smooth muscle cells of matrix PG with a higher capacity to retain apoB-lipoproteins.

LDL complex formation with proteoglycans and its possible clinical significance

If we accept that exaggerated LDL entrapment in the intima may contribute to atherogenesis, then factors increasing this association may modulate lesion progress. Therefore, if we could measure ex vivo some of these properties they may correlate with disease progress. As early as 1949, Mogen Faber, studying human lesions, suggested that the affinity of cholesterol-transporting proteins in plasma for chondroitin sulfate in the intima might control cholesterol deposition and contribute to atheroma formation [54]. This hypothesis was extended by Gero et al. and was put into a more precise context by Srinivasan et al. and Hollander [40,55,56]. Based on these seminal studies, our laboratory searched for evidence of this presumed contribution by comparing the affinity of LDL in serum for isolated human arterial versican in groups with clinical manifestations of atherosclerosis. We measured the affinity LDL-PGs in male subjects that were classified as apparently ischemics (77) or nonischemics (214) by exercise electrocardiography. High affinity of LDL for arterial PGs was clearly more frequent in the apparently ischemics than in the controls. To further evaluate the hypothesis that the affinity of LDL for arterial PGs may discriminate against patients with coronary artery disease, we studied patients that have suffered a myocardial infarction before they were 50 years of age. The apparently healthy controls were randomly selected from a similar population in Göteborg, Sweden, and were age- and sex-matched. In multiple regression analysis, with patient or control as the dependent variable, LDL-PG reactivity, plasma apoB-content and serum triglycerides appeared as the stronger independent contributors to the regression [57]. Taken together, these studies suggest that the LDL of subjects with clinical manifestations of atherosclerosis have a higher affinity for the versican of human arteries than that of apparently healthy subjects. A question arising from the above results is whether a higher affinity of LDL in serum for arterial PGs was the result of the presence of LDL subfractions with special high affinity or if the entire range of LDL particles shared this property.

Anber et al. [58] studied the affinity for arterial proteoglycans of lipoproteins from subjects that have the "atherogenic lipoprotein phenotype" (ALP). This is the most common lipoprotein disorder associated with coronary heart disease. It is characterized by moderately elevated VLDL triglycerides, low HDL, preponderance of small dense LDL and is associated with insulin resistance and type II diabetes. Their results show a significant correlation between the presence of high amounts of small, dense LDL-III and a tendency for the total LDL fraction to form complexes with the arterial PGs. The same laboratory found that the reactivity of all the particles containing apoB-100 of subjects with the atherogenic lipoprotein phenotype (ALP) was greater than the lipoproteins from subjects with a normal phenotype. The authors concluded that the overall reactivity of apoB-containing particles is greatest in individuals with small, dense LDL. Interestingly, they found that IDL has also a high tendency to form complexes with arterial PG and suggested that this may also contribute to the atherogenicity of this common phenotype [59]. The affinity of LDL or PGs can be altered by drugs.

Wiklund et al. [60] found that treatment with Gemfibrozil®, a compound that is known to increase the size of LDL, reduced in dyslipidemic patients the reactivity of LDL for arterial proteoglycans. However, statins that are known not to affect the size distribution of LDL did not change the LDL-PGs reactivity.

Response-to-retention: a possible self-perpetuating ethio-pathogenic cycle

Most of the observations discussed originate from in vitro models and we must be cautious on their interpretation. However, they provide consistent evidence supporting the hypothesis that retention of apoB-lipoproteins by PGs of the intima extracellular matrix causes their structural alteration. Additionally, the cited evidence suggests that this entrapment and subsequent modifications potentiate hydrolytic and oxidative changes of the lipoproteins that generate products with diverse cellular effects. These substances, which may include NEFA, lysophospholipids, ceramides and oxidation products of polyunsaturated fatty acids and of the apoB-100 protein, could cause the metabolic "injury" that triggers the

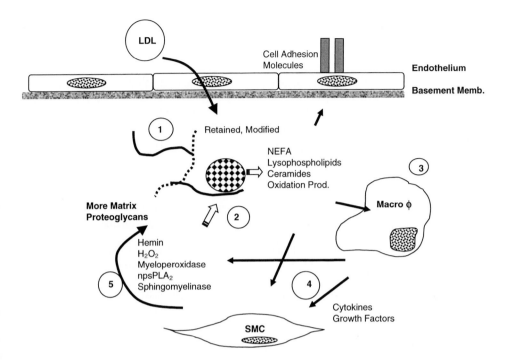

Fig. 1. Hypothetical atherogenic cycle initiated by retention of apoB lipoproteins in the intima extracellular matrix. 1. Binding of LDL by extracellular proteoglycans (PGs). 2. Structural and hydrolytic modification of LDL by PGs and enzymes residing in the extracellular matrix. 3. Uptake of modified lipoproteins by macrophages and cellular effects of products of LDL modification. 4. Macrophage induction of matrix production by smooth muscle cells that could retain more lipoproteins. 5. Further modification of retained lipoproteins by products of macrophages and smooth muscle cells.

atherogenic cell response. Such a response may be accompanied by overproduction of matrix that induces further focal lipoprotein retention and modification.

As in any cyclic sequence, it is difficult to discriminate which could be the initiating step. It is possible that, in most cases, elevated levels of apoB-lipoproteins retained may be the initiator. However, it is also feasible that, at given lesion-prone sites, excessive accumulation of extracellular PG with a high affinity for apoB-lipoproteins may be produced by cells conditioned by hemodynamic factors. These sites may cause lipoprotein entrapment even with "normal" levels of apoB-100. The diagram in Fig. 1 represents this hypothetical self-perpetuating cycle caused by entrapment and modification of apoB-lipoproteins in the intima.

References

1. Ross R. Atherosclerosis: an inflammatory disease. N Engl J Med 1999;340:115–126.
2. Williams KJ, Tabas I. The response-to-retention hypothesis of early atherogenesis. Arterioscl Thromb Vasc Biol 1995;15:551–561.

3. Williams K, Tabas I. The response-to-retention hypothesis of atherogenesis reinforced. Curr Opin Lipidol 1998;9:471—474.

4. Wight TN. The vascular extracellular matrix. In: Fuster V, Ross R, Topol E (eds) Atherosclerosis and Coronary Artery Disease. Philadelphia: Lippincott-Raven, 1996;421—440.

5. Hurt-Camejo E, Camejo G, Rosengren B, López F, Wiklund O, Bondjers G. Differential uptake of proteoglycan-selected subfractions of low density lipoprotein by human macrophages. J Lipid Res 1990;31:1387—1398.

6. Olsson U, Camejo G, Hurt-Camejo E, Elfsber K, Wiklund O, Bondjers G. Possible functional interactions of apolipoprotein B-100 segments that associate with cell proteoglycans and the apoB/E receptor. Arterioscl Thromb Vasc Biol 1997;17:149—155.

7. Hirose N, Blankenship DT, Krivanek MA, Jackson RL, Cardin AD. Isolation and characterization of four heparin-binding cyanogen bromide peptides of human plasma apolipoprotein B. Biochemistry 1987;26(17):5505—5512.

8. Camejo G, Olofsson S-O, López F, Carlsson P, Bondjers G. Identification of apoB-100 segments mediating the interaction of low density lipoproteins with arterial proteoglycans. Arteriosclerosis 1988;8:368—377.

9. Camejo G, Rosengren B, Olsson U, López F, Olofsson S-O, Westerlund C, Bondjers G. Molecular basis of the association of arterial proteoglycans with low density lipoproteins: its effect on the structure of the lipoprotein particle. Eur Heart J 1990;11(Suppl. E):164—173.

10. Olsson U, Camejo G, Olofsson S-O, Bondjers G. Molecular parameters that control the association of low density lipoprotein apoB-100 with chondroitin sulphate. Biochim Biophys Acta 1991;1097:37—44.

11. Olsson U, Camejo G, Bondjers G. Binding of a synthetic apolipoprotein B-100 peptide and peptide analogues to chondroitin 6-sulfate: effects of the lipid environment. Biochemistry 1993; 32(7):1858—1865.

12. Wiklund O, Matsson L, López F, Bondjers G. Cationic polypeptides modulate in vitro the association of low density lipoproteins with arterial proteoglycans, fibroblasts and arterial tissue. Arteriosclerosis 1990;10:695—702.

13. Chan L. Apolipoprotein B, the major protein component of triglyceride-rich and low density lipoproteins. J Biol Chem 1992;267:25621—25624.

14. Segrest J, Jones M, Mishra V, Pierotti V, Young S, Borén J, Innerarity T, Dashti N. Apolipoprotein B-100: conservation of lipid-associating amphipathic secondary structural motifs in nine species of vertebrates. J Lipid Res 1998;39:85—102.

15. Chatterton J, Phillips M, Curtiss LK, Milne R, Fruchart J-C, Schumaker V. Immunoelectron microscopy of low density lipoproteins yield a ribbon and bow model for the conformation of apolipoprotein B on the lipoprotein surface. J Lipid Res 1995;36:2027—2037.

16. Borén J, Olin K, Lee I, Chait A, Wight T, Innerarity T. Identification of the principal proteoglycan-binding site in LDL: a single point mutation in apoB-100 severely affects proteoglycan interaction without affecting LDL receptor binding. J Clin Invest 1998;101:2658—2664.

17. Borén J, Olin K, O'Brien K, Kay A, Ludwig E, Wight T, Innerarity T. Engineering non-atherogenic low density lipoproteins — direct evidence for the "Response-to-Retention Hypothesis". Circulation 1998;97(Suppl. I):I-314.

18. Nielsen L, Stender S, Jauhianien M, Nordestgaard B. Preferential influx and decreased fractional loss of lipoprotein(a) in atherosclerosis compared with nonlesioned rabbit aorta. J Clin Invest 1996;98:563—571.

19. Lundstam U, Hurt-Camejo E, Olsson G, Sartipy P, Camejo G, Wiklund O. Proteoglycans contribution to association of lipoprotein(a) and low density lipoprotein with smooth muscle cell extracellular matrix. Arterioscl Thromb Vasc Biol 1999;19:1162—1167.

20. Mateu L, Avila EM, León V, Liscano N. The structural stability of low density lipoprotein: a kinetic X-ray scattering study of its interaction with arterial wall proteoglycans. Biochim Biophys Acta 1984;795:525—534.

21. Bihari-Varga M, Camejo G, Horn C, Szabo D, López F, Gruber E. Structure of low density lipo-

protein complexes formed with arterial matrix components. Int J Biol Macromol 1983;5:59–62.

22. Camejo G, Hurt E, Wiklund O, Rosengren B, López F, Bondjers G. Modifications of low density lipoprotein induced by arterial proteoglycans and chondroitin-6-sulfate. Biochim Biophys Acta 1991;1096:253–261.

23. Hurt-Camejo E, Camejo G. Potential involvement of type II phospholipase A2 in atherosclerosis. Atherosclerosis 1997;132:1–8.

24. Sartipy P, Bondjers G, Hurt-Camejo E. Phospholipase A_2 type II binds to extracellular matrix byglycan: modulation of its activity on low density lipoproteins by colocalization in glycosaminoglycan matrixes. Arterioscl Thromb Vasc Biol 1998;18:1934–1941.

25. Schissel S, Tweedie-Hardman J, Rapp J, Graham G, Williams K, Tabas I. Rabbit aorta and human atherosclerotic lesions hydrolyze the sphingomyelin of retained low-density lipoprotein. J Clin Invest 1996;98:1455–1464.

26. Camejo G, Hurt E, Romano M. Properties of lipoprotein complexes isolated by affinity chromatography from human aorta. Biomed Biophys Acta 1985;44:389–401.

27. Hakala J, Öörni K, Ala-Korpela M, Kovanen P. Lypolytic modification of LDL by phospholipase A2 induces particle aggregation in the absence and fusion in the presence of heparin. Arterioscl Thromb Vasc Biol 1999;19:1276–1283.

28. Hauton JC, Lafont H. Lipid biodynamics: new perspectives. Biochimie 1987;69:117–204.

29. McNamara J, Small D, Li Z, Schaefer E. Differences in LDL subspecies involve alterations in lipid composition and conformational changes in apolipoprotein B. J Lipid Res 1996;37: 1924–1935.

30. Hurt E, Camejo G. Effect of arterial proteoglycans on the interaction of LDL with human monocyte-derived macrophages. Atherosclerosis 1987;67:115–126.

31. Hurt E, Bondjers G, Camejo G. Interaction of LDL with human arterial proteoglycans stimulates its uptake by human monocyte-derived macrophages. J Lipid Res 1990;31:443–454.

32. Vijayagopal P, Srinivasan SR, Xu J-H, Dalfere ED, Radhakrishnamurthy B, Berenson GS. Lipoprotein-proteoglycan complexes induce continued cholesteryl ester accumulation in foam cells from rabbit atherosclerotic lesions. J Clin Invest 1993;91:1011–1018.

33. Vijayagopal P. Regulation of the metabolism of lipoprotein-proteoglycan complexes in human monocyte derived macrophages. Biochem J 1994;301:675–681.

34. Bondjers G, Wiklund O, Olofsson S-O, Fager G, Hurt E, Camejo G. Low density lipoprotein interaction with arterial wall proteoglycans: effects on lipoprotein interaction with arterial cells. In: Sukling K, Groot P (eds) Hyperlipidemia and Atherosclerosis. London: Academic Press, 1988;135–148.

35. Camejo G, Hurt-Camejo E, Rosengren B, Wiklund O, López F, Bondjers G. Modification of copper-catalyzed oxidation of low density lipoprotein by proteoglycans and glycosaminoglycans. J Lipid Res 1991;32:1983–1991.

36. Upritchard J, Sutherland W. Oxidation of heparin-treated low density lipoprotein by peroxidases. Atherosclerosis 1999;146:211–219.

37. Hurt-Camejo E, Camejo G, Rosengren B, López F, C. A, Fager G, Bondjers G. Effect of arterial proteoglycans and glycosaminoglycans on low density lipoprotein oxidation and its uptake by human macrophages and arterial smooth muscle cells. Arterioscl Thromb 1992;12:569–583.

38. Bernfeld P, Nisselbaum J. Reaction of human betalipoglobulin with macromolecular polysulfated esters. Fed Proc 1956;15:220–227.

39. Amenta J, Waters L. The precipitation of serum lipoproteins by mucopolysaccharides extracted from aortic tissue. Yale J Biol Med 1960;33:112–121.

40. Gero S, Gergely J, Szérely L, Virag S. Role of mucoid substances of the aorta in the deposition of lipids. Nature 1960;187:152–153.

41. Bihari-Varga M, Vegh M. Quantitative studies on the complexes formed between aortic mucopolysaccharides and serum lipoproteins. Biochim Biophys Acta 1967;144:202–210.

42. Iverius P-H. Possible role of the glycosaminoglycans in the genesis of atherosclerosis. In: Porter R, Knight J (eds) Atherogenesis: Initiating Factors. Amsterdam: Elsevier, 1973;185–196.

52

43. Hollmann J, Thiel J, Schmidt A, Buddecke E. Increased activity of chondroitin sulfate-synthesizing enzymes during proliferation of arterial smooth muscle cells. Exp Cell Res 1986;167: 484–494.

44. Merriles MJ, Campbell JH, Spanidis E, Campbell GR. Glycosaminoglycan synthesis by smooth muscle cells of differing phenotype and their response to endothelial cell conditioned media. Atherosclerosis 1990;81:245–254.

45. Schmidt A, Buddecke E. Changes in heparan sulfate structure during transition from the proliferating to the non-dividing state of cultured arterial smooth muscle cell. Eur J Cell Biol 1990;52:229–235.

46. Schönherr E, Järveläinen HT, Sandell LJ, Wight TN. Effects of platelet-derived growth factor and transforming growth factor β1 on the synthesis of large versican-like chondroitin sulfate proteoglycan by arterial smooth muscle cell. J Biol Chem 1991;266:117640–117647.

47. Alavi M, Richardson M, Moore S. The in vivo interactions between serum lipoproteins and proteoglycans of the neo intima of rabbit aorta after a single balloon catheter injury. Am J Pathol 1989;134:287–294.

48. Cardoso LE, Mourao PA. Glycosaminoglycan fractions from human arteries presenting diverse susceptibilities to atherosclerosis have different binding affinities to plasma LDL. Arterioscl Thromb 1994;14:115–124.

49. Steele R, Wagner W. Lipoprotein interaction with artery wall derived proteoglyvan. Comparisons between atherosclerosis-susceptible WC-2 and resistant Show Racer pigeons. Atherosclerosis 1987;65:63–73.

50. Camejo G, Fager G, Rosengren B, Camejo-Hurt E, Bondjers G. Binding of low density lipoproteins by proteoglycans synthesized by proliferating and quiescent human arterial smooth muscle cells. J Biol Chem 1993;268:14131–14137.

51. Edwards IJ, Xu H, Obunike J, Goldberg I, Wagner WD. Differentiated macrophages synthesize a heparan sulfate proteoglycan and an oversulfated chondroitin sulfate proteoglycan that bind lipoprotein lipase. Arterioscl Thromb Vasc Biol 1995;15:400–409.

52. Henning B, Boissenault G, Lipke D, Ramasamy S. Role of fatty acids and eicosanoids in modulating proteoglycan metabolism in endothelial cells. Prostaglandins Leukotrients Essen Fat Acid 1995;53:315–324.

53. Olsson U, Bondjers G, Camejo G. Fatty acids modulate the composition of extracellular matrix in cultured smooth muscle cells by altering the expression of genes for proteoglycan core proteins. Diabetes 1999;48:616–622.

54. Faber M. The human aorta: sulfate-containing polyuronides and the deposition of cholesterol. Arch Pathol Lab Med 1949;48:342–350.

55. Srinivasan SR, Dolan P, Radhakrishnamurthy B, Pargaonkar PS, Berenson GS. Lipoprotein mucopolysaccharides complexes from human atherosclerotic lesions. Biochim Biophys Acta 1975;388:58–70.

56. Hollander W. Unified concept on the role of acidic mucopolysaccharides and connective tissue proteins in the accumulation of lipids lipoproteins and calcium in the atherosclerotic plaque. Exp Mol Pathol 1976;25:106–120.

57. Lindén T, Bondjers G, Camejo G, Bergstrand R, Wilhelmsen L, Wiklund O. Affinity of LDL to a human arterial proteoglycan among male survivors of myocardial infarction. Eur J Clin Invest 1989;19:38–44.

58. Anber V, Griffin B, McConnell M, Packard C, Sheperd J. Influence of plasma lipid and LDL-subfraction profile on the interaction between low density lipoprotein with human arterial wall proteoglycans. Atherosclerosis 1996;124:261–271.

59. Anber V, Millar J, McConnell M, Sheperd J, Packard C. Interaction of very-low-density, and low density lipoproteins with human arterial proteoglycans. Arterioscl Thromb Vasc Biol 1997;17:2507–2514.

60. Wiklund O, Bondjers G, Wright I, Camejo G. Insoluble complex formation between LDL and arterial proteoglycans in relation to serum lipid levels and effect of lipid lowering drugs. Atherosclerosis 1996;119:57–68.

© 2000 Elsevier Science B.V. All rights reserved.
Atherosclerosis XII.
S. Stemme and A.G. Olsson, editors.

Inflammation, injury and atherosclerosis — the Russell Ross Memorial Lecture

Göran K. Hansson

Center for Molecular Medicine and Department of Medicine, Karolinska Institutet, Stockholm, Sweden

Abstract. This chapter provides an overview of current knowledge of inflammatory mechanisms in atherosclerosis. It is based on the Russell Ross Memorial Lecture delivered at the XIIth International Symposium on Atherosclerosis. The discovery of the platelet-derived growth factor, the proposal of the response-to-injury hypothesis, and the understanding of atherosclerosis as an inflammatory disease are discussed. Inflammatory cells and mediators identified in atherosclerotic lesions are described and the attempts to deduce their roles in the pathogenesis of disease by analysing gene-targeted murine models are discussed in this chapter.

Keywords: cytokines, growth factors, immunity, low-density lipoprotein, macrophages, T cells.

Introduction

This lecture is dedicated to the memory of Russell Ross, who was at the forefront of atherosclerosis research for nearly three decades before his untimely death in the spring of 1999. Among his many contributions, some of the most important ones were: the discovery of the platelet-derived growth factor (PDGF), the proposal of the response-to-injury hypothesis, and his work on inflammatory aspects of atherosclerosis.

The response-to-injury hypothesis

In 1974, Russell Ross together with John Glomset, Beverly Kariya and Lawrence Harker identified a platelet-derived factor that induced the growth of vascular smooth muscle cells [1]. This finding prompted Ross and Glomset to propose the response-to-injury hypothesis [2]. This was not the first time injury had been suggested to play a role in the initiation of atherosclerosis — such hypotheses had been proposed several times starting with Rudolf Virchow in the 1850s [3]. The importance of the Ross-Glomset hypothesis was that it linked the disease process to a specific molecule, PDGF. By doing so, Ross and Glomset helped transferring atherosclerosis research into the molecular era. The discovery of PDGF and the proposal of the response-to-injury hypothesis therefore played a

Address for correspondence: Göran K. Hansson, MD, PhD, Center for Molecular Medicine L8:03, Karolinska Hospital, SE-17176 Stockholm, Sweden. Fax: +46-8-313147.
E-mail: Goran.Hansson@cmm.ki.se

similar role for vascular pathobiology as Brown and Goldstein's discovery of the LDL receptors and elucidation of the cellular cholesterol metabolism [4] had for lipid metabolism.

The response-to-injury hypothesis stated that denuding injury to the vascular endothelium leads to platelet adhesion and aggregation; adhering platelets release PDGF, which induces proliferation of smooth muscle cells, which in turn leads to the formation of an intimal lesion with smooth muscle cells. This lesion may regress and the normal arterial histology be restored. However, repeated or chronic injury such as vascular damage caused by hypercholesterolemia will stimulate lesion formation to such an extent that regression will no longer be possible. Instead, an atherosclerotic lesion with smooth muscle cells and cholesterol forms at the site of injury.

Inflammatory cells in atherosclerosis

The original response-to-injury hypothesis soon had to be modified. In 1985—1986, we and others determined the cellular composition of human atherosclerosis plaques with the use of cell type-specific monoclonal antibodies and found that the smooth muscle cell was far from dominating in the disease process [5—8]. In addition, there were abundant inflammatory cells, particularly macrophages and T cells.

The role of the macrophage was obvious from Brown and Goldstein's discovery of the scavenger receptors and the cholesterol cycle in the macrophage [9]. A large proportion of cholesterol-laden foam cells was found to express molecular markers of the monocyte-macrophage lineage [6,10,11] and the presence of oxidatively modified lipoproteins in the lesion [12] suggested that uptake through scavenger receptors had led to foam cell formation [12,13]. A few years later, the SR-A scavenger receptors were cloned [14,15] and could be detected in atherosclerotic lesions [16]. More recent research has revealed that scavenger receptors are a family of molecules with several members that are multifunctional and may mediate cell adhesion as well as uptake of oxidized lipoproteins and microorganisms [17—22].

Further studies of human lesions clarified that the macrophage not only accumulates cholesterol but also produces a variety of cytokines, growth factors, and enzymes. Ross et al. and other laboratories showed that PDGF is expressed by macrophages as well as vascular cells both in culture [23—25] and throughout the different phases of atherosclerosis [26—28].

Other growth-regulatory molecules were also linked to atherosclerosis. They included the transforming growth factor-β, which regulates smooth muscle growth through an autocrine PDGF loop [29], and IL-1, another macrophage (and endothelial) product that is a smooth muscle mitogen [30]. In addition, macrophages can produce procoagulant activity, which may be important in arterial thrombosis and plaque activation [31,32].

These and other findings stimulated Ross to modify the response-to-injury hypothesis to incorporate the new information concerning the role of macro-phages and growth-regulatory molecules. The modified response-to-injury hypothesis was published in 1986 and emphasized the adherence to and invasion of the arterial intima by monocytes as an important early step in atherosclerosis [33]. Furthermore, it had become clear that endothelial dysfunction rather than overt denudation occurred in early atherogenesis; the latter was observed only at later stages such as the transition phase from fatty streak to fibrofatty lesion [34,35]. In the latter situation, the fibrotic smooth muscle response and the re-modeling of the arterial intima exhibited a striking resemblance to chronic inflammation and it became obvious to many of us that atherosclerosis carried several features of this condition.

The recruitment of monocytes could be elucidated after the discovery of endothelial leukocyte adhesion molecules during the 1980s. In 1991, Cybulsky and Gimbrone reported that cholesterol feeding of rabbits rapidly induced endothelial expression of an adhesion molecule that was later identified as the vascular cell adhesion molecule-1 (VCAM-1) [36]. Subsequent studies in several animal models as well as in human lesions revealed the involvement of several adhesins in the atherosclerotic process, including VCAM-1, ICAM-1 and E-selectin [37–41]. However, adhesion was probably insufficient to cause monocyte migration into the intima and differentiation into macrophages. The observation of significant amounts of chemoattractant cytokines called chemokines as well as of macrophage colony stimulating factors (CSFs) in lesions [42–45], induction in response to fatty diets [46,47] and expression by vascular cells [48–51] sug-gested that a set of molecular signals may govern the formation of macrophage-rich fatty lesions during early atherogenesis.

Transgenic mouse models permit a dissection of molecular pathogenesis

The development of transgenic and gene-targeted murine models permitted a dissection of the sequence of events leading to atherosclerosis. As described by others in this volume, targeted disruption of the gene for apolipoprotein E (apoE) in the mouse leads to severe, spontaneous atherosclerosis [52–54], while disruption of the LDL receptor gene leads to an increased sensitivity to cholester-ol and to the development of early stages of atherosclerosis when mice are fed a cholesterol-rich diet [55]. Not only did the construction of these mice permit an identification of the role of these cholesterol-regulating genes in atherogenesis, it also made it possible to study the contribution of other genes by cross-breeding apoE or LDL receptor knockout (KO) mice with other KO models.

Compound KO mice that represent crosses between the atherosclerosis-prone apoE KO strain and mice lacking functioning scavenger receptors (SR-A KO mice) showed significant reduction of atherosclerosis [56]. A defective differentia-tion of blood monocytes into macrophages caused by a mutation in the M-CSF gene (the *op* mutation) led to an even more substantial reduction in the develop-ment of atherosclerotic lesions [57]. M-CSF is abundantly expressed in atherosclerotic lesions [58,59], as is the chemokine, monocyte chemoattractant protein-1 (MCP-1), which promotes the recruitment of mononuclear cells to the arterial intima [42,43,49]. Importantly, mice lacking this chemokine or its receptor, CCR-2, also show relative protection from atherosclerosis [60,61]. Recruitment of monocytes, their differentiation into macrophages, and transformation into foam cells through uptake of modified lipoproteins are therefore pivotal in atherogenesis. We can conclude that innate immunity, i.e., the antigen-independent immune activity carried largely by cells of the monocyte-macrophage lineage, is necessary for the development of atherosclerosis. The role of adaptive immunity, i.e., the antigen-specific immune responses carried by T and B cells, has been more controversial.

Adaptive immunity in atherosclerosis

The T cells, although not as common as the macrophages, could play an important regulatory role in atherogenesis due to their capacity to control macrophage activity and inflammation. While the resting T cell is essentially inert, activation leads to the secretion of a host of biological mediators, including the cytokines interferon-γ, interleukin-2 (IL-2), IL-4, TNF-α, TGF-β and others by different subsets of T cells. Among these cytokines, interferon-γ is the major priming signal for macrophage activation. This can lead to production of macrophage-derived cytokines such as IL-1 and TNF-α and also to secretion of matrix metalloproteinases as well as complement and coagulation factors including tissue factor [62]. In addition, interferon-γ downregulates scavenger receptor expression [63–65] apolipoprotein E secretion [66] and expression of the ABC cassette receptor needed for cholesterol elimination [67].

Interferon-γ also has drastic effects on vascular cells. It induces expression of major histocompatibility complex (MHC) class II antigens such as HLA-DR in endothelial (68) and smooth muscle cells [5,69], inhibits their proliferation [69–71] and reduces angiogenesis [72]. The fibrinolytic activity of endothelial cells is modulated by interferon-γ [73,74], as is the expression of adhesion molecules [75].

The in vivo effects of interferon-γ on the vessel wall are equally striking. The formation of a neointima after mechanical injury is inhibited [76,77] but the development of lesions during chronic rejection of vascular grafts is greatly increased [78]. When mice deficient in interferon-γ receptors are bred with apoE KO mice, the doubly deficient offspring exhibits significantly reduced atherosclerosis [79]. This suggests that interferon-γ accelerates atherosclerosis in spite of its growth-inhibitory action.

In addition to interferon-γ T cells produce a large number of other cytokines that regulate inflammation, antibody production, and cell proliferation. The pattern of cytokine expression, and hence of effector function, differs between subsets of T cells. The interferon-γ producing CD4$^+$ T cells are usually called Th1 cells; their activation induces macrophage activation and formation of an inflammatory lesion dominated by macrophages, T cells, and intracellular degradation, i.e., a DTH-like reaction. Th2 cells produce IL-4, IL-5, IL-10 and other cytokines and induce allergy type responses, while Th3 cells make TGF-β. The naive CD4$^+$ T cell that is activated by its cognate antigen through the mechanism of antigen presentation can differentiate into either of these subsets depending on the cytokines present in its milieu. The presence of IL-12 promotes Th1 differentiation while IL-10 inhibits Th1 and promotes Th2 development. The advanced human plaque is dominated by T cells of the Th1 type [80], possibly due to the production of IL-12 in this lesion [81]. Th1 cells appear to carry proatherogenic activity since IL-10 deficient mice show increased fatty streak formation [82].

Adaptive immune responses require the recognition by T and B cells of specific antigens that are bound to their specific antigen receptors. The T cell antigen receptor (TCR) as well as the B cell receptor, which is a cell-surface immunoglobulin are unique for each cell and formed by somatic rearrangement of gene fragments during lymphoblast differentiation. Those T cells that express TCRs recognizing molecules present in the thymus during early life are removed by the clonal selection process, as are those that cannot interact with MHC molecules on antigen-presenting cells. The remaining cells (approx 1%) escape clonal deletion and are released into the circulation. When any of these T cells encounter an antigen (often a peptide fragment of a protein), it responds by proliferation, cytokine secretion and sometimes also development of cytotoxic activity. The repeated cell divisions of activated T cells leads to the formation of a clone of cells with identical TCR. Consequently, the identification of a T cell clone in a tissue implies the expansion of cells, usually due to antigen-specific activation.

When T cell infiltrates of advanced human plaques were analyzed, a heterogeneous pattern of TCR rearrangements were detected [83]. This would argue against antigen-specific mechanisms in disease development. However, antigen-specific T cells could be cloned from plaques [84] and we speculated that clonal expansion could be limited to certain earlier phases of disease and followed by an infiltration of heterogeneous T cells into the advanced plaque. We therefore examined TCR rearrangement in early lesions of apoE KO mice. This revealed a very restricted heterogeneity, with selective expression of certain TCR β chains in oligoclonal patterns [85]. Interestingly, similar TCR types that are overrepresented in lesions are common in T cell lines reactive towards oxidized LDL (A. Nicoletti, G. Paulsson and G.K. Hansson, unpublished observations). These data together with the evidence for T cell activation support a role for antigen-specific cellular immune reactions in atherosclerosis.

The immune specificity of plaque T cells has been characterized by cloning T cells from human plaques and exposing them to candidate antigens. Using this approach, it was determined that a significant proportion of plaque CD4$^+$ T cells recognize oxidized LDL as an HLA-DR dependent antigen [84]. This indicates that oxidized LDL not only activates and is internalized by macrophages but also is recognized as a local antigen by immune cells of the plaque. Subsequent studies have identified T cells reactive towards other local antigens, including heat shock protein 60 (hsp60) [86] in animal models of disease.

How important are adaptive immune responses for the development of atherosclerosis? This question was first addressed experimentally by Dansky et al., who constructed a compound KO mouse that lacked T and B cells due to a defect in the recombinase activating gene-1 (RAG-1) as well as apoE [87]. These mice exhibited a significant reduction of atherosclerosis, however, the difference reduced when the mice were fed large amounts of cholesterol [87,88]. These findings were first interpreted as indicating a minor role for T (and B) cells in atherosclerosis. However, it was later clarified that immune effector functions are modulated by cholesterol levels: while Th1 immunity dominates at moderate levels of hypercholesterolemia, excessive cholesterol levels lead to a switch towards Th2 activity [89]. Therefore, adaptive immune responses may play an important role in atherogenesis under pathophysiologically relevant experimental conditions, in line with the finding that apoE KO mice lacking interferon-γ receptors as well as mice lacking the CD40 ligand (CD154) needed for immune activation exhibit reduced atherosclerosis [79,90]. This conclusion was supported by our recent findings in another immune-deficient mouse model. The apoExS-CID mouse carries a mutation that leads to severe combined immunodeficiency; it exhibits a 70% reduction of atherosclerosis when compared to immunocompetent apoE KO mice [91]. Transfer of CD4$^+$ T cells from immunocompetent apoE KO mice into apoExSCID mice accelerated disease development drastically, indicating a proatherogenic role for these cells [91].

Recent studies that show antiatherosclerotic effects of immunomodulating therapy are particularly encouraging for investigators of the immunopathogenesis of atherosclerosis. Inhibition of cellular immunity by injections of polyclonal immunoglobulins reduced atherosclerosis in apoE KO mice significantly [92] and administration of blocking antibodies to CD40 ligand reduced lesion development in LDL receptor KO mice [93]. Equally interesting, protective immunization with the candidate antigen, oxidized LDL, has been shown to inhibit atherogenesis in several models [94–96]. It will be interesting to see whether immunomodulation and/or antigen-specific immunization may develop into useful therapy against atherosclerosis.

LDL oxidation promotes inflammation and immune reactions

A wealth of data point to oxidized LDL as a culprit in atherosclerosis [97]. LDL oxidation renders the particle susceptible to uptake by scavenger receptors, leading to foam cell formation [98,99]. Such oxidized LDL particles are found in atherosclerotic lesions [100] and elicit antibody formation [101,102]. They promote macrophage activation [103] and can act as chemoattractants [104,105]. Oxidized LDL contains T cell antigens that induce T-cell dependent B cell activation [96]. In addition, it carries oxidized lipid species that are recognized by T-cell independent IgM antibodies [106]. Bioactive lipids derived from LDL oxidation can also modulate adhesion molecule expression and intracellular signal transduction [107–109]. In conclusion, oxidized LDL particles carry a host of different proinflammatory, immunogenic and immune-modulating molecules that are likely to affect the process of atherosclerosis.

Antioxidants that prevent the formation of such molecules reduce atherogenesis in animal models [110,111], however, clinical trials of antioxidants in patients have yielded contradictory results. Further work may be needed to clarify the precise type of oxidative modification that takes place in the artery during atherogenesis in man and use agents that prevent this particular kind of modification rather than "general" inhibitors of nonenzymatic oxidation.

In addition to oxidized LDL, proinflammatory and immunogenic agents that increase atherosclerosis may include endogenous "stress" proteins such as hsp60 as well as exogenous microbes such as *Chlamydia pneumoniae* [112]. Although atherosclerosis develops in experimental animals bred in a completely microbe-free environment [113], it is possible that microbes increase the risk for plaque activation and ischemic events. In fact, plaque fissuring and the formation of mural thrombi in "culprit lesions" of coronary arteries show increased immune and inflammatory activation [114,115].

Patients with acute coronary syndromes exhibit signs of systemic immune activation, with circulating activated T cells, inflammatory cytokines, and acute phase reactants [116–118]. The lack of suitable experimental models has prevented scientists from following the transition from silent atherosclerotic plaques to occlusion, ischemia and infarction. Our recent development of a model to study myocardial infarction in hypercholesterolemic, atherosclerotic mice [119] may offer new opportunities to dissect this process and clarify whether inflammatory mechanisms are important also at this stage of the atherosclerotic disease.

The legacy of Russell Ross

In his last review article, Russell Ross elegantly summarized our understanding of the intricate interplay between lipid metabolic, hemodynamic, inflammatory, and local factors in atherogenesis [120]. He wrote: "The lesions of atherosclerosis represent a series of highly specific cellular and molecular responses that can best be described, in aggregate, as an inflammatory disease". This paper, which was entitled "Atherosclerosis — an inflammatory disease", was published in January 1999, less than 3 months before Dr Ross' death.

Our understanding of atherosclerosis as an inflammatory disease is in no small part thanks to Russell Ross. By proposing the response-to-injury hypothesis, he played a key role in the transfer of atherosclerosis research into the molecular era. By summarizing current knowledge and pointing out new directions in cardiovascular science, he led its development for many years. And by daring to propose novel, brave and testable hypotheses, he pointed out a path for scientific investigation that remains for all of us to follow. For all this, we are greatly indebted to Russell Ross as a friend, scientist, and scholar.

60

Acknowledgements

I am grateful to my colleagues Sten Stemme, Yong-jian Geng, Xinghua Zhou, Gabrielle Paulsson, Antonino Nicoletti and Giuseppina Caligiuri for their collaboration in some of the studies described in this chapter.

Our work is supported by the Swedish Medical Research Council (project 6816), Heart-Lung Foundation, and the Söderberg Foundation.

References

1. Ross R, Glomset JA, Kariya B, Harker LA. A platelet dependent serum factor that stimulates the proliferation of arterial smooth muscle cells in vitro. Proc Natl Acad Sci USA 1974;71: 1207–1211.
2. Ross R, Glomset JA. The pathogenesis of atherosclerosis. N Engl J Med 1976;295:420–425.
3. Virchow R. Der atheromatose Prozess der Arterien. Wien Med Wochenschr 1856;6:825–828.
4. Brown MS, Goldstein JL. A receptor-mediated pathway for cholesterol homeostasis. Science 1986;232:34–47.
5. Jonasson L, Holm J, Skalli O, Gabbiani G, Hansson GK. Expression of class II transplantation antigen on vascular smooth muscle cells in human atherosclerosis. J Clin Invest 1985;76:125–131.
6. Jonasson L, Holm J, Skalli O, Bondjers G, Hansson GK. Regional accumulations of T cells, macrophages, and smooth muscle cells in the human atherosclerotic plaque. Arteriosclerosis 1986;6:131–138.
7. Gown AM, Tsukada T, Ross R. Human atherosclerosis. II. Immunocytochemical analysis of the cellular composition of human atherosclerotic lesions. Am J Pathol 1986;125:191–207.
8. van der Wal AC, Das PK, van de Berg DB, van der Loos CM, Becker AE. Atherosclerotic lesions in humans. In situ immunophenotypic analysis suggesting an immune mediated response. Lab Invest 1989;61:166–170.
9. Brown MS, Goldstein JL. Lipoprotein metabolism in the macrophage: implifications for cholesterol deposition in atherosclerosis. Ann Rev Biochem 1983;52:223–261.
10. Aqel NM, Ball RY, Waldmann H, Mitchinson MJ. Monocytic origin of foam cells in human atherosclerotic plaques. Atherosclerosis 1984;53:265–271.
11. Vedeler CA, Nyland H, Matre R. In situ characterization of the foam cells in early human atherosclerotic lesions. Acta Pathol Microbiol Immunol Scand 1984;92:133–137.
12. Steinberg D, Parthasarathy S, Carew TE, Khoo JC, Witztum JL. Beyond cholesterol: modifications of low-density lipoprotein that increase its atherogenicity. N Engl J Med 1989;320:915–924.
13. Fogelman AM, Van Lenten BJ, Warden C, Haberland ME, Edwards PA. Macrophage lipoprotein receptors. J Cell Sci 1988;9:135–149.
14. Kodama T, Freeman M, Rohrer L, Zabrecky J, Matsudaira P, Krieger M. Type I macrophage scavenger receptor contains alpha-helical and collagen-like coiled coils. Nature 1990;343:531–535.
15. Rohrer L, Freeman M, Kodama T, Penman M, Krieger M. Coiled-coil fibrous domains mediate ligand binding by macrophage scavenger receptor type II. Nature 1990;343:570–572.
16. Naito M, Suzuki H, Mori T, Matsumoto A, Kodama T, Takahashi K. Coexpression of type I and type II human macrophage scavenger receptors in macrophages of various organs and foam cells in atherosclerotic lesions. Am J Pathol 1992;141:591–600.
17. Fraser I, Hughes D, Gordon S. Divalent cation-independent macrophage adhesion inhibited by monoclonal antibody to murine scavenger receptor. Nature 1993;364:343–346.
18. Haworth R, Platt N, Keshav S, Hughes D, Darley E, Suzuki H, Kurihara Y, Kodama T, Gordon S. The macrophage scavenger receptor type A is expressed by activated macrophages and pro-

tects the host against lethal endotoxic shock. J Exp Med 1997;186:1431–1439.

19. Krieger M, Acton S, Ashkenas J, Pearson A, Penman M, Resnick D. Molecular flypaper, host defense, and atherosclerosis. J Biol Chem 1993;268:4569–4572.

20. Elomaa O, Kangas M, Sahlberg C et al. Cloning of a novel bacteria-binding receptor structurally related to scavenger receptors and expressed in a subset of macrophages. Cell 1995;80: 603–609.

21. Endemann G, Stanton LW, Madden KS, Bryant CM, White RT, Protter AA. CD36 is a receptor for oxidized low density lipoprotein. J Biol Chem 1993;268:11811–11816.

22. Febbraio M, Abumrad NA, Hajjar DP, Sharma K, Cheng W, Pearce SF, Silverstein RL. A null mutation in murine CD36 reveals an important role in fatty acid and lipoprotein metabolism. J Biol Chem 1999;274:19055–19062.

23. Seifert RA, Schwartz SM, Bowen PD. Developmentally regulated production of platelet-derived growth factor-like molecules. Nature 1984;311:669–671.

24. Shimokado K, Raines EW, Madtes DK, Barrett TB, Benditt EP. A significant part of macrophage-derived growth factor consists of at least two forms of PDGF. Cell 1985;43:277–286.

25. Sjölund M, Hedin U, Sejersen T, Heldin CH, Thyberg J. Arterial smooth muscle cells express platelet-derived growth factor (PDGF) a chain mRNA, secrete a PDGF-like mitogen, and bind exogenous PDGF in a phenotype- and growth state-dependent manner. J Cell Biol 1988; 106:403–413.

26. Rubin K, Tingstrîm A, Hansson GK et al. Induction of B-type receptors for platelet-derived growth factor in vascular inflammation: possible implications for development of vascular proliferative lesions. Lancet 1988;1:1353–1356.

27. Wilcox JN, Smith KM, Williams LT, Schwartz SM, Gordon D. Platelet derived growth factor mRNA detection in human atherosclerotic plaques by in situ hydribization. J Clin Invest 1988; 82:1134–1139.

28. Ross R, Masuda J, Raines EW et al. Localization of PDGF-B protein in macrophages in all phases of atherogenesis. Science 1990;248:1009–1012.

29. Battegay EJ, Raines EW, Seifert RA, Bowen PD, Ross R. TGF-beta induces bimodal proliferation of connective tissue cells via complex control of an autocrine PDGF loop. Cell 1990;63: 515–524.

30. Libby P, Warner S, Friedman GB. Interleukin-1: a mitogen for human vascular smooth muscle cells that induces the release of growth-inhibitory prostanoids. J Clin Invest 1988;81:487–498.

31. Ryan J, Geczy CL. Characterization and purification of mouse macrophage procoagulant-inducing factor. J Immunol 1986;137:2864–2870.

32. Gregory SA, Kornbluth RS, Helin H, Remold HG, Edgington TS. Monocyte procoagulant inducing factor: a lymphokine involved in the T cell-instructed monocyte procoagulant response to antigen. J Immunol 1986;137:3231–3239.

33. Ross R. The pathogenesis of atherosclerosis — an update. N Engl J Med 1986;1986:488–491.

34. Faggiotto A, Ross R. Studies of hypercholesterolemia in the nonhuman primate. I. Changes that lead to fatty streak formation. Arteriosclerosis 1984;4:323–340.

35. Faggiotto A, Ross R. Studies of hypercholesterolemia in the nonhuman primate. II. Fatty streak conversion to fibrous plaque. Arteriosclerosis 1984;4:341–356.

36. Cybulsky MI, Fries J, Williams AJ et al. Alternative splicing of human VCAM-1 in activated vascular endothelium. Am J Pathol 1992;138:815–820.

37. Li H, Cybulsky MI, Gimbrone MA, Libby P. An atherogenic diet rapidly induces VCAM-1, a cytokine-regulatable mononuclear leukocyte adhesion molecule, in rabbit aortic endothelium. Arterioscl Thromb 1993;13:197–204.

38. Li H, Cybulsky MI, Gimbrone MA, Libby P. Inducible expression of vascular cell adhesion molecule-1 by vascular smooth muscle cells in vitro and within rabbit atheroma. Am J Pathol 1993;143:1551–1559.

39. Poston RN, Haskard DO, Coucher JR, Gall NP, Johnson-Tilney RR. Expression of intercellular adhesion molecule-1 in atherosclerotic plaques. Am J Pathol 1992;140:665–673.

40. O'Brien KD, McDonald TO, Chait A, Allen MD, Alpers CE. Neovascular expression of E-selectin, intercellular adhesion molecule-1, and vascular cell adhesion molecule-1 in human atherosclerosis and their relation to intimal leukocyte content. Circulation 1996;93:672–682.

41. Nakashima Y, Raines EW, Plump AS, Breslow JL, Ross R. Upregulation of VCAM-1 and ICAM-1 at atherosclerosis-prone sites on the endothelium in the apoE-deficient mouse. Arter Thromb Vasc Biol 1998;18:842–851.

42. Ylä-Herttuala S, Lipton BA, Rosenfeld ME et al. Expression of monocyte chemoattractant protein 1 in macrophage-rich areas of human and rabbit atherosclerotic lesions. Proc Natl Acad Sci USA 1991;88:5252–5256.

43. Nelken NA, Coughlin SR, Gordon D, Wilcox JN. Monocyte chemoattractant protein-1 in human atheromatous plaques. J Clin Invest 1991;88:1121–1127.

44. Yu X, Dluz S, Graves DT et al. Elevated expression of monocyte chemoattractant protein 1 by vascular smooth muscle cells in hypercholesterolemic primates. Proc Natl Acad Sci USA 1992; 89:6953–6957.

45. Mach F, Sauty A, Iarossi AS et al. Differential expression of three T lymphocyte-activating CXC chemokines by human atheroma-associated cells. J Clin Invest 1999;104:1041–1050.

46. Liao F, Andalibi A, deBeer FC, Fogelman AM, Lusis AJ. Genetic control of inflammatory gene induction and NF-kappa B-like transcription factor activation in response to an atherogenic diet in mice. J Clin Invest 1993;91:2572–2579.

47. Terkeltaub R, Banka CL, Solan J, Santoro D, Brand K, Curtiss LK. Oxidized LDL induces monocytic cell expression of interleukin-8, a chemokine with T-lymphocyte chemotactic activity. Arterioscler Thromb 1994;14:47–53.

48. Dixit VM, Green S, Sarma V et al. Tumor necrosis factor-alpha induction of novel gene products in human endothelial cells including a macrophage-specific chemotaxin. J Biol Chem 1990; 265:2973–2978.

49. Wang JM, Sica A, Peri G et al. Expression of monocyte chemotactic protein and interleukin-8 by cytokine-activated human vascular smooth muscle cells. Arterioscler Thromb 1991;11: 1166–1174.

50. Colotta F, Sciacca FL, Sironi M, Luini W, Rabiet MJ, Mantovani A. Expression of monocyte chemotactic protein-1 by monocytes and endothelial cells exposed to thrombin. Am J Pathol 1994;144:975–985.

51. Torzewski J, Oldroyd R, Lachmann P, Fitzsimmons C, Proudfoot D, Bowyer D. Complement-induced release of monocyte chemotactic protein-1 from human smooth muscle cells — A possible initiating event in atherosclerotic lesion formation. Arteriosclerosis, Thromb Vasc Biol 1996;16:673–677.

52. Piedrahita JA, Zhang SH, Hagaman JR, Oliver PM, Maeda N. Generation of mice carrying a mutant apolipoprotein E gene inactivated by gene targeting in embryonic stem cells. Proc Natl Acad Sci USA 1992;89:4471–4475.

53. Plump AS, Smith JD, Hayek T et al. Severe hypercholesterolemia and atherosclerosis in apolipoprotein E-deficient mice created by homologous recombination in ES cells. Cell 1992;71: 343–353.

54. Nakashima Y, Plump AS, Raines EW, Breslow JL, Ross R. ApoE-deficient mice develop lesions of all phases of atherosclerosis throughout the arterial tree. Arterioscler Thromb 1994;14:133–140.

55. Ishibashi S, Goldstein JL, Brown MS, Herz J, Burns DK. Massive xanthomatosis and atherosclerosis in cholesterol-fed low density lipoprotein receptor-negative mice. J Clin Invest 1994; 93:1885–1893.

56. Suzuki H, Kurihara Y, Takeya M, Kamada N, Kataoka M, Jishage K, Ueda O, Sakaguchi H, Higashi T, Suzuki T, Takashima Y, Kawabe Y, Cynshi O, Wada Y, Honda M, Kurihara H, Aburatani H, Doi T, Matsumoto A, Azuma S, Noda T, Toyoda A. A role for macrophage scavenger receptors in atherosclerosis and susceptibility to infection. Nature 1997;386:292–296.

57. Smith JD, Trogan E, Ginsberg M, Grigaux C, Tian J, Miyata M. Decreased atherosclerosis in

mice deficient in both macrophage colony-stimulating factor (op) and apolipoprotein E. Proc Natl Acad Sci USA 1995;92:8264—8268.

58. Clinton SK, Underwood R, Hayes L, Sherman ML, Kufe DW, Libby P. Macrophage colony-stimulating factor gene expression in vascular cells and in experimental and human atherosclerosis. Am J Pathol 1992;140:301—316.

59. Rosenfeld ME, Yla HS, Lipton BA, Ord VA, Witztum JL, Steinberg D. Macrophage colony-stimulating factor mRNA and protein in atherosclerotic lesions of rabbits and humans. Am J Pathol 1992;140:291—300.

60. Gu L, Okada Y, Clinton SK, Gerard C, Sukhova GK, Libby P, Rollins BJ. Absence of monocyte chemoattractant protein-1 reduces atherosclerosis in low density lipoprotein receptor-deficient mice. Molecular Cell 1998;2:275—281.

61. Boring L, Gosling J, Cleary M, Charo IF. Decreased lesion formation in CCR2–/– mice reveals a role for chemokines in the initiation of atherosclerosis. Nature 1998;394:894—897.

62. Moon DK, Geczy CL. Recombinant IFN-gamma synergizes with lipopolysaccharide to induce macrophage membrane procoagulants. J Immunol 1988;141:1536—1542.

63. Fong LG, Fong AT, Cooper AD. Inhibition of mouse macrophage degradation of acetyl-low density lipoprotein by interferon-γ. J Biologic Chem 1990;265:11751—11760.

64. Geng YJ, Hansson GK. Interferon-γ inhibits scavenger receptor expression and foam cell formation in human monocyte-derived macrophages. J Clin Invest 1992;89:1322—1330.

65. Geng YJ, Holm J, Nygren S, Bruzelius M, Stemme S, Hansson GK. Expression of macrophage scavenger receptor in atherosclerosis. Relationship between scavenger receptor isoforms and the T cell cytokine, interferon-γ. Arterioscler Thromb Vasc Biol 1995;15:1195—1202.

66. Brand K, Mackman N, Curtiss LK. Interferon-gamma inhibits macrophage apolipoprotein E production by posttranslational mechanisms. J Clin Inv 1993;91:2031—2039.

67. Panousis CG, Zuckerman SH. Interferon-gamma induces downregulation of Tangier disease gene (ATP-binding-cassette transporter 1) in macrophage-derived foam cells [see comments]. Arterioscler Thromb Vasc Biol 2000;20:1565—1571.

68. Pober JS, Gimbrone MA, Cotran RS et al. Ia expression by vascular endothelium is inducible by activated T cells and by human gamma interferon. J Exp Med 1983;157:1339—1353.

69. Hansson GK, Jonasson L, Holm J, Clowes MM, Clowes AW. Gamma-interferon regulates vascular smooth muscle proliferation and Ia antigen expression in vivo and in vitro. Circ Res 1988;63:712—719.

70. Friesel R, Komoriya A, Maciag T. Inhibition of endothelial cell proliferation by gamma-interferon. J Cell Biol 1987;104:689—696.

71. Hansson GK, Hellstrand M, Rymo L, Rubbia L, Gabbiani G. Interferon-γ inhibits both proliferation and expression of differentiation-specific α-smooth muscle actin in arterial smooth muscle cells. J Exp Med 1989;170:1595—1608.

72. Arenberg DA, Kunkel SL, Polverini PJ et al. Interferon-γ-inducible protein 10 (IP-10) is an angiostatic factor that inhibits human non-small cell lung cancer (NSCLC) tumorigenesis and spontaneous metastasis. J Exp Med 1994;184:981—992.

73. Niedbala MJ, Stein Picarella M. Tumor necrosis factor induction of endothelial cell urokinase-type plasminogen activator mediated proteolysis of extracellular matrix and its antagonism by γ-interferon. Blood 1992;79:678—687.

74. Arnman V, Stemme S, Rymo L, Risberg B. Interferon-γ modulates the fibrinolytic response in cultured human endothelial cells. Thromb Res 1995;77:431—440.

75. Lechleitner S, Gille J, Johnson DR, Petzelbauer P. Interferon enhances tumor necrosis factor-induced vascular cell adhesion molecule 1 (CD106) expression in human endothelial cells by an interferon-related factor-1 dependent pathway. J Exp Med 1998;187:2023—2030.

76. Hansson GK, Holm J. Interferon-γ inhibits arterial stenosis after injury. Circulation 1991;84:1266—1272.

77. Hansson GK, Holm J, Holm S, Fotev Z, Hedrich HJ, Fingerle J. T lymphocytes inhibit the vascular response to injury. Proc Natl Acad Sci USA 1991;88:10530—10534.

78. Tellides G, Tereb DA, Kirkiles-Smith NC et al. Interferon-gamma elicits arteriosclerosis in the absence of leukocytes [In Process Citation]. Nature 2000;403:207–211.

79. Gupta S, Pablo AM, Jiang X-c, Wang N, Tall AR, Schindler C. IFN-γ potentiates atherosclerosis in apoE knock-out mice. J Clin Invest 1997;99:2752–2761.

80. Frostegård J, Ulfgren AK, Nyberg P et al. Cytokine expression in advanced human athero-sclerotic plaques: dominance of pro-inflammatory (Th1) and macrophage-stimulating cyto-kines. Atherosclerosis 1999;145:33–43.

81. Uyemura K, Demer L, Castle SC et al. Cross-regulatory roles of interleukin (IL)-12 and IL-10 in atherosclerosis. J Clin Invest 1996;97:2130–2138.

82. Mallat Z, Besnard S, Duriez M et al. Protective role of interleukin-10 in atherosclerosis [In Pro-cess Citation]. Circ Res 1999;85:e17–24.

83. Stemme S, Rymo L, Hansson GK. Polyclonal origin of T lymphocytes in human atherosclerotic plaques. Lab Invest 1991;65:654–660.

84. Stemme S, Faber B, Holm J, Wiklund O, Witztum JL, Hansson GK. T lymphocytes from human atherosclerotic plaques recognize oxidized LDL. Proc Natl Acad Sci USA 1995;92:3893–3897.

85. Paulsson G, Zhou X, Törnquist E, Hansson GK. Oligoclonal T cell expansions in atherosclerotic lesions of apoE-deficient mice. Arterioscler Thromb Vasc Biol 2000;20:10–17.

86. Xu Q, Kleindienst R, Waitz W, Dietrich H, Wick G. Increased expression of heat shock protein 65 coincides with a population of infiltrating T lymphocytes in atherosclerotic lesions of rabbits specifically responding to heat shock protein 65. J Clin Invest 1993;91:2693–2702.

87. Dansky HM, Charlton SA, Harper MM, Smith JD. T and B lymphocytes play a minor role in atherosclerotic plaque formation in the apolipoprotein E-deficient mouse. Proc Natl Acad Sci USA 1997;94:4642–4646.

88. Daugherty A, Puré E, Delfel-Butteiger D, Leferovich J, Roselaar SE. The effects of total lympho-cyte deficiency on the extent of atherosclerosis in apolipoprotein E-/- mice. J Clin Invest 1997; 100:1575–1580.

89. Zhou X, Paulsson G, Stemme S, Hansson GK. Hypercholesterolemia is associated with a Th1/ Th2 switch of the autoimmune response in atherosclerotic apo E-knockout mice. J Clin Invest 1998;101:1717–1725.

90. Lutgens E, Gorelik L, Daemen MJ et al. Requirement for CD154 in the progression of athero-sclerosis. Nat Med 1999;5:1313–1316.

91. Nicoletti A, Paulsson G, Caligiuri G, Zhou X, Hansson GK. Induction of neonatal tolerance to oxidized lipoprotein reduces atherosclerosis in ApoE knockout mice [In Process Citation]. Mol Med 2000;6:283–290.

92. Nicoletti A, Kaveri S, Caligiuri G, Bariéty J, Hansson GK. Immunoglobulin treatment reduces atherosclerosis in apo E knockout mice. J Clin Invest 1998;102:910–918.

93. Mach F, Schönbeck U, Sukhova GK, Atkinson E, Libby P. Reduction of atherosclerosis in mice by inhibition of CD40 signalling. Nature 1998;394:200–203.

94. Palinski W, Miller E, Witztum JL. Immunization of low density lipoprotein (LDL) receptor-defi-cient rabbits with homologous malondialdehyde-modified LDL reduces atherogenesis. Proc Natl Acad Sci USA 1995;92:821–825.

95. Ameli S, Hultgårdh-Nilsson A, Regnström J et al. Effect of immunization with homologous LDL and oxidized LDL on early atherosclerosis in hypercholesterolemic rabbits. Arterioscler Thromb Vasc Biol 1996;16:1074–1079.

96. Zhou X, Caligiuri G, Hamsten A, Hansson GK. Protection against atherosclerosis by LDL immunization is associated with T cell dependent IgG antibodies in apoE-deficient mice. Arter-ioscler Thromb Vasc Biol 2000;in press.

97. Steinberg D. Low density lipoprotein oxidation and its pathobiological significance. J Biologic Chem 1997;272:20963–20966.

98. Fogelman AM, Shechter I, Seager J, Hokom M, Child JS, Edwards PA. Malondialdehyde altera-tion of low density lipoproteins leads to cholesteryl ester accumulation in human monocyte-macrophages. Proc Natl Acad Sci USA 1980;77:2214–2218.

99. Quinn MT, Parthasarathy S, Fong LG, Steinberg D. Oxidatively modified low density lipoproteins: a potential role in recruitment and retention of monocyte/macrophages during atherogenesis. Proc Natl Acad Sci USA 1987;84:2995–2998.

100. Ylä-Herttuala S, Palinski W, Rosenfeld ME et al. Evidence for the presence of oxidatively modified low density lipoprotein in atherosclerotic lesions of rabbit and man. J Clin Invest 1989; 84:1086–1095.

101. Palinski W, Rosenfeld ME, Ylä-Herttuala S et al. Low density lipoprotein undergoes oxidative modification in vivo. Proc Natl Acad Sci USA 1989;86:1372–1376.

102. Palinski W, Ylä-Herttuala S, Rosenfeld ME et al. Antisera and monoclonal antibodies specific for epitopes generated during oxidative modification of low density lipoprotein. Arterioscl Thromb 1990;10:325–335.

103. Frostegård J, Nilsson J, Haegerstrand A, Hamsten A, Wigzell H, Gidlund M. Oxidized low density lipoprotein induces differentiation and adhesion of human monocytes and the monocytic cell line U937. Proc Natl Acad Sci USA 1990;87:904–908.

104. McMurray HF, Parthasarathy S, Steinberg D. Oxidatively modified low density lipoprotein is a chemoattractant for human T lymphocytes. J Clin Invest 1993;92:1004–1008.

105. Berliner JA, Schwartz DS, Territo MC et al. Induction of chemotactic cytokines by minimally oxidized LDL. Adv Exp Med Biol 1993;351:13–18.

106. Shaw PX, Horkko S, Chang MK et al. Natural antibodies with the T15 idiotype may act in atherosclerosis, apoptotic clearance, and protective immunity [In Process Citation]. J Clin Invest 2000;105:1731–1740.

107. Shih PT, Elices MJ, Fang ZT, Ugarova TP, Strahl D, Territo MC, Frank JS, Kovach NL, Cabanas C, Berliner JA, Vora DK. Minimally modified low-density lipoprotein induces monocyte adhesion to endothelial connecting segment-1 by activating β1 integrin. J Clin Invest 1999;103: 613–625.

108. Mattsson-Hultén L, Lindmark H, Diczfalusy U, Björkhem I, Ottosson M, Liu Y, Bondjers G, Wiklund O. Oxysterols present in atherosclerotic tissue decrease the expression of lipoprotein lipase messenger RNA in human monocyte-derived macrophages. J Clin Invest 1996;97: 461–468.

109. Ohlsson BG, Englund MCO, Karlsson ALK, Knutsen E, Erixon C, Skribeck H, Liu Y, Bondjers G, Wiklund O. Oxidized low density lipoprotein inhibits lipopolysaccharide-induced binding of nuclear factor-kappa B to DNA and the subsequent expression of tumor necrosis factor-alpha and interleukin-1 beta in macrophages. J Clin Invest 1996;98:78–89.

110. Ferns G, Forster L, Stewart LA, Konneh M, Nourooz ZJ, ÉnggÜrd EE. Probucol inhibits neointimal thickening and macrophage accumulation after balloon injury in the cholesterol-fed rabbit. Proc Natl Acad Sci USA 1992;89:11312–11316.

111. Freyschuss A, Stiko RA, Swedenborg J et al. Antioxidant treatment inhibits the development of intimal thickening after balloon injury of the aorta in hypercholesterolemic rabbits. J Clin Invest 1993;91:1282–1288.

112. Saikku P. Chlamydia pneumoniae and atherosclerosis — an update. Scand J Infect Dis Suppl 1997;104:53–56.

113. Wright SD, Burton C, Hernandez M et al. Infectious agents are not necessary for murine atherogenesis. J Exp Med 2000;191:1437–1442.

114. van der Wal AC, Becker AE, van der Loos CM, Das PK. Site of intimal rupture or erosion of thrombosed coronary atherosclerotic plaques is characterized by an inflammatory process irrespective of the dominant plaque morphology. Circulation 1994;89:36–44.

115. Libby P. Molecular bases of the acute coronary syndromes. Circulation 1995;91:2844–2850.

116. Biasucci LM, Vitelli A, Liuzzo G, Altamura S, Caligiuri G, Monaco C, Rebuzzi AG, Ciliberto G, Maseri A. Elevated levels of interleukin-6 in unstable angina. Circulation 1996;94:874–877.

117. Caligiuri G, Summaria F, Liuzzo G, Maseri A. Time course of T-lymphocyte activation and of C-reactive protein in unstable angina: relation to prognosis. Circulation 1996;94:I-571.

118. Caligiuri G, Paulsson G, Nicoletti A, Maseri A, Hansson GK. Evidence for antigen-driven T-

cell response in unstable angina. Circulation 2000;in press.

119. Caligiuri G, Lévy B, Pernow J, Thorén P, Hansson GK. Myocardial infarction mediated by endothelin receptor signaling in hypercholesterolemic mice. Proc Natl Acad Sci USA 1999;96: 6920–6924.

120. Ross R. Atherosclerosis — an inflammatory disease. N Engl J Med 1999;340:115–126.

Inflammation and plaque stability

Peter Libby, Masanori Aikawa, Uwe Schönbeck, Galina K. Sukhova, François Mach, Nikolaus Marx and Jorge Plutzky

Brigham and Women's Hospital, Boston, Massachussetts, USA

Atherosclerosis is an indolent disease whose seeds are sown in infancy [1]. Adolescents in Western societies have surprisingly high prevalence of atherosclerotic lesions [2,3]. Risk factors for atherosclerosis measured early in life influence later coronary heart disease morbidity and mortality [4]. By middle age, this disease is virtually endemic. Yet, for most of its course, atherosclerosis causes no symptoms. Atherosclerosis has one of the longest incubation periods of any human disease. Eventually, some patients with fixed lesions may develop various ischemic syndromes in the coronary circulation, manifested by unstable angina or acute myocardial infarction. However, we must bear in mind the systemic nature of atherosclerosis. Acute complications of atheroma in the arteries perfusing the central nervous system can cause transient ischemic attacks or strokes. In the peripheral arteries, acute occlusions can give rise to critical limb ischemia.

Inflammation and the pathophysiology of acute manifestations of atherosclerosis

Pathologists have taught us much regarding the micro-anatomical causes of the transition from asymptomatic or chronic stable atherosclerosis to the acute thrombotic complications that cause the manifestations mentioned above [5]. We now recognize that thrombosis of a disrupted atheroma causes most acute coronary syndromes. We further have learned that physical disruption of atherosclerotic plaques is the most common precursor to thrombotic complications. Some three-quarters of acute myocardial infarction result from fracture of the plaque's fibrous cap. The remainder usually results from superficial erosion of the endothelial layer [6]. In both cases, the disruption triggers thrombosis. In the case of fibrous cap rupture, coagulation induced by Tissue Factor in the plaque's lipid core incites thrombus formation. In the case of superficial erosion, platelet aggregation and activation by subendothelial von Willebrand factor and collagen may instigate the thrombus.

Some years ago, we proposed a pathophysiologic model of plaque rupture that

---

Address for correspondence: Peter Libby MD, Brigham and Women's Hospital, 221 Longwood Avenue, LMRC 307, Boston, MA 02115, USA. Tel.: +1-617-732-6628. Fax: +1-617-732-6961. E-mail: plibby@rics.bwh.harvard.edu

was predicated on the primordial role interstitial collagen plays in determining the tensile strength of the plaque's fibrous cap [7]. Laboratory findings emerging from our group over the last decade suggested a role for the lymphokine gamma interferon (γ-IFN) in inhibiting collagen synthesis by smooth muscle cells [8]. Our laboratory and others further characterized a series of matrix-degrading proteinases capable of catabolizing the collagen in the plaque's fibrous cap [9—11]. Our contribution to the last volume in these series provides more details regarding the experimental underpinnings of this concept of plaque stability [12].

One outstanding question that has now been elucidated by our subsequent work relates to the demonstration of an actual excess of active matrix metalloproteinase (MMP) in situ. We and others had previously immunolocalized one interstitial collagenase, MMP-1, in atheroma [10,11]. However, cells in human atheroma secrete a number of tissue inhibitors of MMPs (TIMPs 1—4) able to neutralize MMP activity [10,13,14]. Furthermore, none of the antibodies currently available reliably distinguish the inactive zymogen form of MMPs from their processed, catalyticly active forms.

Using newly developed and validated reagents that detect the new epitope formed by cleavage of the collagen fibril by interstitial collagenase [15], we have documented the presence of cleaved collagen in extracts of human atherosclerotic plaques (Fig. 1) [16]. Uninvolved arteries had little or no cleaved collagen (Fig. 1). Plaques categorized a priori on the basis of inspection as having a predominantly fibrous vs. atheromatous (lipid-rich) morphology had variable levels of the cleaved collagen. In situ, the cleaved collagen epitope colocalized with macrophages expressing interstitial collagenases, not only the previously described MMP-1 but also collagenase-3 (MMP-13). Extracts of plaques also displayed increased levels of MMP-1 and MMP-13, with higher levels in atheromatous vs. fibrous plaques (Fig. 1). Levels of intact fibrillar collagen varied inversely with the amounts of collagenases and cleaved collagen (Figs. 1 and 2). These observations reinforced our hypothesis regarding the dynamic nature of collagen in the plaque's fibrous cap.

Recent work has also helped resolve another outstanding question regarding mechanisms of plaque thrombosis. Overexpression of Tissue Factor by a subpopulation of macrophages within human atheroma was first identified in the 1980s [17,18]. However, the common soluble cytokines previously described in human atheroma stimulate Tissue Factor gene expression little if at all. Pathological studies disclosed close approximation of T cells and macrophages in human atherosclerotic plaques whose rupture causes fatal coronary thromboses in humans [19]. We recently described the expression of a cell surface cytokine, CD154 (CD40 ligand), by T lymphocytes and other cells within human atherosclerotic plaques [20]. We therefore tested the hypothesis that CD40 ligation might provide the elusive missing link between the activated T cell and the macrophage in terms of Tissue Factor gene expression in atheroma. In vitro studies bore out the ability of CD40 ligation to enhance Tissue Factor gene expression, with changes in both protein level and biological activity (Fig. 3) [21]. In

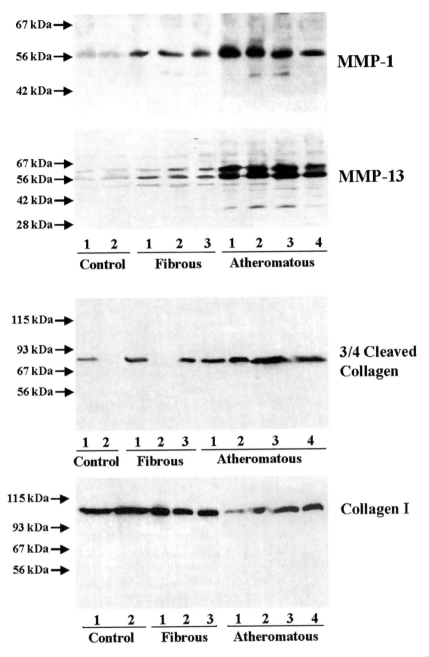

Fig. 1. Collagen cleavage and overexpression of the interstitial collagenases MMP-1 and –13 in atheromatous plaques. Tissue extracts (50 μg/lane) from two nonatherosclerotic arteries (Control), three fibrous, and four atheromatous (lipid-rich) plaques were analyzed by Western blotting for MMP-1 and MMP-13. Western blot analysis of the same tissue extracts indicated increased levels of collagenase-cleaved type I collagen and reciprocal decrease of collagen type I. The molecular weight markers are indicated. Analyses were repeated at least twice, yielding similar results. (From [16], adapted with permission.)

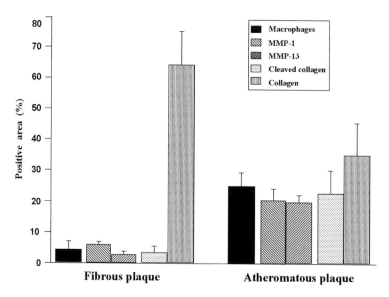

Fig. 2. Elevated expression of macrophage-derived MMP-1, MMP-13, and collagenase-cleaved collagen type I as well as reciprocal decrease of interstitial collagen type I in atheromatous vs. fibrous lesions. The expression of the above-mentioned proteins was determined immunohistochemically. Photomicrographs were employed for quantitative color image analysis of the percent positive areas. Values represent mean ± SD (n = 10/group). (From [16], adapted with permission.)

situ studies colocalized CD40, the receptor for CD154, and the target gene product, Tissue Factor, within human atherosclerotic plaques, suggesting their potential interaction.

Strategies for limiting inflammatory activation yielding stabilization of human atherosclerotic plaques

So far, we have addressed the mechanisms leading to destabilization of the atheroma. The rest of this essay will consider strategies for limiting inflammation with the ultimate goal of rendering atherosclerotic plaques more stable, and hence less likely to cause thrombotic complications. We will discuss three possible strategies: lipid lowering, interruption of CD154 signaling, and activation of peroxisomal proliferation activating receptor alpha (PPAR-α).

Lipid lowering improves features of atherosclerotic plaques associated with stability

A series of animal experiments have examined the proposition that lipid lowering can improve characteristics of atherosclerotic plaques associated with stability, and hence resistance to rupture and thrombosis. To address this, we generated experimental atheroma in rabbits by a combination of balloon injury and atherogenic diet. Atheroma in the rabbit aorta produced by such treatment share several

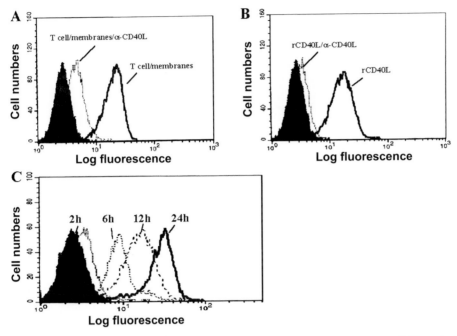

Fig. 3. CD40 ligation induces tissue factor expression in human macrophages. FACS analysis of monocytes/macrophages cultured in RPMI medium supplemented with 10% human serum stained for TF (open histograms) or the isotype control (solid histograms). **A:** Monocytes/macrophages stimulated (12 h) with cell membranes isolated from activated CD4$^+$ T cells in the presence or absence of an anti-CD40L mAb (α-CD40L, 1 μg/ml). **B:** Monocytes/macrophages were stimulated (12 h) with rCD40L (5 μg/ml) in the presence or absence of an anti-CD40L mAb (α-CD40L, 1 μg/ml). **C:** Monocytes/macrophages were stimulated with rCD40L (5 μg/ml) for the indicated time. (From [21] reproduced with permission.)

characteristics in common with advanced human atherosclerotic plaques. These lesions have a fibrous cap rich in smooth muscle cells. A lipid pool replete with macrophage-derived foam cells lurks underneath the fibrous cap. As in human atheroma, the macrophages in these experimentally produced lesions markedly overexpress interstitial collagenase (MMP-1). After 16 months of persistent hypercholesterolemia due to continued consumption of an atherogenic diet, abundant macrophages bearing MMP-1 populated the aortic intima in the control group of rabbits [22]. In the group shifted to a low cholesterol chow diet at the end of 16 months, the aorta showed much less inflammation and marked reduction in inflammatory cells and levels of MMP-1 (Fig. 4). Consistent with the role of collagenase in collagen catabolism, analysis of the collagenous skeleton of the plaques of the persistently hypercholesterolemic group showed a filamentous and scant collagen skeleton. In contrast, we observed a marked reinforcement in the interstitial collagen fibrillar structure of the intima in the aortic lesions of the rabbits shifted to the low cholesterol diet.

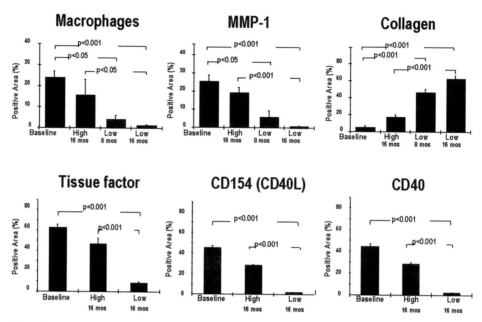

Fig. 4. Quantitative analysis of macrophage accumulation, MMP-1 (collagenase-1) expression, interstitial collagen accumulation, tissue factor, CD154 (CD40 ligand) and CD40 expression in atheroma of hypercholesterolemic rabbit aorta during dietary lipid lowering. Data is reported as a percentage of positive areas for immunostaining or picrosirius red polarization within the intima using a computer-assisted color image analysis. We produced experimental atheroma in New Zealand White rabbits by balloon injury and a cholesterol-enriched diet for 4 months. At that time 15 rabbits were sacrificed (Baseline group). A hyperlipemic group continued an atherogenic diet for 16 further months (High 16 mos, n = 5), while a lipid-lowering group consumed a purified chow diet with no added cholesterol or fat for 8 (Low 8 mos, n = 3) or 16 months (Low 16 mos, n = 10). Dietary lipid lowering for 8 or 16 months substantially decreased macrophage accumulation and MMP-1 (collagenase-1) expression and, in parallel, increased interstitial collagen content in rabbit atheroma. Lipid lowering by diet also reduced expression of tissue factor and its inducers, CD154 and CD40, in rabbit atheroma. Statistical testing used one-way ANOVA followed by post-hoc test. Bars represent SEM. (From [22,23], reproduced with permission.)

In addition to testing features of plaque stability in this series of animals, we also assessed the effect of dietary lipid lowering on Tissue Factor activity [23]. As in human atheroma, the baseline lesions displayed prominent macrophage Tissue Factor expression. In animals with continued hypercholesterolemia, a Tissue Factor expression persisted. However, animals shifted to a low cholesterol diet showed a marked diminution in the level of Tissue Factor in the intima (Fig. 4). The decrease in immunoreactive Tissue Factor accompanied decreases in the binding of factor VIIa and factor X in situ, corresponding to a decrease in Tissue Factor activity [23].

Because ligation of CD40 may contribute to Tissue Factor gene expression by intimal macrophages, we tested the effect of modulations in lipid levels on CD154 and its receptor, CD40. Baseline lesions in those from the aortae of rabbits continued on the high cholesterol diet showed considerable expression of both CD154 and its receptor [23]. However, CD154 and CD40 levels dropped markedly in animals that had undergone dietary intervention to lower lipids (Fig. 4). Taken together, these results indicate that lipid lowering can induce molecular changes that should render plaques more stable. Furthermore, such interventions can also reduce inflammation and limit the procoagulant potential within the atheromatous plaque.

Interruption of CD40 signaling promotes features of plaques associated with stability

The surface-based signaling dyad, CD154/CD40, shares the ability to induce adhesion molecules on the surface of endothelial cells (e.g., E-selectin, vascular cell adhesion molecule-1, intracellular adhesion molecule-1) with soluble cytokines such as TNF-α or IL-1β [24,25]. CD40 ligation, like soluble proinflammatory cytokines, can enhance the production of various matrix metalloproteinases (e.g., MMP-1, -2, -3, -9, and -13) and even stimulate further cytokine production [20,26,27]. In addition to these features shared by soluble cytokines, CD40 ligation has several particular effects. For example, CD154 can induce expression of the unusual metalloproteinase, stromelysin-3 (MMP-11) [28]. CD40 ligation activates caspase-1, promoting the release of the mature form of the inflammatory mediator interleukin-1β from vascular smooth muscle cells [29]. As noted above, CD154, but not the traditional soluble cytokines, can augment Tissue Factor gene expression by macrophages [20]. Given this intriguing palette of biological activities, we have tested the hypothesis that interruption of CD40 signaling can retard atherogenesis, prevent the progression of established lesions, and promote a qualitative shift in plaques toward those exhibiting features of stability.

In one series of experiments, LDL-receptor-deficient animals consumed a high cholesterol diet for a 12-week period [30]. During the entire period of exposure to hyperlipidemia, the mice received twice-weekly injections of one of three regimens: antibody that neutralizes CD154, a type and class matched irrelevant rat IgG, or saline. At the end of the 12-week period, quantitative image analysis delineated the amount of lipid deposition and atheroma formation. When compared to either control group, treatment with the neutralizing antibody significantly reduced the area of aortic wall involved by fatty lesions, the thickness of the intima, and the amount of lipid deposition. Additionally, the number of macrophages and T lymphocytes per section decreased significantly. Further indication of the efficacy of the CD154 neutralization strategy derived from the decrease in MMP-11 expression in the lesions from the treated mice [28]. Subsequent results from another group confirmed this result using mice bearing a targeted inactivation of CD154 [31].

A subsequent study tested whether interruption of CD154 signaling could not only retard initiation of atherosclerosis, but could influence the evolution of established lesions. In these experiments, lesion formation occurred during a 13-week period of diet-induced hypercholesterolemia before an additional 13-

week period of treatment with the anti-CD154 antibody or controls [32]. In this experiment, animals receiving the irrelevant rat IgG or saline alone showed progression of the atheroma from the 13th through the 26th week of hypercholesterolemia. However, the animals treated with the anti-CD154 antibody exhibited a markedly attenuated evolution of the lesions (Fig. 5). Furthermore, the animals treated with anti-CD154 antibody showed more abundant smooth muscle cells in the aortic arch, a decreased number of T-lymphocytes and macrophages, and an increased level of collagen. As discussed above, the better-developed collagenous skeleton of these atheromatous lesions should increase their tensile strength. In humans, one would consider lesions containing more abundant collagen as more stable, and less prone to rupture and cause thrombosis. Thus, interruption of CD154 action in hypercholesterolemic mice yielded reduced formation of atherosclerotic lesions and limited the evolution of established atheroma. Moreover, this treatment promoted processes expected to render a plaque more biomechanically stable and therefore less likely to undergo disruption and attendant complication. Others simultaneously reported complementary results [33].

PPAR-α agonism, a further anti-inflammatory strategy in atherosclerosis

Convergence of clinical trial data and basic scientific advances has stimulated interest in the peroxisome proliferator-activated receptors (PPARs) in the context of atherosclerosis. The appellation "PPARs", derived from early observations regarding peroxisome proliferation in rodents, is especially unfortunate since activation of this family of nuclear receptors does not appear to cause peroxisomal proliferation in humans.

PPARs belong to the nuclear receptor superfamily, joining other better known family members such as receptors for steroid hormones, thyroid hormones, and retinoids. Nuclear receptors typically bind low molecular weight lipophilic ligands, either natural or synthetically derived, that readily permeate cells. Once bound to ligands, PPARs, like other nuclear receptors, pair with retinoid X-receptors to form a heterodimer, which constitutes an active transcriptional complex. By binding to cognate sequences in the promoter regions of various genes, PPAR/RXR heterodimers can influence their transcription either positively or negatively. One member of the PPAR family, PPAR-α, has particular interest in the context of atherosclerosis because it can augment the transcription of apolipoprotein A-1, yielding increased levels of HDL, an atheroprotective lipoprotein.

Our group became interested in PPAR-α when we sought a mechanistic explanation for the anti-inflammatory effects of certain polyunsaturated fatty acids, notably docosahexaneoic acid (DHA). Previous studies by DeCaterina in our laboratory had shown that DHA could limit cytokine-induced expression of VCAM-1 and other proinflammatory functions in human endothelial cells [34–37]. Because certain fatty acids can bind PPAR-α, we tested the hypothesis that human atherosclerotic lesions express PPAR-α and that activation of this transcriptional regulator could have anti-inflammatory actions on vascular cells.

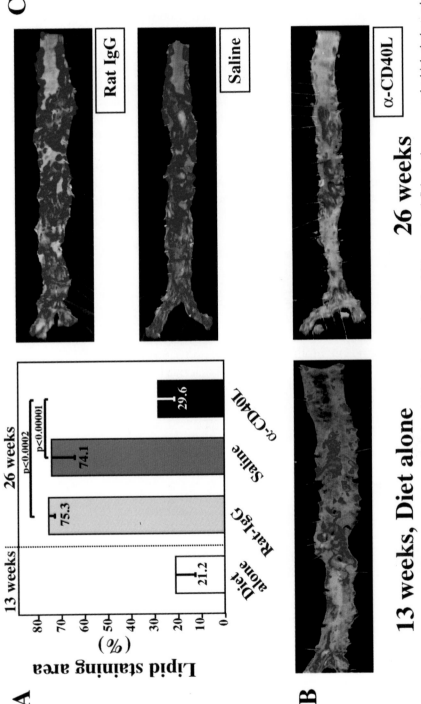

Fig. 5. Interruption of CD40 signaling limits the progression of established atheroma in mice. LDL-receptor-deficient mice consumed a high cholesterol diet for 13 weeks (**A**, white bar; **B**) before treatment with either rat IgG (**A**, light gray bar; **C**), saline (**A**, dark gray bar; **C**), or anti-CD40L antibody (**A**, dark gray bar; **C**) for 13 weeks during continued regimen of the diet. Photomicrographs of tissue sections of longitudinally cut abdominal aortas stained for lipid deposition with Sudan IV (**B**,**C**), were analyzed by computer-assisted image quantification for percent positive areas (**A**). Representative specimens from each group are shown.

Indeed, immunohistochemical studies showed immunoreactive PPAR-α (and another isoform, PPAR-γ in the nuclei of endothelial and smooth muscle cells in human atherosclerotic plaques [38,39] Thus convinced of the potential relevance of PPAR-α signaling to atherogenesis, we proceeded to a series of in vitro experiments. Drugs of the fibric acid class are thought to activate PPAR-α. Our cell culture studies revealed that PPAR-α ligands such as fenofibrate markedly diminished the increase in VCAM-1 induced by tumor necrosis factor-α in human endothelial cells (Fig. 6) [39]. This effect appeared selective, as PPAR-α stimulation did not alter the expression of intercellular adhesion molecule-1 (ICAM-1) or of E-selectin (Fig. 6). Moreover, several structurally distinct PPAR-gamma agonists did not share this anti-inflammatory actions.

The inhibitory effect of fenofibrate on cytokine induced endothelial activation

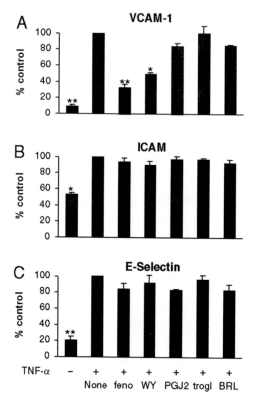

Fig. 6. PPARα but not PPARγ activators inhibit cytokine-induced cell surface expression of VCAM-1 in human EC. Cells were pretreated with PPARα [100μM fenofibrate (feno), 250μM WY14643 (WY)] or PPARγ activators [10 μM troglitazone (trogl), 10 μM 15d-PGJ2 (PGJ2), 10 μM rosiglitazone (BRL)] for 24 h and then stimulated with TNF-α (10 μg/l) for 8 h before performing cell surface enzyme immunoassays for VCAM-1 (A), ICAM-1 (B), and E-selectin (C). Results were expressed as a percentage of TNF-α-stimulated cells (% control). Bars represent mean ± SEM (VCAM-1 n = 8; ICAM-1/E-selectin n = 4); * indicates p < 0.05, and ** p < 0.01 compared to control. (From [39], reproduced with permission.)

depended on agonist dose and time of exposure. Decreases in VCAM protein levels on the surface of endothelial cells corresponded to decreased levels of VCAM-1 messenger RNA in cells treated with PPAR-α agonists. This effect did not result from an altered stability of VCAM-1 messenger RNA as shown by experiments with RNA synthase inhibitors. Further studies with promoter-reporter constructs indicated the essential nature of the tandem NF-κB elements in the VCAM-1 promoter for the PPAR-α-dependent inhibition of VCAM-1 gene expression. Electromobility shift assays confirmed that PPAR-α agonism inhibited TNF-stimulated activation of NF-κB.

To assess the functional relevance of these biochemical molecular changes, we performed studies of leukocyte adhesion to endothelial monolayers in vitro. Fluorescently labeled monocytoid cells of the U-937 line bound less well to endothelial monolayers stimulated with TNF-α in the presence of fenofibrate than TNF-α stimulated monolayer in the absence of the PPAR-α agonist. Taken together, these results show that PPAR-α agonists, such as the fibric acid derivatives, may have actions beyond their effects on the lipoprotein profile.

These results take on particular significance in view of the findings of recent clinical trials with fibric acid derivatives. The Veteran's Administration HDL Intervention Trial (VA-HIT) showed a marked reduction in atherosclerotic complications in a series of patients receiving gemfibrozil [40]. In the VA-HIT study, LDL levels, which were near target levels at baseline, were unchanged by treatment, suggesting that the beneficial effect on atherosclerotic events in this study did not depend on reductions in plasma LDL concentration. The Diabetes Atherosclerosis Intervention Study (DAIS), presented at this meeting, further showed a modulation of angiographic progression of coronary atherosclerosis due to fenofibrate treatment [41,42]. Although not powered for events, there was a trend toward decreased atherosclerotic events in the DAIS study due to fenofibrate treatment. This finding heightens interest in potential direct arterial wall effects of fibric acid derivatives mediated through PPAR-α.

Conclusion

The last decade has witnessed a remarkable advance in our understanding of the relationship between inflammation and the thrombotic complications of atherosclerosis. This enhanced insight of pathophysiology allows us to hone our anti-atherosclerotic interventions more keenly. The foregoing discussion illustrates three different strategies for interrupting inflammatory signaling operative during atherogenesis. Such targeting of proinflammatory pathways offers a novel approach to the therapy of atherosclerosis. The ensemble of data summarized above suggests that therapies that attenuate arterial inflammation may not only limit lesion formation and evolution, but also forestall the dreaded thrombotic complications that lead to the acute manifestations of this insidious systemic disease.

References

1. Ikari Y, McManus BM, Kenyon J, Schwartz SM. Neonatal intima formation in the human coronary artery. Arterioscl Thromb Vasc Biol 1999;19:2036—2040.

2. Tuzcu EM, Hobbs RE, Rincon G, Bott-Silverman C, De Franco AC, Robinson K, McCarthy PM, Stewart RW, Guyer S, Nissen SE. Occult and frequent transmission of atherosclerotic coronary disease with cardiac transplantation. Insights from intravascular ultrasound. Circulation 1995;91:1706—1713.

3. McGill HC Jr, McMahan CA, Herderick EE, Tracy RE, Malcom GT, Zieske AW, Strong JP. Effects of coronary heart disease risk factors on atherosclerosis of selected regions of the aorta and right coronary artery. PDAY research group. Pathobiological determinants of atherosclerosis in youth. Arterioscl Thromb Vasc Biol 2000;20:836—845.

4. Stamler J, Daviglus ML, Garside DB, Dyer AR, Greenland P, Neaton JD. Relationship of baseline serum cholesterol levels in 3 large cohorts of younger men to long-term coronary, cardiovascular, and all-cause mortality and to longevity. JAMA 2000;284:311—318.

5. Davies MJ. Stability and instability: the two faces of coronary atherosclerosis. The Paul Dudly White lecture, 1995. Circulation 1996;94:2013—2020.

6. Farb A, Burke A, Tang A, Liang Y, Mannan P, Smialek J, Virmani R. Coronary plaque erosion without rupture into a lipid core. A frequent cause of coronary thrombosis in sudden coronary death. Circulation 1996;93:1354—1363.

7. Libby P. The molecular bases of the acute coronary syndromes. Circulation 1995;91:2844—2850.

8. Amento EP, Ehsani N, Palmer H, Libby P. Cytokines positively and negatively regulate interstitial collagen gene expression in human vascular smooth muscle cells. Arteriosclerosis 1991; 11:1223—1230.

9. Henney AM, Wakeley PR, Davies MJ, Foster K, Hembry R, Murphy G, Humphries S. Localization of stromelysin gene expression in atherosclerotic plaques by in situ hybridization. Proc Natl Acad Sci USA 1991;88:8154—8158.

10. Galis Z, Sukhova G, Lark M, Libby P. Increased expression of matrix metalloproteinases and matrix degrading activity in vulnerable regions of human atherosclerotic plaques. J Clin Invest 1994;94:2493—2503.

11. Nikkari ST, O'Brien KD, Ferguson M, Hatsukami T, Welgus HG, Alpers CE, Clowes AW. Interstitial collagenase (MMP-1) expression in human carotid atherosclerosis. Circulation 1995;92: 1393—1398.

12. Lee R, Libby P. The increasing significance of the unstable atheroma. In: Jacotot B, Mathé D, Fruchart J-C (eds) Atherosclerosis. Singapore: Elsevier Science, 1998;83—88.

13. Fabunmi RP, Sukhova GK, Sugiyama S, Libby P. Expression of tissue inhibitor of metalloproteinases-3 in human atheroma and regulation in lesion-associated cells: a potential protective mechanism in plaque stability. Circ Res 1998;83:270—278.

14. Dollery CM, Humphries SE, McClelland A, Latchman DS, McEwan JR. Expression of tissue inhibitor of matrix metalloproteinases 1 by use of an adenoviral vector inhibits smooth muscle cell migration and reduces neointimal hyperplasia in the rat model of vascular balloon injury. Circulation 1999;99:3199—3205.

15. Billinghurst RC, Dahlberg L, Ionescu M, Reiner A, Bourne R, Rorabeck C, Mitchell P, Hambor J, Diekmann O, Tschesche H, Chen J, Van Wart H, Poole AR. Enhanced cleavage of type II collagen by collagenases in osteoarthritic articular cartilage. J Clin Invest 1997;99:1534—1545.

16. Sukhova GK, Schonbeck U, Rabkin E, Schoen FJ, Poole AR, Billinghurst RC, Libby P. Evidence for increased collagenolysis by interstitial collagenases-1 and -3 in vulnerable human atheromatous plaques. Circulation 1999;99:2503—2509.

17. Wilcox JN, Smith KM, Schwartz SM, Gordon D. Localization of tissue factor in the normal vessel wall and in the atherosclerotic plaque. Proc Natl Acad Sci USA 1989;86:2839—2843.

18. Drake TA, Morrissey JH, Edgington TS. Selective cellular expression of tissue factor in human

tissues. Implications for disorders of hemostasis and thrombosis. Am J Pathol 1989;134: 1087–1097.

19. Van der Wal AC, Becker AE, Van der Loos CM, Das PK. Site of intimal rupture or erosion of thrombosed coronary atherosclerotic plaques is characterized by an inflammatory process irrespective of the dominant plaque morphology. Circulation 1994;89:36–44.

20. Mach F, Schönbeck U, Sukhova GK, Bourcier T, Bonnefoy J-Y, Pober JS, Libby P. Functional CD40 ligand is expressed on human vascular endothelial cells, smooth muscle cells, and macrophages: implications for CD40-CD40 ligand signaling in atherosclerosis. Proc Natl Acad Sci USA 1997;94:1931–1936.

21. Mach F, Schoenbeck U, Bonnefoy J-Y, Pober J, Libby P. Activation of monocyte/macrophage functions related to acute atheroma complication by ligation of CD40. Induction of collagenase, stromelysin, and tissue factor. Circulation 1997;96:396–399.

22. Aikawa M, Rabkin E, Okada Y, Voglic S, Clinton S, Brinckerhoff C, Sukhova G, Libby P. Lipid lowering by diet reduces matrix metalloproteinase activity and increases collagen content of rabbit atheroma: a potential mechanism of lesion stabilization. Circulation 1998;97:2433–2444.

23. Aikawa M, Voglic SJ, Sugiyama S, Rabkin E, Taubman MB, Fallon JT, Libby P. Dietary lipid lowering reduces tissue factor expression in rabbit atheroma. Circulation 1999;100:1215–1222.

24. Schonbeck U, Mach F, Libby P. CD154 (CD40 ligand). Int J Biochem Cell Biol 2000;32:687–693.

25. Phipps RP. Atherosclerosis: the emerging role of inflammation and the CD40-CD40 ligand system. Proc Natl Acad Sci USA 2000;97:6930–6932.

26. Mach F, Schonbeck U, Fabunmi RP, Murphy C, Atkinson E, Bonnefoy JY, Graber P, Libby P. T lymphocytes induce endothelial cell matrix metalloproteinase expression by a CD40L-dependent mechanism: implications for tubule formation. Am J Pathol 1999;154:229–238.

27. Schoenbeck U, Mach F, Sukhova GK, Murphy C, Bonnefoy JY, Fabunmi RP, Libby P. Regulation of matrix metalloproteinase expression in human vascular smooth muscle cells by T lymphocytes: a role for CD40 signaling in plaque rupture? Circ Res 1997;81:448–454.

28. Schoenbeck U, Mach F, Sukhova GK, Atkinson E, Levesque E, Herman M, Graber P, Basset P, Libby P. Expression of stromelysin-3 in atherosclerotic lesions: regulation via CD40-CD40 ligand signaling in vitro and in vivo. J Exp Med 1999;189:843–853.

29. Schoenbeck U, Mach F, Bonnefoy JY, Loppnow H, Flad HD, Libby P. Ligation of CD40 activates interleukin 1beta-converting enzyme (caspase-1) activity in vascular smooth muscle and endothelial cells and promotes elaboration of active interleukin 1beta. J Biol Chem 1997;272: 19569–19574.

30. Mach F, Schonbeck U, Sukhova GK, Atkinson E, Libby P. Reduction of atherosclerosis in mice by inhibition of CD40 signalling. Nature 1998;394:200–203.

31. Lutgens E, Gorelik L, Daemen MJ, de Muinck ED, Grewal IS, Koteliansky VE, Flavell RA. Requirement for CD154 in the progression of atherosclerosis. Nat Med 1999;5:1313–1316.

32. Schonbeck U, Sukhova GK, Shimizu K, Mach F, Libby P. Inhibition of CD40 signaling limits evolution of established atherosclerosis in mice. Proc Natl Acad Sci USA 2000;97:7458–7463.

33. Lutgens E, Cleutjens KB, Heeneman S, Koteliansky VE, Burkly LC, Daemen MJ. Both early and delayed anti-CD40L antibody treatment induces a stable plaque phenotype. Proc Natl Acad Sci USA 2000;97:7464–7469.

34. De Caterina R, Cybulsky MI, Clinton SK, Gimbrone MJ, Libby P. The omega-3 fatty acid docosahexaenoate reduces cytokine-induced expression of proatherogenic and proinflammatory proteins in human endothelial cells. Arterioscl Thromb 1995;14:1829–1836.

35. De Caterina R, Cybulsky MI, Clinton SK, Gimbrone MJ, Libby P. Omega-3 fatty acids and endothelial leukocyte adhesion molecules. Prostaglandins Leukotrients Essen Fat Acid 1995; 52:191–195.

36. De Caterina R, Bernini W, Carluccio MA, Liao JK, Libby P. Structural requirements for inhibition of cytokine-induced endothelial activation by unsaturated fatty acids. J Lipid Res 1998; 39:1062–1070.

37. De Caterina R, Spiecker M, Solaini G, Basta G, Bosetti F, Libby P, Liao J. The inhibition of endothelial activation by unsaturated fatty acids. Lipids 1999;34 Suppl:S191—S194.

38. Marx N, Sukhova G, Murphy C, Libby P, Plutzky J. Macrophages in human atheroma contain PPARgamma: differentiation-dependent peroxisomal proliferator-activated receptor gamma(P-PARgamma) expression and reduction of MMP-9 activity through PPARgamma activation in mononuclear phagocytes in vitro. Am J Pathol 1998;153:17—23.

39. Marx N, Sukhova GK, Collins T, Libby P, Plutzky J. PPARalpha activators inhibit cytokine-induced vascular cell adhesion molecule-1 expression in human endothelial cells. Circulation 1999;99:3125—3131.

40. Rubins HB, Robins SJ, Collins D, Fye CL, Anderson JW, Elam MB, Faas FH, Linares E, Schaefer EJ, Schectman G, Wilt TJ, Wittes J. Gemfibrozil for the secondary prevention of coronary heart disease in men with low levels of high-density lipoprotein cholesterol. Veterans affairs high-density lipoprotein cholesterol intervention trial study group. N Engl J Med 1999;341:410—418.

41. Steiner G. The Diabetes Atherosclerosis Intervention Study (DAIS): a study conducted in co-operation with the World Health Organization. The DAIS Project Group. Diabetologia 1996;39:1655—1661.

42. Steiner G, Stewart D, Hosking JD. Baseline characteristics of the study population in the Diabetes Atherosclerosis Intervention Study (DAIS). World Health Organization collaborating centre for the study of atherosclerosis in diabetes. Am J Cardiol 1999;84:1004—1010.

Nitric oxide in cardiovascular function and disease

S. Moncada and E.A. Higgs
The Wolfson Institute for Biomedical Research, University College London, London, UK

In 1980 Furchgott and Zawadzki demonstrated that the relaxation of rabbit aorta in response to acetylcholine (ACh) is entirely dependent on the presence of an intact endothelial cell layer and identified a factor, endothelium-derived relaxing factor (EDRF), responsible for this action [1]. Nitric oxide (NO) was later shown to account for the activity of EDRF and thus to explain endothelium-dependent relaxation [2]. The release of NO from the endothelium has since been demonstrated arteries, arterioles, veins and venules from a wide range of species, including humans, both in vitro and in vivo [3]. Furthermore, the vasorelaxant properties of many other hormones and autacoids, including bradykinin, substance P and serotonin, have also been shown to be endothelium-dependent, as is "flow-dependent dilatation" [3,4].

Nitric oxide is generated from one of the terminal guanidino nitrogen atoms of the semi-essential amino acid L-arginine [5] by a family of enzymes known as NO synthase. There are three isoforms of NO synthase, named according to the cell type or conditions under which they were first identified: endothelial NO synthase (eNOS), neuronal NO synthase (nNOS) and an immunologically-induced NO synthase (iNOS). eNOS is also found in other cell types including platelets and the endocardium and nNOS is found in the brain and in "nitrergic" nerves throughout the peripheral nervous system. Both eNOS and nNOS occur constitutively, whereas iNOS requires de novo synthesis and is induced in nearly all tissues following exposure to certain microbial products and cytokines [3].

Nitric oxide synthase is inhibited by substrate analogues such as N^G-mono-methyl-L-arginine (L-NMMA) which impairs the response to "endothelium-dependent" dilators and causes endothelium-dependent vasoconstriction of isolated vascular tissue [3]. Administration of L-NMMA in vivo causes widespread vasoconstriction and elevation in blood pressure [6], suggesting that an NO-dependent dilator tone is an important component of the regulatory systems of blood flow and blood pressure [3]. This proposal has been strengthened by studies in mice in which the gene for eNOS has been disrupted. Such animals lack eNOS and have an elevated blood pressure compared with their wild-type counterparts [7]. L-NMMA, which does not affect the blood pressure of the eNOS

Address for correspondence: Prof S. Moncada, The Wolfson Institute for Biomedical Research, University College London, Gower Street, London, WC1E 6BT, UK. Tel.: +44-207-679-6789. Fax: +44-207-209-0470. E-mail: s.mocada@ucl.ac.uk

mutant animals, increases the blood pressure of wild-type animals to that of the mutants.

The discovery of the NO-dependent vasodilator tone indicated the existence of an endogenous system for the regulation of blood pressure and flow, whose actions are imitated by compounds such as glyceryl trinitrate and sodium nitroprusside which act as NO donors [8,9]. In addition to its vasodilator actions, NO also contributes to the control of platelet aggregation [10] and the regulation of cardiac contractility [11]. These physiological effects of NO are largely mediated by activation of the soluble guanylate cyclase and the consequent enhanced synthesis of cyclic GMP. Other cardiovascular actions of NO include inhibition of white cell activation [12] and inhibition of smooth muscle cell proliferation [13].

Nitric oxide is now known to be the mediator released in the peripheral nervous system by a widespread network of nerves, previously recognized as nonadrenergic and noncholinergic [14−16]. Nitric oxide released by such nitrergic nerves in blood vessels may contribute to the control of vascular tone, with NO acting as a direct vasodilator or a neuromodulator altering the release of other transmitters [16]. In the cerebral circulation nitrergic nerves may be important in vasoneuronal coupling – the process by which blood flow is increased to active areas of the brain [17]. In the corpus cavernosum, NO released from nitrergic nerves mediates relaxation of the smooth muscle and increased blood flow, leading to penile erection [18].

Thus, NO is a physiological homeostatic regulator of the vessel wall, playing a role in the maintenance of a vasodilator tone, inhibition of platelet and white cell activation, and maintaining vascular smooth muscle in a nonproliferative state. Impaired production of NO has been implicated in several cardiovascular disorders, including hypertension, vasospasm and atherosclerosis [19].

Studies in humans indicate that essential hypertension may be associated with a decrease in NO generation [20]. Impaired production of NO has also been demonstrated in some animal models of hypertension [21,22]. One example of experimental hypertension in which there is evidence for an impairment in the generation of NO is the Sabra hypertension-prone (salt-sensitive) rat in which vasorelaxant responses to ACh are diminished, the constrictor responses to L-NMMA are reduced, less eNOS is present in the vasculature, and the circulating levels of nitrite and nitrate (breakdown products of NO) are lower than in its hypertension-resistant strain [23]. Because NO plays a role in the excretion of sodium in the kidney it is likely that a reduction in production of NO leads to a dual effect, namely, an increase in vascular reactivity and reduced excretion of sodium, both of which play a role in the hypertensive state of these animals.

Some animal models such as spontaneously hypertensive rats, however, have been shown to exhibit a normal or enhanced responsiveness to bradykinin and to inhibitors of NO synthase [24,25], which indicates that production of NO by these animals is unimpaired or even increased. Results in animal models have led to the hypothesis that in relation to NO there may be two types of hypertension. In one type, increased vasoconstrictor activity (which may be caused by different factors) leads to an increase in NO generation as a compensatory mechanism; in this situation there may be normal or increased sodium excretion. The other type may depend on a deficiency in NO generation in the vessel wall that would be accompanied by abnormal renal sodium handling [26,27]. Thus the first type of hypertension would be associated with abnormally high vasoconstrictor activity, whereas in the second type, normal levels of vasoconstrictors will in effect behave as excessive due to the lack of counteracting NO-dependent vasodilator tone.

Animal studies suggest that impairment of the L-arginine:NO system may also predispose to atherogenesis [28]; for example, pharmacological inhibition of NO synthesis causes accelerated atherogenesis in hypercholesterolaemic rabbits [29] and eNOS mutant mice develop larger proliferative lesions following mechanical damage to vascular tissue [30]. Furthermore, in rings of atherosclerotic human coronary arteries, the endothelium-dependent relaxation is decreased and the responses to vasoconstrictors are often greater than in rings of normal coronary arteries [31]. Vasodilatation induced by increased blood flow or ACh is impaired in the coronary circulation of patients with atherosclerosis [32], smokers and children with familial hypercholesterolaemia [33]. The increased basal NO-mediated dilatation in women compared to men disappears after the menopause, a time at which cardiovascular risk increases [34]. Thus changes in the L-arginine:NO pathway due to disease states, oestrogen concentrations or smoking habit may provide a common mechanism for the promotion of atheroma formation and vessel occlusion. Interestingly, certain polymorphisms of the eNOS gene may be associated with increased risk of severe coronary artery disease [35] and with atherosclerosis linked to cigarette smoking [36].

L-arginine, the substrate for synthesis of NO, has been shown to normalize the vascular dysfunction in patients and animals with hypercholesterolaemia [37,38]. In animals the effect is accompanied by a reduction in the thickness of the intimal lesions [38]. Administration of L-arginine may be beneficial in preventing restenosis after balloon angioplasty, since it attenuates intimal hyperplasia in rabbits [39]. In a study in low-density lipoprotein (LDL) receptor knockout mice, dietary arginine supplementation markedly reduced the number of intimal lesions that these animals normally develop in response to a high cholesterol diet [40]. These effects were prevented by co-administration of an inhibitor of NO synthase, suggesting that they were caused by the conversion of L-arginine to NO. Donors of NO have also been shown to possess anti-atherosclerotic actions [41] as have inhibitors of angiotensin-converting enzyme [42] which prevent the breakdown of bradykinin which stimulates the synthesis of NO.

eNOS mRNA is increased during pregnancy and following treatment with oestradiol [43,44]. This oestrogen-induced enhancement of NO synthesis could contribute to the decrease in vascular tone and contractility that occurs during pregnancy and the reduced incidence of heart disease in premenopausal women. Interestingly, studies in a mouse model of neointimal growth have shown that females have a smaller intimal response than males to placement of a cuff around the femoral artery and that this response to injury is abolished in pregnant animals [30].

The induction of both eNOS mRNA and protein has also been demonstrated following exposure of cultured vascular endothelial cells to shear stress [45]. Shear stress-induced generation of NO accounts for the phenomenon of flow-mediated dilatation and might be a mechanism by which vessels keep shear forces constant despite changes in flow. Chronic exercise has also been shown to enhance eNOS gene expression in the aortic endothelium [45].

One approach to the treatment of cardiovascular disorders involving impaired production of NO is the use of gene therapy. Transfer of recombinant eNOS, normally using a viral vector, has been successfully achieved in cardiovascular beds both ex vivo and in vivo [46,47]. Enhanced relaxation has been reported in canine basilar arteries following ex vivo exposure to recombinant eNOS [48], and in vivo in rat carotid arteries after intraluminal administration [49]. Intravenous injection of recombinant eNOS to spontaneously hypertensive rats produces prolonged reduction of blood pressure [50] while its administration via aerosol reduces pulmonary arterial pressure in a rat model of acute hypoxia [51]. As well as its vasorelaxant effects the recombinant eNOS inhibits smooth muscle cell proliferation in vitro [52] and reduces injury-induced formation of neointima [49]. Recently, recombinant eNOS administered to the corpora cavernosa of aged rats has been shown to enhance cavernosal pressure and erectile responses [53]. Gene delivery of iNOS to injured vascular tissue in animals has also been used successfully [54,55]. Such treatment has been shown to reduce smooth muscle proliferation and intimal hyperplasia and may prove useful in the prevention of allograft atherosclerosis in aortic and vein transplantation. Gene therapy using eNOS or iNOS may therefore provide a novel approach to the treatment of a variety of cardiovascular diseases when safe techniques for its administration have been developed.

Inducible stimuli such as endotoxin lipopolysaccharide and cytokines induce iNOS in many cells and tissues. This enzyme was identified originally in macrophages and contributes to the cytotoxic actions of these cells [56—58]. The NO produced by iNOS in the vasculature is involved in the profound vasodilatation of septic shock as well as the myocardial damage that occurs in some inflammatory conditions of the heart [59]. Endotoxin induces iNOS in the myocardium [60] and endocardium, and studies in rat myocytes in culture [61] and in isolated working hearts [62] indicate the involvement of iNOS induction in cytokine-induced myocardial contractile dysfunction. Enhanced synthesis of NO by this enzyme may therefore contribute to the cardiac dysfunction associated with endotoxaemia [63]. The cardiac dysfunction of dilated cardiomyopathy also may be associated with induction of this enzyme [63]. Thus, in the heart as in the vasculature, NO may have a physiological role when generated by the constitutive enzyme that is present normally in the myocardium and may become pathological, causing dilatation and tissue damage, when generated in large quantities and for long periods by the inducible enzyme. L-NMMA, when used at low doses in animals and man, reverses the hypotension and the hyporeactivity to vasoconstriction characteristic of shock [59]. Selective inhibitors of the inducible NOS may prove beneficial for the treatment of the hypotension of shock or cytokine therapy and may also provide a new approach to anti-inflammatory therapy.

iNOS has also been shown to be induced in macrophages and smooth muscle cells of atherosclerotic vessels in animals [64] and in humans [65]. In human advanced atherosclerotic plaques the iNOS was found to colocalise with nitrotyrosine, a marker for peroxynitrite-induced damage [66]. The oxidation of low-density lipoprotein (LDL) is thought to be a key factor in the formation of atherosclerotic lesions and it has been shown that peroxynitrite can modify LDL to a potentially atherogenic form [67]. Peroxynitrite, which originates from the interaction between NO and superoxide anion [68–70], is now emerging as a key substance to explain a wide range of pathological effects of NO [71]. Thus, it may be that low concentrations of NO generated by eNOS protect against atherosclerosis by promoting vasodilatation, inhibiting leukocyte and platelet adhesion and/or aggregation and smooth muscle cell proliferation, while higher concentrations of NO generated by iNOS promote atherosclerosis either directly or via the formation of NO adducts, notably peroxynitrite.

One way in which NO may change from being a physiological mediator to a pathological entity is through its actions on mitochondrial respiration. Nitric oxide is a potent inhibitor of cytochrome oxidase (complex IV) [72], the terminal enzyme of the mitochondrial respiratory chain. It has been shown that NO generated by vascular endothelial cells under basal and stimulated conditions modulates the respiration of these cells in response to changes in oxygen concentration. This action occurs at the level of complex IV and depends on the influx of calcium [73]. Thus, NO plays a physiological role in adjusting the capacity of this enzyme to use oxygen, allowing the endothelial cells to adapt to acute changes in their environment. The effect of long-term exposure to NO on different enzymes of the respiratory chain in a variety of cell lines has also been studied. These studies have shown that, although NO inhibits complex IV in a way that is always reversible, prolonged exposure to NO results in a gradual and persistent inhibition of complex I that is concomitant with a reduction in the intracellular concentration of reduced glutathione. This inhibition appears to result from S-nitrosylation of critical thiols in the enzyme complex [74,75]. These results suggest that, although NO may regulate cell respiration physiologically by its action on complex IV, long-term exposure to higher concentrations of NO leads to oxidative stress secondary to the release of superoxide in the respiratory chain, persistent inhibition of complex I and potentially to cell pathology.

The discovery of the L-arginine: NO pathway has had a great impact in our understanding of the physiology and pathophysiology of the cardiovascular system. It is likely that this knowledge will lead to novel therapies for the treatment and prevention of cardiovascular disease.

86

References

1. Furchgott RF, Zawadzki JV. The obligatory role of endothelial cells in the relaxation of arterial smooth muscle by acetylcholine. Nature 1980;288:373–376.
2. Palmer RM, Ferrige AG, Moncada S. Nitric oxide release accounts for the biological activity of endothelium-derived relaxing factor. Nature 1987;327:524–526.
3. Moncada S, Palmer RM, Higgs EA. Nitric oxide: physiology, pathophysiology and pharmacology. Pharmacol Rev 1991;43:109–142.
4. Furchgott RF. Role of endothelium in responses of vascular smooth muscle. Circ Res 1983;53:557–573.
5. Palmer RM, Ashton DS, Moncada S. Vascular endothelial cells synthesize nitric oxide from L-arginine. Nature 1988;333:664–666.
6. Rees DD, Palmer RM, Moncada S. Role of endothelium-derived nitric oxide in the regulation of blood pressure. Proc Natl Acad Sci USA 1989;86:3375–3378.
7. Huang PL, Huang Z, Mashimo H et al. Hypertension in mice lacking the gene for endothelial nitric oxide synthase. Nature 1995;377:239–242.
8. Moncada S, Palmer RM, Higgs EA. The discovery of nitric oxide as the endogenous nitrovasodilator. Hypertension 1988;12:365–372.
9. Feelisch M, Stamler J. Donors of nitrogen oxides. In: Feelisch M, Stamler JS (eds) Methods in Nitric Oxide Research. New York: John Wiley & Sons, 1996;71–115.
10. Radomski MW, Moncada S. Biological role of nitric oxide in platelet function. In: Moncada S, Higgs EA et al. (eds) Clinical Relevance of Nitric Oxide in the Cardiovascular System. Madrid: EDICOMPLET 1991:45–56.
11. Kelly RA, Balligand JL, Smith TW. Nitric oxide and cardiac function. Circ Res 1996;79:363–380.
12. Kubes P, Suzuki M, Granger DN. Nitric oxide: an endogenous modulator of leukocyte adhesion. Proc Natl Acad Sci USA 1991;884651–884655.
13. Garg UC, Hassid A. Nitric oxide-generating vasodilators and 8-bromo-cyclic guanosine monophosphate inhibit mitogenesis and proliferation of cultured rat vascular smooth muscle cells. J Clin Invest 1989;83:1774–1777.
14. Gillespie JS, Liu X, Martin W. The neurotransmitter of the non-adrenergic non-cholinergic inhibitory nerves to smooth muscle of the genital system. In: Moncada S, Higgs EA (eds) Nitric Oxide from arginine: A Bioregulatory System. Amsterdam: Elsevier Science Publishers BV, 1990:147–164.
15. Rand MJ. Nitrergic transmission: Nitric oxide as a mediator of non-adrenergic, non-cholinergic neuro-effector transmission. Clin Exp Pharmacol Physiol 1992;19:147–169.
16. Toda N. Nitric oxide and the regulation of cerebral arterial tone. In: Vincent S (ed) Nitric Oxide in The Nervous System. Orlando: Academic Press Ltd, 1995:207–225.
17. Toda N, Yoshida K, Okamura T. Involvement of nitroxidergic and noradrenergic nerves in the relaxation of dog and monkey temporal veins. J Cardiovasc Pharmacol 1995;25:741–747.
18. Rajfer J, Aronson WJ, Bush PA, Dorey FJ, Ignarro LJ. Nitric oxide as a mediator of relaxation of the corpus cavernosum in response to non-adrenergic, non-cholinergic neurotransmission. N Engl J Med 1992;326:90–94.
19. Moncada S, Higgs A. The arginine-nitric oxide pathway. N Engl J Med 1993;329:2002–2012.
20. Panza JA, Quyyumi AA, Brush JE Jr, Epstein SE. Abnormal endothelium-dependent vascular relaxation in patients with essential hypertension. N Engl J Med 1990;323:22–27.
21. Osugi S, Shimamura K, Sunano, S. Decreased modulation by endothelium of noradrenaline-induced contractions in aorta from stroke-prone spontaneously hypertensive rats. Arch Int Pharmacodyn 1990;305:86–99.
22. Maruyama J, Maruyama K. Impaired nitric oxide-dependent responses and their recovery in hypertensive pulmonary arteries of rats. Am J Physiol 1994;266:H2476–H2488.
23. Rees D, Ben Ishay D, Moncada S. Nitric oxide and the regulation of blood pressure in the hyper-

tension-prone and hypertension-resistant Sabra rat. Hypertension 1996;28:367–371.

24. Yamazaki J, Fujita N, Nagao T. N^G-monomethyl-arginine-induced pressor response at developmental and established stages in spontaneously hypertensive rats. J Pharmacol Exp Ther 1991; 259:52–57.

25. Kelm M, Feelisch M, Krebber T, Deussen A, Motz W, Strauer BE. Role of nitric oxide in the regulation of coronary vascular tone in hearts from hypertensive rats. Maintenance of nitric oxide-forming capacity and increased basal production of nitric oxide. Hypertension 1995;25: 186–193.

26. Navarro J, Sanchez A, Saiz J et al. Hormonal, renal and metabolic alterations during hypertension induced by chronic inhibition of NO in rats. Am J Physiol 1994;267:R1516–R1521.

27. Lahera V, Salom MG, Miranda Guardiola F, Moncada S, Romero JC. Effects of N^G-nitro-arginine methyl ester on renal function and blood pressure. Am J Physiol 1991;261:F1033–F1037.

28. Verbeuren TJ, Jordaens FH, Van Hove CE, Van Hoydonck AE, Herman AG. Release and vascular activity of endothelium-derived relaxing factor in atherosclerotic rabbit aorta. Eur J Pharmacol 1990;191:173–184.

29. Naruse K, Shimizu K, Muramatsu M et al. Long-term inhibition of NO synthesis promotes atherosclerosis in the hypercholesterolemic rabbit thoracic aorta. PGH$_2$ does not contribute to impaired endothelium-dependent relaxation. Arterioscl Thromb 1994;14:746–752.

30. Moroi M, Zhang L, Yasuda T et al. Interaction of genetic deficiency of endothelial nitric oxide, gender and pregnancy in vascular response to injury in mice. J Clin Invest 1998;101:1225–1232.

31. Forstermann U. Properties and mechanisms of production and action of endothelium-derived relaxing factor. J Cardiovasc Pharmacol 1986;8(Suppl 10):S45–S51.

32. Cox DA, Vita JA, Treasure CB et al. Atherosclerosis impairs flow-mediated dilation of coronary arteries in humans. Circulation 1989;80:458–465.

33. Celermajer DS, Sorensen KE, Gooch VM et al. Non-invasive detection of endothelial dysfunction in children and adults at risk of atherosclerosis. Lancet 1992;340:1111–1115.

34. Stampfer MJ, Colditz GA. Estrogen replacement therapy and coronary heart disease: a quantitative assessment of the epidemiologic evidence. Prev Med 1991;20:47–63.

35. Hingorani AD, Liang CF, Fatibene J et al. A common variant of the endothelial nitric oxide synthase gene is a risk factor for coronary atherosclerosis in the East Anglian region of the UK. Circulation 1997;96:I–545.

36. Wang XL, Sim AS, Badenhop RF, McCredie RM, Wilcken DE. A smoking-dependent risk of coronary artery disease associated with a polymorphism of the endothelial nitric oxide synthase gene. Nat Med 1996;2:41–45.

37. Drexler H, Zeiher AM, Meinzer K et al. Correction of endothelial dysfunction in coronary microcirculation of hypercholesterolaemic patients by arginine. Lancet 1991;338:1546–1550.

38. Cooke JP, Tsao P. Cellular mechanisms of atherogenesis and the effects of nitric oxide. Curr Opin Cardiol 1992;7:799–804.

39. McNamara DB, Bedi B, Aurora H et al. arginine inhibits balloon catheter-induced intimal hyperplasia. Biochem Biophys Res Commun 1993;193:291–296.

40. Aji W, Ravalli S, Szabolcs M et al. arginine prevents xanthoma development and inhibits atherosclerosis in LDL receptor knockout mice. Circulation 1997;95:430–437.

41. Lefer AM, Lefer DJ. Therapeutic role of nitric oxide donors in the treatment of cardiovascular disease. Drugs Future 1994;19:665–672.

42. Farhy RD, Carretero OA, Ho KL et al. Role of kinins and nitric oxide in the effects of angiotensin converting enzyme inhibitors on neointima formation. Circ Res 1993;72:1202–1210.

43. Weiner CP, Lizasoain I, Baylis SA et al. Induction of calcium-dependent nitric oxide synthases by sex hormones. Proc Natl Acad Sci USA 1994;91:5212–5216.

44. Nathan L, Chaudhuri G. Estrogens and atherosclerosis. Annu Rev Pharmacol Toxicol 1997;37: 477–515.

45. Sessa WC. The nitric oxide synthase family of proteins. J Vasc Res 1994;31:131–143.

46. Chen AF, O'Brien T, Katusic ZS. Transfer and expression of recombinant nitric oxide synthase genes in the cardiovascular system. Trends Pharmacol Sci 1998;19:276−286.

47. Kibbe M, Billiar T, Tzeng E. Nitric oxide synthase gene transfer to the vessel wall. Curr Opin Nephrol Hypertens 1999;8:75−81.

48. Chen AF, O'Brien T, Tsutsui M, Kinoshita H, Pompili VJ, Crotty TB, Spector DJ, Katusic ZS. Expression and function of recombinant endothelial nitric oxide synthase gene in canine basilar artery. Circ Res 1997;80:327−335.

49. Von der Leyen HE, Gibbons GH, Morishita R, Lewis NP, Zhang L, Nakajima M, Kaneda Y, Cooke JP, Dzau VJ. Gene therapy inhibiting neointimal vascular lesion: in vivo transfer of endothelial cell nitric oxide synthase gene. Proc Natl Acad Sci USA 1995;92:1137−1141.

50. Lin KF, Chao L, Chao J. Prolonged reduction of high blood pressure with human nitric oxide synthase gene delivery. Hypertension 1997;30:307−313.

51. Janssens SP, Bloch KD, Nong Z, Gerard RD, Zoldhelyi P, Collen D. Adenoviral-mediated transfer of the human endothelial nitric oxide synthase gene reduces acute hypoxic pulmonary vasoconstriction in rats. J Clin Invest 1996;98:317−324.

52. Kullo IJ, Schwartz RS, Pompili VJ, Tsutsui M, Milstein, S, Fitzpatrick LA, Katusic ZS, O'Brien T. Expression and function of recombinant endothelial NO synthase in coronary artery smooth muscle cells. Arterioscl Thromb Vasc Biol 1997;17:2405−2412.

53. Champion HC, Bivalacqua TJ, Hyman AL, Ignarro LJ, Hellstrom WJ, Kadowitz PJ. Gene transfer of endothelial nitric oxide synthase to the penis augments erectile responses in the aged rat. Proc Natl Acad Sci USA 1999;96:11648−11652.

54. Shears LL, Kawaharada N, Tzeng E, Billiar TR, Watkins SC, Kovesdi I, Lizonova A, Pham SM. Inducible nitric oxide synthase suppresses the development of allograft arteriosclerosis. J Clin Invest 1997;100:2035−2042.

55. Kibbe MR, Tzeng E. Nitric oxide synthase gene therapy in vascular pathology. Sem Perinatol 2000;24:51−54.

56. Hibbs JB Jr, Taintor RR, Vavrin Z et al. Nitric oxide: a cytotoxic activated macrophage effector molecule. Biochem Biophys Res Commun 1988;157:87−94.

57. Marletta MA, Yoon PS, Iyengar R et al. Macrophage oxidation of arginine to nitrite and nitrate: Nitric oxide is an intermediate. Biochemistry 1988;27:8706−8711.

58. Stuehr DJ, Gross SS, Sakuma I et al. Activated murine macrophages secrete a metabolite of arginine with the bioactivity of endothelium-derived relaxing factor and the chemical reactivity of nitric oxide. J Exp Med 1989;169:1011−1020.

59. Vallance P, Moncada S. Role of endogenous nitric oxide in septic shock. New Hor 1993;1:77−86.

60. Schulz R, Nava E, Moncada S. Induction and potential biological relevance of a Ca(2+) independent nitric oxide synthase in the myocardium. Br J Pharmacol 1992;105:575−580.

61. Ungureanu Longrois D, Balligand JL, Kelly RA et al. Myocardial contractile dysfunction in the systemic inflammatory response syndrome: role of a cytokine-inducible nitric oxide synthase in cardiac myocytes. J Mol Cell Cardiol 1995;27:155−167.

62. Schulz R, Panas DL, Catena R et al. The role of nitric oxide in cardiac depression induced by interleukin-1 beta and tumour necrosis factor-alpha. Br J Pharmacol 1995;114:27−34.

63. de Belder A, Moncada S. Cardiomyopathy: a role for nitric oxide? Int J Cardiol 1995;50:263−268.

64. Behr D, Rupin A, Fabiani JN, Verbeuren TJ. Distribution and prevalence of inducible nitric oxide synthase in atherosclerotic vessels of long-term cholesterol-fed rabbits. Atherosclerosis 1999;142:335−344.

65. Luoma JS, Yla-Herttuala S. Expression of inducible nitric oxide synthase in macrophages and smooth muscle cells in various types of human atherosclerotic lesions. Virchows Arch 1999;434:561−568.

66. Cromheeke KM, Kockx MM, De Meyer GR, Bosmans JM, Bult H, Beelaerts WJ, Vrints CJ, Herman AG. Inducible nitric oxide synthase colocalizes with signs of lipid oxidation/peroxida-

tion in human atherosclerotic plaques. Cardiovasc Res 1999;43:744—754.

67. Hogg N, Darley-Usmar VM, Graham A, Moncada S. Peroxynitrite and atherosclerosis. Biochem Soc Trans 1993;21:358—362.

68. Gryglewski RJ, Palmer RM, Moncada S. Superoxide anion is involved in the breakdown of endothelium-derived vascular relaxing factor. Nature, 1986;320:454—456.

69. McCall TB, Boughton-Smith NK, Palmer RM, Whittle BJ, Moncada S. Synthesis of nitric oxide from arginine by neutrophils. Release and interaction with superoxide anion. Biochem J 1989; 261:293—296.

70. Beckman JS, Beckman TW, Chen J, Marshall PA, Freeman BA. Apparent hydroxyl radical production by peroxynitrite: implications for endothelial injury from nitric oxide and superoxide. Proc Natl Acad Sci USA 1990;87:1620—1624.

71. Murphy MP, Packer MA, Scarlet JL, Martin SW. Peroxynitrite: a biologically significant oxidant. Gen Pharmacol,1998;31:179—186.

72. Brown GC, Cooper CE. Nanomolar concentrations of nitric oxide reversibly inhibit synaptosomal respiration by competing with oxygen at cytochrome oxidase. FEBS Lett 1994;356:295—298.

73. Clementi E, Brown GC, Foxwell N, Moncada S. On the mechanism by which vascular endothelial cells regulate their oxygen consumption. Proc Natl Acad Sci USA 1999;96:1559—1562.

74. Clementi E, Brown GC, Feelisch M, Moncada S. Persistent inhibition of cell respiration by nitric oxide: crucial role of S-nitrosylation of mitochondrial complex I and protective action of glutathione. Proc Natl Acad Sci USA 1998;95:7631—7636.

75. Beltran B, Orsi A, Clementi E, Moncada S. Oxidative stress and S-nitrosylation of proteins in cells. Br J Pharmacol 2000;129:953—960.

Atherosclerosis XII.
S. Stemme and A.G. Olsson, editors.

Proteinases in the vessel wall and the heart: the challenging balance between tissue destruction and healing

Peter Carmeliet

The Center for Transgene Technology and Gene Therapy, Flanders Interuniversity Institute for Biotechnology, KU Leuven, Leuven, Belgium

Abstract. Proteinases are able to destroy but at the same also to heal tissues. Gene inactivation studies in mice over the last decade have revealed their distinct roles in these apparently opposite processes. These processes need to be tightly controlled and balanced. When the balance is disturbed, excess proteolysis may cause life-threatening destruction of the atherosclerotic aorta or ischemic myocardium, or destabilization of atherosclerotic plaques. Conversely, when healing proceeds in an uncontrolled manner, it may lead to occluding arterial restenosis or atherosclerotic plaques. In contrast, when healing is impaired, it predisposes to cardiac failure after myocardial infarction. It is now becoming obvious that proteinases have distinct roles depending on their spatio-temporal and cell-specific expression. For example, urokinase-type plasminogen activator (u-PA), when excessively expressed by infiltrating neutrophils, may contribute to cardiac rupture whereas the same proteinase is essential for proper cardiac healing and function after myocardial infarction by activation of fibrogenic growth factors. These highly regulated and context-dependent functions of the distinct proteinases pose a challenge to unravel their contribution to cardiovascular disorders. However, we are starting to obtain the necessary insights to develop the appropriate drugs to modulate the role of these proteinases in cardiovascular disorders.

Introduction

Various families of proteinases, mainly cysteine, serine, and metalloproteinases, have been implicated in cardiovascular disease, influencing cellular migration, cytokine activation, extracellular matrix turn-over, growth factor availability and angiogenesis. Cardiovascular diseases constitute the leading cause of mortality in Western Societies causing more than 2,600 deaths every day in the United States alone (http://www.americanheart.org/statistics/03cardio.html). Consequently, the development of efficient strategies to prevent or remedy cardiovascular disorders are of major medical importance. This requires a thorough understanding of the processes and their underlying molecular mechanisms, leading to the disease. The development of transgene technologies in mice has allowed the study of the consequences of genetic alterations on cardiovascular (patho)-physiology, and gene transfer studies have contributed to evaluate the therapeutic potential of gene products for gene therapy of cardiovascular disorders.

Address for correspondence: P. Carmeliet MD, PhD, Center for Transgene Technology & Gene Therapy, Campus Gasthuisberg, Herestraat 49, University of Leuven, Leuven, B-3000, Belgium. Tel.: +32-16-34-57-72. Fax: +32-16-34-59-90. E-mail: peter.carmeliet@med.kuleuven.ac.be

The plasminogen and MMP (matrix metalloproteinase) systems can degrade most components of the extracellular matrix in the vessel wall and the myocardium. Matrix degradation in the context of cell migration and remodeling is essential in numerous biological and pathological processes, including cardiovascular pathology. The plasminogen system [1] consists of an inactive zymogen plasminogen (Plg) which can be converted to plasmin by two types of plasminogen activators (PAs), tissue-type PA (t-PA), generally believed to be mainly associated with fibrinolysis due to its fibrin specificity, and urokinase-type PA (u-PA), which binds to its receptor u-PAR and is implicated in cell migration and tissue remodeling. The system is controlled by plasminogen activator inhibitor-1 (PAI-1), the main physiological inhibitor of u-PA and t-PA, as well as by α_2-antiplasmin (directly inhibiting plasmin).

The MMP system is a growing family of Zn^{2+}- and Ca^{2+}-dependent proteinases able to degrade most extracellular matrix proteins [2]. Based on substrate specificity and structural features, different groups can be distinguished. Collagenases (MMP-1, 8, 13 and 18) mostly degrade fibrillar collagens while gelatinases (MMP-2 and MMP-9) mainly degrade collagen type IV and denatured collagens. Stromelysin-1 and 2 (MMP-3 and MMP-10) and matrilysin (MMP-7) have a broad substrate specificity including proteoglycan core proteins, laminin, fibronectin, gelatin, nonhelical collagens and elastin, whereas stromelysin-3 (MMP-11) does not degrade any of the major extracellular matrix components but targets serine proteinase inhibitors (serpins) like α-1 proteinase inhibitor [3]. Metalloelastase (MMP-12) primarily degrades elastin, and the membrane-type metalloproteinases (MT-MMPs; MMP-14-17) have an additional transmembrane domain anchoring them to the cell surface. The system is controlled at several levels: (i) transcriptional control by growth factors and cytokines, (ii) activation of the inactive zymogens (pro-MMPs); u-PA-generated plasmin is a likely pathological activator of several pro-MMPs [4], and (iii) tissue- and substrate-specific inhibition of the active enzymes by tissue inhibitors of MMPs (TIMPs) of which four members are known to date. This review focuses on the involvement of the plasminogen and the MMP systems in cardiovascular biology and disorders as unveiled by gene targeting and gene transfer studies, with the exception of bleeding and thrombotic phenotypes which have been reviewed previously [5,6].

Tissue destruction

Atherosclerotic aneurysm formation

Atherosclerosis is a slow, progressive disease that usually remains asymptomatic until middle age. However, plaque rupture and the resultant formation of an occluding thrombus can precipitate sudden clinical syndromes of myocardial infarction and stroke. Another life-threatening complication, killing more than 2% of elderly patients, is rupture of an aneurysmally dilated artery due to excessive extracellular matrix breakdown [7]. The pathogenetic mechanisms contributing to aneurysm formation have remained largely undefined until recently. A possible role for the plasminogen activators and MMPs in atherosclerotic aneurysms was suggested by the elevated levels of u-PA, t-PA [8] and of several MMPs in excess of their inhibitors in atherosclerotic lesions [9]. However, conclusive evidence for a precipitating role of these factors in aneurysm fomration in vivo was lacking, as homozygous deficiencies for these proteinases are extremely rare in humans. Mice with a combined deficiency of one of the plasminogen or MMP system components in the atherosclerosis-prone apolipoprotein-E (apoE) or LDL (low density lipoprotein) receptor-deficient background offer an opportunity to study such processes.

Significant genotypic differences were observed in the integrity of the atherosclerotic aortic wall. Indeed, destruction of the media with resultant erosion, transmedial ulceration, necrosis of medial SMCs, aneurysmal dilatation and rupture of the vessel wall were more prevalent and severe in mice lacking apoE or apoE:t-PA than in mice lacking apoE:u-PA [4]. Macrophages only infiltrated the media of atherosclerotic arteries after destruction of elastin fibers. Plaque macrophages (and especially those infiltrating into the media) expressed abundant amounts of u-PA similar to that in patients. Since plasmin by itself is unable to degrade insoluble elastin or fibrillar collagen, it most likely activated other matrix proteinases, such as the MMPs. Wild-type and t-PA-deficient, but not u-PA-deficient, cultured macrophages activated secreted pro-MMP-3, 9, 12 and 13, but only in the presence of plasminogen, indicating that u-PA-generated plasmin was responsible for the activation of these pro-MMPs [4]. These plasmin-activatable metalloproteinases colocalized with u-PA in plaque macrophages. Another possible mechanism of action of plasmin is that it mediates the degradation of glycoproteins in the stroma of the aortic wall, thereby exposing the highly insoluble elastin to elastases and facilitating elastolysis in vivo. Taken together, these results implicate an important role of u-PA in the structural integrity of the atherosclerotic vessel wall, likely via triggering activation of matrix metalloproteinases. A gene transfer study revealed that local overexpression of TIMP-1 in a rat aneurysm model prevents aneurysm degeneration and rupture [10]. In mice with an LDL receptor deficiency, aortic medial elastin degradation was reduced using a broad-spectrum MMP inhibitor [11]. However, direct proof of how and which MMPs are involved in media destruction, aneurysm formation and atherosclerotic lesion formation requires further analysis in mice that are deficient for each of these MMPs. A recent study revealed that loss of MMP-9 partially protected mice against aneurysmal dilatation of the aorta after elastase perfusion [12]. Surprisingly, single loss of MMP-12 had no effect, while combined loss of both MMP-9 and MMP-12 further protected mice. Since rupture of aneurysms in this nonatherosclerotic model does not occur, the role of these MMPs, as well as of others, (interstitial collagenases) remains to be defined [7].

Cardiac rupture after myocardial ischemia

More than 1.5 million people suffer acute myocardial infarction (AMI) annually in the USA alone. About 30% of them die within the first 24 h, due to arrhythmias or pump failure. With improved treatments, cardiac rupture has become a serious complication, accounting for 5—31% of in-hospital mortality after AMI. Several risk factors, including hypertension, diabetes, cardiac hypertrophy, fatty infiltration, infarct expansion, and delayed thrombolysis with streptokinase, have been related to rupture, but their relevance remains controversial. In addition, genetic predisposition factors or criteria for identifying patients at risk of cardiac rupture after AMI remain undetermined. A better understanding of the mechanisms underlying cardiac rupture might lead to prevention strategies, but this has been precluded by lack of reproducible animal models. Both plasminogen activators and matrix metalloproteinases have been implicated in coronary or myocardial remodeling after AMI [13], but their precise role and their involvement in cardiac rupture still is unclear.

A combination of gene inactivation and gene transfer techniques in mice was applied to address these issues, using a model for AMI based on ligation of the left anterior descending coronary artery causing an infarct of 45% of the left ventricular wall [14]. In male mice, cardiac rupture after AMI was observed in 30% of wild-type mice and mice lacking t-PA, the urokinase receptor, stromelysin-1 (MMP-3) or metalloelastase (MMP-12). In contrast, deficiency of u-PA completely protected against rupture, while lack of gelatinase-B (MMP-9) generally (24 of 26) protected against cardiac rupture. A close correlation was observed between the number of neutrophils infiltrating the infarcts and rupture. Further, these inflammatory cells produced increased levels of u-PA and MMPs. Thus, neutrophils require proteinases to migrate into the infarct and, once arrived, contribute to myocardial destruction by generating uncontrolled proteolysis, oxidative stress and cytokine release [14]. Adenoviral gene transfer of PAI-1 or TIMP-1 completely protected wild-type mice against rupture without aborting infarct healing (myocardial healing resumed beyond 14 days resulting in normal scar formation by 5 weeks after infarction; see below). Thus, proteinase inhibitors could constitute a new approach to prevent cardiac rupture after AMI [14].

Tissue healing

Myocardial healing

Healing of tissues typically involves initial removal of necrotic debris by infiltrating macrophages, subsequent revascularization by invading endothelial and smooth muscle cells, finally followed by accumulation of fibroblasts producing a dense collagen-rich scar. Wound cells require proteinases such as u-PA and MMPs to migrate into wounds. Not surprisingly therefore, removal of necrotic cardiomyocytes was complete by 14 days after AMI in wild-type mice, but not in u-PA deficient mice, in which necrotic cardiomyocytes persisted for up to 5 weeks as mummified ghosts embedded in laminin-rich basement membrane [14]. Ultrastructurally, these necrotic u-PA-deficient cardiomyocytes exhibited signs found in cells that die of severe acute ischemia. This likely resulted from the reduced macrophage accumulation in u-PA-deficient infarcts. u-PA was also essential for capillary angiogenesis and growth of collateral arteries during infarct revascularization. During revascularization, u-PA is expressed by migrating endothelial and smooth muscle cells (SMCs), but inflammatory cells, which produce angiogenic factors, also express u-PA. The greater requirement for u-PA in revascularization of the myocardium as compared to other tissues may relate to its greater content of interstitial collagen. Defective revascularization of ischemic myocardium might provide an additional explanation for the increased incidence of reinfarction in patients suffering impaired fibrinolysis [15]. Importantly, VEGF (vascular endothelial growth factor) could not improve infarct revascularization in the absence of u-PA, possibly because its action depends on endothelial u-PA expression. This implicates that therapeutic angiogenesis is determined by genetic predisposition factors, such as u-PA, justifying genetic pre-screening of patients, eligible for angiogenic treatment. It will be interesting to explore whether decreased fibrinolysis in patients also impairs therapeutic myocardial angiogenesis as in u-PA-deficient mice. Conversely, impaired revascularization of ischemic myocardial zones at risk could also explain why PAI-1 is a risk factor for ischemic heart disease, independently or additionally to its role in thrombosis.

u-PA-deficient myofibroblasts also failed to infiltrate the infarct. Since these cells produce a collagen-rich extracellular matrix, scar formation was impaired in u-PA-deficient mice. Furthermore, lack of u-PA impaired activation of latent TGFβ-1 (transforming growth factor-beta 1), a strong stimulus for matrix production. The apparent paradox that lack of proteinase reduces the collagen content of a wound can be explained by the impaired accumulation of collagen-producing fibroblasts and the reduced activation of growth factors involved in collagen production. Thus, proteinases are initially required for wound cells to migrate into the wound. On arriving in the wounds, they play a role in activating growth factors.

A remarkable finding was that the impaired infarct healing/scar formation in u-PA-deficient mice significantly suppressed cardiac performance and resulted in cardiac failure after adrenergic stress. Hemodynamic performance was comparable in infarcted wild-type and u-PA-deficient mice under baseline conditions [14]. However, the adrenergic agent dobutamine failed to increase contractility and stroke volume in u-PA-deficient mice after AMI. Electrocardiographic (ECG) recordings revealed comparable polarity of repolarization and prolongation of the QTc interval in both genotypes within 2 days of AMI. By 14 days after AMI, ECG signs normalized in wild-type mice but deteriorated in u-PA-deficient mice. In addition, ventricular extrasystoles and atrioventricular conduction disturbances occurred in infarcted u-PA-deficient mice. The genotypic differences became more apparent after stressing infarcted mice with isoproterenol, an adrenergic agonist known to induce arrhythmias after AMI [14]. In contrast to wild-type mice, u-PA-deficient mice developed severe repolarization disturbances, ventricular extrasystoles and arrhythmias, and died in cardiogenic shock within 15 min of isoproterenol administration. Impaired infarct healing in u-PA-deficient mice also caused ischemia in the remote noninfarcted myocardium. The depressed cardiac function in infarcted u-PA-deficient mice may be due to impaired revascularization and increased systolic dyskinesis of the necrotic segment which, because of its reduced collagen content, is more compliant. This imposes a greater work load on and induces ischemia in the residual viable cardiomyocytes and results in cardiac failure. Thus, caution should be used to treat patients for prolonged or uncontrolled periods with proteinase inhibitors for postinfarct remodeling [16], inflammation, or cancer [17].

Atherosclerosis

Epidemiologic studies indicate that high levels of plasma PAI-1 are a risk factor for recurrent myocardial infarction and atherosclerosis progression in middle aged patients, most likely because of impaired lysis of fibrin-rich thrombi [15,18]. Indeed, incorporation of fibrin-rich thrombi could contribute to lesion progression not only because their bulky mass increases plaque size, but also because it chemoattracts inflammatory, endothelial, or SMCs. In addition, PAI-1 could promote the formation of fatal occluding thrombi after plaque rupture. Therefore, we anticipated that the absence of PAI-1 would reduce plaque growth because of the increased levels of u-PA-mediated plasmin and resultant matrix degradation. However, when plaque size was determined, plaques were significantly larger at advanced stages of atherosclerosis in mice with a combined deficiency of apoE and PAI-1 as compared to apoE-deficient mice, both in the thoracic and in the abdominal aorta (unpublished observations). The unexpected effects of PAI-1 deficiency on plaque size might be explained by the fact that PAI-1, expressed by cells within the atherosclerotic plaque, may affect plaque progression by influencing cellular migration, or by modulating the activation and liberation of growth factors sequestered within the extracellular matrix [19,20]. One possibility which we are currently investigating is whether PAI-1 inhibits excessive activation of latent TGF-β1. These findings are consistent with the reduction of atherosclerotic lesions after adenoviral-mediated overexpression of TIMP-1 in another study [21].

Arterial restenosis

Vascular interventions for the treatment of atherothrombosis (balloon angioplasty, stenting) induce restenosis of the vessel within 3–6 months in 30–50% of treated patients. Arterial stenosis may result from remodeling of the vessel wall and/or from accumulation of cells and extracellular matrix in the intimal layer. Several candidate molecules involved in these responses to injury have been identified based on correlative expression studies, but their in vivo role and importance has frequently remained obscure. Proteinases participate in the proliferation and migration of SMCs, and in the matrix remodeling during arterial wound healing. In a mouse model of arterial wound healing, we demonstrated that u-PA, but not t-PA, mediates vascular wound healing and arterial neointima formation in mice. Indeed, the degree and rate of arterial neointima formation was reduced in u-PA-deficient mice 4—6 weeks after injury, most likely due to impairment of cellular migration [22]. Neointima formation was also reduced in plasminogen-deficient, but not in u-PAR-deficient, mice. This indicates that, in this model, u-PA-mediated plasmin proteolysis was independent of u-PA binding to its receptor [23]. Neointima formation was accelerated in PAI-1-deficient arteries and could be inhibited by adenoviral gene transfer of human PAI-1 [13,24]. Surprisingly, α_2-antiplasmin, the major inhibitor of plasmin, does not play an essential role in SMC migration and neointima formation during arterial wound healing, as demonstrated by the comparable results obtained with α_2-antiplasmin-deficient and wild-type mice [25].

The involvement of the MMP system in vascular wound healing was shown by the fact that TIMP-1 overexpression (by seeding retrovirally transduced SMCs onto balloon-injured rat carotid arteries) inhibited intimal thickening [26]. Consistent with this, neointima formation was increased in TIMP-1-deficient mice after electrical injury of the femoral artery [27]. In addition, after balloon injury in rat carotid arteries, MMP inhibition by a broad spectrum inhibitor delayed (but did not prevent) intimal lesion formation by reducing SMC migration [11]. An analogous effect was seen by adenoviral gene transfer of TIMP-2 after balloon angioplasty in rat carotid arteries [28], whereby early SMC migration was blocked but neointima formation at later points in time was not prevented. This lack of effect in neointima formation at later time points by both synthetic inhibitors and adenoviral gene transfer of TIMP-2 could be due to compensatory smooth muscle cell proliferation [11]. In a recent study, overexpression of gelatinase-B (MMP-9) by seeding of stably transfected SMCs after balloon denudation increased SMC migration and influenced vessel remodeling, as was evident from vessel wall thinning and lower intimal matrix content [29]. A role for stromelysins in neointima formation was suggested by thinner neointimas in cultured balloon-injured rat carotid arteries treated with antisense oligonucleotides to stromelysin mRNA [30]. However, in stromelysin-3 (MMP-11)-deficient mice, neointima formation was increased — not decreased — after electrical injury of the femoral artery due to enhanced elastin degradation and cellular migration [31]. The mechanisms by which MMP-11 would impair cellular migration and elastin degradation require further investigation.

Vein graft stenosis

Coronary artery bypass surgery is a frequent intervention in patients with multivessel coronary artery disease. Although arterial grafts are preferred, the saphenous vein is still used because of several advantages such as convenient harvesting and sufficient yield of graft material. However, vein graft failure occurs in 30–50% of the cases within 10 years [32], due to the combined effects of thrombosis, neointima formation and graft atherosclerosis. The role of plasminogen in intimal hyperplasia after vein grafting was recently studied in plasminogen-deficient mice, using a model that shares many features with the human saphenous vein graft [33]. Implantation of a vein segment on the carotid artery caused substantial intimal hyperplasia in both wild-type and plasminogen-deficient mice, but no significant differences in the extent of neointima formation were detected between the two genotypes. This lack of effect is in contrast with the reduced neointima formation observed after arterial injury in plasminogen-deficient mice [34]. The most likely explanation for this is the absence of well-developed elastic laminae in veins, which constitute an important barrier for smooth muscle cell migration in arteries. This hypothesis is further underscored by findings that inflammatory and smooth muscle cells can only cross degraded elastic laminae in atherosclerotic plaques or transplanted allografts (see below).

A role for metalloproteinases in vein graft stenosis was recently suggested by inhibition of neointima formation after adenoviral gene transfer of TIMP-1, 2, or 3 in cultured human saphenous veins [35]. However, in an in vivo model in pigs only TIMP-3 overexpression was able to inhibit late neointima formation, due to both MMP inhibition and induction of SMC apoptosis, whereas TIMP-2 was not [35]. The lack of an in vivo effect of TIMP-2 in late neointima formation is possibly due to the time-limited effect of adenoviral gene transfer and to the fact that TIMP-2 affects smooth muscle cell migration more than proliferation [11]. Conclusive evidence for the involvement of TIMP-2 and other components of the MMP system can be generated using the above-mentioned vein graft model in gene-deficient mice.

Transplant arteriosclerosis

Accelerated coronary arteriosclerosis is an important limitation to the long-term survival of patients with heart transplantation. The role of the plasminogen system in allograft transplant stenosis was studied using a mouse model of transplant arteriosclerosis that in many ways mimics the accelerated arteriosclerosis in coronary arteries of transplanted cardiac allografts in humans. In this model, host-derived leukocytes adhere to and infiltrate beneath the endothelium and form a predominantly leukocyte-rich neointima within 15 days of transplantation, whereas at later times, SMCs, derived from the donor graft, accumulate in the neointima. The role of leukocyte adhesion in the pathogenesis of transplant arteriosclerosis was recently highlighted by reduced neointimal lesions in mice deficient for intercellular adhesion molecule-1 (ICAM-1) [36]. Since previous targeting studies had shown that migration of leukocytes and SMCs is dependent on plasmin proteolysis, carotid arteries from B.10A (2R) wild-type mice were transplanted in C57BL6:129 plasminogen-deficient or wild-type recipient mice. Briefly, graft arteriosclerosis was largely prevented in plasminogen-deficient recipients due to the inability of inflammatory cells to infiltrate the media and of SMCs to migrate into the intima. Fragmentation of the elastic laminae and neoadventitia formation were less severe in plasminogen-deficient than in wild-type mice, where significantly increased expression of MMPs was measured during active cell migration. Since plasmin can directly degrade some but not all matrix components in the media, it presumably activates other matrix-degrading proteinases, most probably of the MMP family, that then contribute to extracellular matrix degradation [37].

Conclusion

These genetic studies emphasize the complexity and diversity of the distinct proteinase systems in cardiovascular disorders. Proteinases may have dual — even opposite — effects, depending on their level and spatio-temporal expression. In addition, tissue architecture may have important influences on the eventual effects of proteinases. Given the medical importance of the various cardiovascular pathologies, further analysis by genetic and other strategies is clearly warranted. Proteinase inhibitors are currently being considered for the treatment of atherosclerotic aneurysm formation and cardiac rupture after myocardial infarction. However, such proteinase inhibitors would not be indicated in patients prone to cardiac failure. In addition, proteinase inhibitors might reduce the efficacy of therapeutic angiogenesis in ischemic heart disease. Finally, while proteinase inhibitors are being considered for the treatment of unstable plaques, they may disregulate the local homeostasis of matrix remodeling within plaques.

References

1. Collen D. The plasminogen (fibrinolytic) system. Thromb Haemost 1999;82:259—270.
2. Nagase H. Activation mechanisms of matrix metalloproteinases. Biol Chem 1997;378:151—160.
3. Pei D, Majmudar G, Weiss SJ. Hydrolytic inactivation of a breast carcinoma cell-derived serpin by human stromelysin-3. J Biol Chem 1994;269:25849—25855.
4. Carmeliet P et al. Urokinase-generated plasmin activates matrix metalloproteinases during aneurysm formation. Nat Genet 1997;17:439—444.
5. Dahlback B. Blood coagulation. Lancet 2000;355:1627—1632.
6. Carmeliet P, Collen D. Development and disease in proteinase-deficient mice: role of the plasminogen, matrix metalloproteinase and coagulation system. Thromb Res 1998;91:255—285.
7. Carmeliet P. Proteinases in cardiovascular aneurysms and rupture: targets for therapy? J Clin Invest 2000;105:1519—1520.
8. Lupu F et al. Plasminogen activator expression in human atherosclerotic lesions. Arterioscl Thromb Vasc Biol 1995;15:1444—1455.
9. George SJ. Tissue inhibitors of metalloproteinases and metalloproteinases in atherosclerosis. Curr Opin Lipidol 1998;9:413—423.
10. Allaire E, Forough R, Clowes M, Starcher B, Clowes AW. Local overexpression of TIMP-1 prevents aortic aneurysm degeneration and rupture in a rat model. J Clin Invest 1998;102:1413—1420.

11. Prescott MF et al. Effect of matrix metalloproteinase inhibition on progression of atherosclerosis and aneurysm in LDL receptor-deficient mice overexpressing MMP-3, MMP-12, and MMP-13 and on restenosis in rats after balloon injury. Ann NY Acad Sci 1999;878:179—190.
12. Pyo R et al. Targeted gene disruption of matrix metalloproteinase-9 (gelatinase B) suppresses development of experimental abdominal aortic aneurysms. J Clin Invest 2000;105:1641—1649.
13. Carmeliet P, Collen D. Transgenic mouse models in angiogenesis and cardiovascular disease. J Pathol 2000;190:387—405.
14. Heymans S et al. Inhibition of plasminogen activators or matrix metalloproteinases prevents cardiac rupture but impairs therapeutic angiogenesis and causes cardiac failure. Nat Med 1999;5:1135—1142.
15. Hamsten A et al. Plasminogen activator inhibitor in plasma: risk factor for recurrent myocardial infarction. Lancet 1987;2:3—9.
16. Rohde LE et al. Matrix metalloproteinase inhibition attenuates early left ventricular enlargement after experimental myocardial infarction in mice. Circulation 1999;99:3063—3070.
17. Kleiner DE, Stetler-Stevenson WG. Matrix metalloproteinases and metastasis. Cancer Chemo Pharmacol 1999;43:S42—S51.
18. Cortellaro M et al. Increased fibrin turnover and high PAI-1 activity as predictors of ischemic events in atherosclerotic patients. A case-control study. The PLAT Group. Arterioscl Thromb 1993;13:1412—1417.
19. Loskutoff DJ, Curriden SA, Hu G, Deng G. Regulation of cell adhesion by PAI-1. APMIS 1999;107:54—61.
20. Rifkin DB, Mazzieri R, Munger JS, Noguera I, Sung J. Proteolytic control of growth factor availability. APMIS 1999;107:80—85.
21. Rouis M et al. Adenovirus-mediated overexpression of tissue inhibitor of metalloproteinase-1 reduces atherosclerotic lesions in apolipoprotein E-deficient mice. Circulation 1999;100:533—540.
22. Carmeliet P et al. Urokinase but not tissue plasminogen activator mediates arterial neointima formation in mice. Circ Res 1997;81:829—839.
23. Carmeliet P et al. Receptor-independent role of urokinase-type plasminogen activator in arterial wound healing and intima formation in mice. J Cell Biol 1998;140:233—245.
24. Carmeliet P et al. Inhibitory role of plasminogen activator inhibitor-1 in arterial wound healing and neointima formation: a gene targeting and gene transfer study in mice. Circulation 1997; 96:3180—3191.
25. Lijnen HR, Van Hoef B, Dewerchin M, Collen D. α_2-Antiplasmin gene deficiency in mice does not affect neointima formation after vascular injury. Arterioscl Thromb Vasc Biol 2000;20:1488—1492.
26. Forough R et al. Overexpression of tissue inhibitor of matrix metalloproteinase-1 inhibits vascular smooth muscle cell functions in vitro and in vivo. Circ Res 1996;79:812—820.
27. Lijnen HR, Soloway P, Collen D. Tissue inhibitor of matrix metalloproteinases-1 impairs arterial neointima formation after vascular injury in mice. Circ Res 1999;85:1186—1191.
28. Cheng L et al. Adenovirus-mediated gene transfer of the human tissue inhibitor of metalloproteinase-2 blocks vascular smooth muscle cell invasiveness in vitro and modulates neointimal development in vivo. Circulation 1998;98:2195—2201.
29. Mason DP et al. Matrix metalloproteinase-9 overexpression enhances vascular smooth muscle cell migration and alters remodeling in the injured rat carotid artery. Circ Res 1999;85:1179—1185.
30. Lovdahl C et al. Antisense oligonucleotides to stromelysin mRNA inhibit injury-induced proliferation of arterial smooth muscle cells. Histol Histopathol 1999;14:1101—1112.
31. Lijnen HR et al. Accelerated neointima formation after vascular injury in mice with stromelysin-3 (MMP-11) gene inactivation. Arterioscl Thromb Vasc Biol 1999;19:2863—2870.
32. Campeau L et al. Atherosclerosis and late closure of aortocoronary saphenous vein grafts: sequential angiographic studies at 2 weeks, 1 year, 5 to 7 years, and 10 to 12 years after surgery.

Circulation 1983;68:II1—7.

33. Shi C et al. Plasminogen is not required for neointima formation in a mouse model of vein graft stenosis. Circ Res 1999;84:883—890.

34. Carmeliet P, Moons L, Ploplis V, Plow E, Collen D. Impaired arterial neointima formation in mice with disruption of the plasminogen gene. J Clin Invest 1997;99:200—208.

35. George SJ, Lloyd CT, Angelini GD, Newby AC, Baker AH. Inhibition of late vein graft neointima formation in human and porcine models by adenovirus-mediated overexpression of tissue inhibitor of metalloproteinase-3. Circulation 2000;101:296—304.

36. Dietrich H et al. Mouse model of transplant arteriosclerosis: role of intercellular adhesion molecule-1. Arterioscl Thromb Vasc Biol 2000;20:343—352.

37. Moons L et al. Reduced transplant arteriosclerosis in plasminogen-deficient mice. J Clin Invest 1998;102:1788—1797.

Atherosclerosis XII.
S. Stemme and A.G. Olsson, editors.

Cardiovascular angiogenesis

Karen Moulton and Judah Folkman
Children's Hospital Hunnewell 103, Boston, Massachusetts, USA

Introduction

Angiogenesis, the growth of new microvessels, is critical to many biological processes, including reproduction, development, and repair. Furthermore, diseases which are angiogenesis-dependent cover a wide spectrum and are the subject of almost every medical specialty, including ophthalmology, dermatology, gynecology, rheumatology, cardiology and oncology, to name just a few. The field of angiogenesis research itself is currently growing rapidly — approximately 30 papers on the subject are published each week.

This field began in the 1960s as an attempt to understand how tumors induce their own private blood supply and to determine if the switch to the angiogenic phenotype is critical for tumor growth. The hypothesis that tumors are angiogenesis-dependent, first proposed in 1971 [1], has now been confirmed by genetic methods as well by the demonstration that specific angiogenesis inhibitors will suppress or regress tumors [2]. From the efforts of many laboratories in this field have come discoveries of novel proteins which stimulate angiogenesis, as well as proteins and other molecules which inhibit angiogenesis.

At least 20 angiogenesis inhibitors for the treatment of advanced cancer are currently in clinical trials, in the USA. Seven have reached Phase III. Another five angiogenesis inhibitors are in clinical trial for eye diseases, such as diabetic retinopathy and macular degeneration. More than 100 pharmaceutical and biotechnology companies worldwide work in this field.

Prior to the initiation of clinical trials of angiogenesis inhibitors, approximately 5 years ago, we asked whether long-term antiangiogenic therapy for cancer could interfere with coronary collateral formation, especially in those cancer patients who also had ischemic heart disease. The following hypothesis was proposed: if growth, bleeding, or rupture of a coronary atherosclerotic plaque are dependent upon plaque neovascularization, and if this neovascularization can be blocked by an angiogenesis inhibitor, would the need for coronary collaterals be obviated?

Evidence for angiogenesis in atherosclerotic plaques

Before this hypothesis could be tested, it was necessary to examine previous

Address for correspondence: Judah Folkman MD, Children's Hospital Hunnewell 103, 300 Longwood Avenue, Boston, MA 02115, USA. Tel.: +1-617-355-7661. Fax: +1-617-355-7662.

104

reports for evidence of the presence of angiogenesis in plaques and to develop a good animal model. In 1984 Barger et al. had demonstrated neovascularization within coronary artery plaques in the human heart (Fig. 1) [3]. In 1988, Williams et al. showed that the vasa vasorum in atherosclerotic coronary arteries of monkeys with high cholesterol was significantly increased, but was decreased when cholesterol was lowered [4]. In 1994, O'Brien et al. showed that most plaque microvessels are invisible in conventional histological sections unless they are highlighted by immuno-labelling techniques. These authors further demonstrated endothelial cell proliferation in the microvessels within human atherosclerotic plaques, indicating the presence of new vessels [5]. In 1998, Kwon et al. reported intense neovascularization in atherosclerotic plaques of pigs fed a cholesterol diet. Microvessel density was increased by 2.5-fold [6].

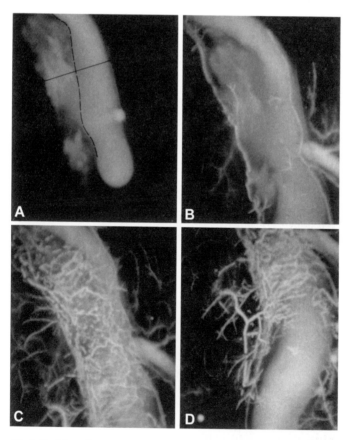

Fig. 1. Serial angiograms on a postmortem human heart after perfusion of the coronary arteries with microfil (a silicone based radio-opaque polymer). **A:** Filling defect in the coronary artery lumen identifies an atherosclerotic plaque which occludes approximately 50% of the lumen. **B:** Later image shows vasa vasorum beginning to fill. **C:** Intense neovascularization in the area of a plaque extends into the interior of the plaque. **D:** The neovascularization is more intense in the region of the plaque as compared to a contiguous noninvolved segment of artery [3].

Development of an animal model of plaque angiogenesis

To develop an animal model of plaque angiogenesis, Karen Moulton fed a diet of 0.15% cholesterol to APO lipoprotein E-deficient mice (Jackson Labs) for up to 6 months [7]. Serum cholesterol levels rose to an average of 790 mg/dl. Opaque plaques developed in the aorta at the branch sites of major arteries in a distribution pattern similar to the pattern in humans (Fig. 2). Increased vasa vasorum in the area of the plaque could also be seen on the external surface of the aorta. Forty histological cross-sections which began at the aortic sinus were then made at 10 μm intervals and stained with antibody to CD31 or von Willebrand factor (vWF) to highlight microvessels. Marked intimal neovascularization was identified in plaques from the aortic sinus and descending aorta (Fig. 3). When intimal thickness exceeded 250 microns there was a sharp increase in the number of plaques that had become neovascularized, e.g., 28% of 114 plaques > 250 microns were neovascularized vs. 2% of plaques less than 250 microns thick which were neovascularized (Table 1). This finding suggested that growth of plaque thickness could not exceed the tissue oxygen diffusion limit without initiation of angiogenesis.

Aortic rings were then cultured in vitro in collagen type I matrix and serum-free media for 8 days as previously described by Nicosia [8]. Capillary sprouts

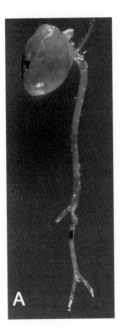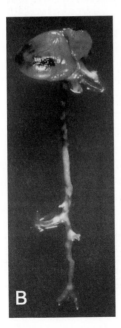

Fig. 2. **A**: Wild-type C57Bl/6 mouse on a normal diet, showing the normal translucent aorta without atherosclerotic plaques. **B**: Aorta removed from an Apo E−/− mouse fed 0.15% cholesterol diet for 6 months. Opaque plaques are observed through the entire aorta at the sites of major branches, as well as at the aortic arch.

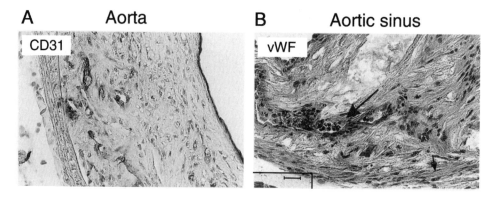

Fig. 3. Lesions from Apo E−/− mice fed cholesterol diet for 6 months. **A**: CD31 positive microvessels in a plaque from the descending aorta, predominately toward the media. **B**: Plaque from the aortic sinus shows microvessel filled with red blood cells identified by vWF staining [7].

grew out radially from aortic rings containing plaques from ApoE −/− mice. In contrast, aortic rings from the same ApoE −/− mice, but without plaques, did not grow out capillary sprouts, or sprout growth was minimal. (Fig. 4).

Inhibition of angiogenesis in murine atherosclerotic plaques

To determine if plaque angiogenesis could be inhibited pharmacologically, two angiogenesis inhibitors (Fig. 5) which are currently in clinical trial, were tested in the aortic ring bioassay. TNP-470 is a synthetic analogue of fumagillin [9]. Endostatin is a 20 kD internal fragment of collagen XVIII [10]. Both molecules significantly inhibited outgrowth of microvascular sprouts from plaque-containing aortic rings which had been isolated from ApoE −/− mice (Fig. 6).

Endostatin and TNP-470 were then administered systemically to ApoE −/− mice. The mice were maintained on a cholesterol diet for 12−14 weeks and then received antiangiogenic therapy for 16 weeks beginning at age 20 weeks, while continuing on the high cholesterol diet. Endostatin was administered at 20 mg/kg subcutaneously daily or TNP-470 was administered at 30 mg/kg subcuta-

Table 1. Incidence of neovascularization in advanced lesions of ApoE−/− mice fed a 0.15% cholesterol diet for 6 months.

Plaque depth	Vessel +	Vessel −	Incidence
> 250 μm	13	33	0.283*
100−250 μm	2	66	0.029*
Total	15	99	0.132

Methods described in [7]. Intimal vessels were counted if they stained positive for CD31 or vWF and were also observed on adjacent histologic sections. *$p < 0.0005$, Fisher's exact.

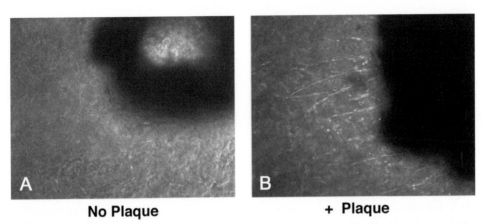

Fig. 4. Aortic rings from Apo E−/− mice cultured in vitro collagen I gel without serum or added growth factors, day 8. **A**: Aortic ring from area without a plaque. There are no capillary sprouts. **B**: Aortic ring from a plaque-containing area. Multiple microvascular sprouts grow in a radial direction from the aortic wall.

neously every other day. Control animals received daily injections of vehicle. There were 10 mice in each group. Plaque area was measured at the aortic origin at 36 weeks. At the conclusion of the 16 week treatment period the median

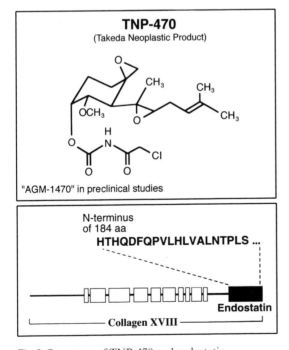

Fig. 5. Structures of TNP-470 and endostatin.

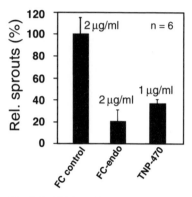

Fig. 6. Inhibition of plaque-induced microvascular sprouts from in vitro aortic rings as depicted in Fig. 4 on day 8. FC-endostatin inhibits sprout formation by approximately 75%. TNP-470 inhabits sprout formation by approximately 60%. Endostatin was produced as a fusion protein between endostatin and the murine FC domain of $IgG_{2a-\gamma}$ [13].

plaque area was significantly reduced by 85% in the endostatin-treated mice and by 70% in the TNP-470-treated mice (Table 2). Furthermore, the total number of microvessels per plaque was reduced. After 16 weeks of treatment, seven out of 24 untreated plaques (29%) were neovascularized. However, only one out of 22 endostatin-treated plaques (5%) and none of the 27 TNP-470-treated plaques (0%) were neovascularized.

Discussion

These studies show significant inhibition of plaque growth by inhibitors of plaque angiogenesis. The inhibitors do not lower cholesterol. Furthermore, the angiogenesis inhibitors have little effect on early plaque growth at the stage of fatty streaks, before the appearance of neovascularization. In ApoE $-/-$ mice on a high cholesterol diet, fatty streaks appear between 8 and 20 weeks of age and plaques

Table 2. Plaque area at aortic origin during treatment with an angiogenesis inhibitor. Apolipoprotein E-deficient mice, aged 20 weeks at start.

Therapy	Median plaque area (mm^2)	Range	% Inhibition of plaque growth	No. of subjects
Before therapy	0.250	0.170–0.348	—	10
After 16 weeks				
Untreated	0.751	0.503–0.838	0	12
TNP-470	0.402	0.248–0.533	70	15
Endostatin	0.321	0.238–0.412	85	10

Data from Moulton et al. [7] showing relative inhibition of plaque growth by TNP-470 or endostatin therapy; $p < 0.001$.

with smooth muscle are not observed until approximately 15 weeks of age. We conclude that neither endostatin nor TNP-470 significantly affect plaques at the very earliest stages before the onset of neovascularization. Plaque growth at advanced stages is more susceptible to inhibition by an angiogenesis inhibitor, presumably by blocking the proliferation of intimal microvessels.

The high correlation between inhibition of angiogenesis in atherosclerotic plaques and suppression of plaque growth suggest that growth beyond a critical plaque thickness, i.e., > 250 µm, is angiogenesis-dependent. If these results apply to human atherosclerosis several speculations can be made. First, chronic anti-angiogenic therapy for cancer may not have an adverse effect on myocardial ischemia, but could, by suppressing plaque growth, have a beneficial effect. In other words, chronic suppression of plaque growth could possibly obviate the need for coronary collaterals. These results indicate that it may be important to follow the cardiac status of cancer patients who are on long-term antiangiogenic therapy to look for improvement in cardiac function or decrease in cardiac-related symptoms, (e.g., reduction of angina, or ischemic complications, etc.). Second, long-term antiangiogenic therapy, could be used to inhibit the growth of coronary atherosclerotic plaques, or perhaps regress them sufficiently to "set back" coronary disease by a decade or more in a given patient. An example could be an orally available cycloxygenase 2 inhibitor which has been demonstrated to be an angiogenesis inhibitor [11]. Third, these results may provide an additional mechanism to explain how aspirin and other inhibitors of platelet adhesion could interfere with progressive growth of atherosclerotic plaques. Platelets contain at least 13 positive regulators of blood vessel growth. When these are released during platelet adhesion they could overcome the fewer negative regulators of vessel growth and stimulate plaque angiogenesis (Table 3). Thus, chronic low dose aspir-

Table 3. Positive and negative regulators of angiogenesis in platelets.

Positive	Negative
VEGF-A (VPC)	PF-4
VEGF-C	Thrombospondin
bFGF	NK1, NK2, NK3 fragments of HGF
HGF	
Angiopoietin-1	TGF-β1
PDGF	Plasminogen (angiostatin)
EGF	High molecular weight kininogen (domain 5)
IGF-1	Fibronectin
IGF BP3	
Vitronectin	EGF (fragment)
Fibronectin	α2 antiplasmin (fragment)
Fibrinogen	β-thromboglobulin
Heparanase	

in could act as a mild inhibitor of angiogenesis in atherosclerotic plaques [12]. Finally, there remains the possibility that these results may be part of a larger picture in the field of angiogenesis research. If it turns out that a wide variety of non-neoplastic diseases are angiogenesis-dependent as tumors are, then antiangiogenic drugs developed to treat cancer may also be useful to treat nonneoplastic disease. These would include diabetic retinopathy, macular degeneration, retinopathy of prematurity, psoriasis, endometriosis and rheumatoid arthritis, to name just a few. For clinical investigators in cardiology, a future goal will be to determine if the new class of drugs called angiogenesis inhibitors can be of practical use to improve the treatment of atherosclerotic coronary disease.

Acknowledgements

Studies were supported by a Physician Scientist Award (K 11 HL-02563) from the National Heart, Lung, and Blood Institute, and the Harvard Medical School 50th Anniversary Program (K.S.M.) and by a grant from EntreMed Inc, (Frederick, Maryland) to Children's Hospital.

References

1. Folkman J. Tumor angiogenesis: therapeutic implications. N Engl J Med 1971;285:1182–1186.
2. Folkman J. Tumor angiogenesis. In: Holland JF, Frei E III, Bast RC Jr, Kufe DW, Pollock RE, Weichelsbaum RR (eds) Cancer Medicine, 5th edn. Burlington, ON, Canada: B.C. Decker Inc, 2000;132–152.
3. Barger AC, Beeuwker R, Lainey L, Silverman KJ. Hypothesis: vasa vasorum and neovascularization of human coronary arteries. N Engl J Med 1984;310:175–177.
4. Williams JK, Armstrong ML, Heistad DD. Vasa vasorum in atherosclerotic coronary arteries: response to vasoactive stimuli and regression of atherosclerosis. Circ Res 1988;62:515–523.
5. O'Brien ER, Garvin MR, Dev R, Stewart DK, Hinohara T, Simpson JB, Schwartz SM. Angiogenesis in human coronary atherosclerotic plaques. Am J Pathol 1994;145:883–894.
6. Kwon HM, Sangiorgi G, Ritman EL, McKenna C, Holmes DR Jr, Schwartz RS, Lerman A. Enhanced coronary vasa vasorum neovascularization in experimental hypercholesteremia. J Clin Invest 1998;101:1551–1556.
7. Moulton KS, Heller E, Konerding MA, Flynn E, Palinski W, Folkman J. Angiogenesis inhibitors endostatin or TNP-470 reduce intimal neovascularization and plaque growth in apolipoprotein E-deficient mice. Circulation 1999;99:1726–1732.
8. Nicosia RF, Ottinetti A. Modulation of microvascular growth and morphogenesis by reconstituted basement membrane gel in three dimensional cultures of rat aorta: a comparative study of angiogenesis in matrigel, collagen, fibrin, and plasma clot. In Vitro Cell Dev Biol 1990;26: 119–128.
9. Ingber DM, Fujita T, Kishimoto S, Sudo K, Kanamaru T, Brem H, Folkman J. Synthetic analogues of fumagillin that inhibit angiogenesis and suppress tumor growth. Nature 1990; 348: 555– 557.
10. O'Reilly MS, Boehm T, Shing Y, Fukai N, Vasios G, Lane WS, Flynn E, Birkhead JR, Olsen BR, Folkman J. Endostatin: an endogenous inhibitor of angiogenesis and tumor growth. Cell 1997; 88:277–285.
11. Masferrer JL, Leahy KM, Koki AT, Zweifel BS, Settle SL, Woerner BM, Edwards DA, Flickin-

ger AG, Moore RJ, Seibert K. Antiangiogenic and antitumor activities of cyclooxygenase-2 inhibitors. Cancer Res 2000;60:1306–1311.

12. Shiff D, Rigas B. Aspirin for cancer. Nature Med 1999;5:1348–1349.
13. Bergers G, Javaherian K, Lo K-M, Folkman J, Hanahan D. Effects of angiogenesis inhibitors on multistage carcinogenesis in mice. Science 1999;284:808–812.

What have we learned from the lipid-lowering trials and where are we going?

Antonio M. Gotto
Weill Medical College of Cornell University, New York, USA

Introduction

The body of evidence supporting the benefits of lipid modification illustrates several important lessons about pharmacologic treatment of lipid disorders. Clinical trials confirm that cholesterol control in a broad range of at-risk patients will help reduce the risk across the spectrum of clinical cardiovascular events, including stroke in secondary prevention. Treatment with the HMG-CoA reductase inhibitors (or statins) is associated with few adverse events and improved survival in some studies. Bucher et al. assessed the risk for total and coronary heart disease (CHD) mortality across 59 randomized, controlled clinical trials of various lipid-modifying strategies involving a total of 85,431 participants in the intervention and 87,729 participants in the control groups [1]. The trials were categorized into seven groups: statins (13 trials), fibrates (12 trials), resins (eight trials), hormones (eight trials), nicotinic acid (two trials), n-3 fatty acids (three trials), and dietary interventions (16 trials). Only statins showed a large and statistically significant reduction in both mortality from CHD (risk ratio, 0.66; 95% confidence interval (CI), 0.54–0.79) and from all causes (risk ratio, 0.75; 95% CI, 0.65–0.86). The difference between statins and the combined estimate of the other classes of agents was unlikely to be due to chance ($p < 0.02$ for both comparisons). Therefore, for the majority of patients with mild to severe elevations in total and low-density lipoprotein (LDL) cholesterol, statins appear to be effective therapy.

Although treatment with fibric acid derivatives (fibrates) appeared to be associated with a mild increase in deaths (Fig. 1), the inclusion of the early World Health Organization trial of clofibrate, which suggested a significant increase in all deaths with that agent, may have biased the analysis [2]. As clofibrate is no longer in wide use, the issue of the safety of other fibrates remains open, although the Helsinki Heart Study of gemfibrozil generated minor controversy regarding a nonsignificant increase in cancer deaths in the gemfibrozil group 3.5 years after the trial ended [3].

Address for correspondence: Antonio M. Gotto Jr, MD, DPhil, c/o Mr. Jesse Jou, Weill Medical College of Cornell University, 445 E. 69th Street, Olin Hall 205, New York, NY 10021, USA. Tel.: +1-212-746-6014. Fax: +1-212-746-8200. E-mail: amg.editorial@med.cornell.edu

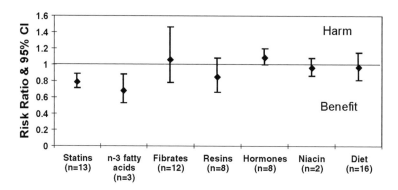

Fig. 1. Meta-analysis of lipid-lowering trials suggests statins reduce both coronary and all-cause mortality. Adapted from Bucher et al. [1].

The recent publication of two additional large-scale clinical trials of fibrates may contribute additional safety information about this drug class. Coronary patients treated with gemfibrozil in the Veterans' Affairs HDL Intervention Trial (VA-HIT) experienced a 22% reduction in risk for nonfatal myocardial infarction (MI) and coronary death (Table 1) [4]. However, the Bezafibrate Infarction Prevention (BIP) study reported no statistically significant reduction in fatal and nonfatal MI and coronary death in a similar cohort, despite an increase in HDL cholesterol of 18% and reduction in triglycerides of 21%. The frequency of the primary endpoint was 13.6% on bezafibrate vs. 15.0% on placebo (p = 0.26). After 6.2 years, the reduction in the cumulative probability of the primary endpoint was 7.3%, (p = 0.24). However, a substantial risk reduction with bezafibrate (39.5%, p = 0.02) was observed post hoc in the small cohort of patients

Table 1. Recent endpoint trials of low HDL patients.

	VA-HIT	BIP	AFCAPS
Drug	Gemfibrozil	Bezafibrate	Lovastatin
Duration (years)	5.1	6.2	5.2
N (M/W)	2531/10	2825/265	5608/997
Baseline lipids, mg/dl (mmol/l)/% change with treatment			
Total cholesterol	175 (4.5)/−4	213 (5.5)/−4.5	221 (5.7)/−18
Triglyceride	160 (1.8)/−31	145 (1.6)/−21	158(1.8)/−15
LDL cholesterol	112 (2.9)/0	149 (3.8)/−6.5	150 (3.9)/−25
HDL cholesterol	32 (0.8)/+6	35 (0.9)/+18	M36 (0.9)
			W40 (1.0)/+6
RRR (%) in 1° endpoint	−22	−9	−37
ARR (%) in 1° endpoint	−4.4	−1.4	−4.1

VA-HIT: Veterans' Affairs HDL Intervention Trial; BIP: Bezafibrate Infarction Prevention Study; AFCAPS: Air Force/Texas Coronary Atherosclerosis Prevention Study; M: men; W: women; RRR: relative risk reduction; ARR: absolute risk reduction.

with elevated triglycerides at baseline (>200 mg/dl (2.26 mmol/l)) [5]. In neither study did clinically adverse experiences differ significantly between treatment groups.

As the contributions of high-density lipoprotein (HDL) cholesterol and triglycerides to coronary risk become better understood, another controversy has arisen as to whether patients with low HDL cholesterol should receive statins or fibrates (Table 1). In the large-scale, primary prevention Air Force/Texas Coronary Atherosclerosis Prevention Study (AFCAPS/TexCAPS), participants with average cholesterol and below-average HDL cholesterol experienced a highly significant 37% reduction in the combined risk for fatal and nonfatal MI, sudden cardiac death, and unstable angina with lovastatin, 20—40 mg/day [6]. The differences in outcomes and lipid responses in these three studies suggest that cardiovascular risk reduction with fibrates and statins may be mediated by different mechanisms.

Where do we go from here?

Although progress in elucidating the benefits of lipid modification has been substantial, clinicians and investigators will now need to address several challenges and questions that will affect the future applications of statin therapy. First, in the clinical setting, a renewed emphasis on applying the clinical research to the at-risk population must be achieved. Second, now that the benefits in stable coronary disease are clearly established, investigations are necessary to determine the viability of statins in the acute coronary syndrome. Finally, a growing database has suggested a number of hypothetical applications of statins beyond lipid modification.

Emphasizing the application of clinical research in the at-risk population

Policy-makers must resolve who should receive treatment when faced with limited healthcare resources and a diversity of treatment options. While these issues are controversial and will, without doubt, influence future guidelines, such discussions should not obscure the consistent deficit between clinical knowledge and clinical practice.

The recent multicenter Lipid Treatment Assessment Project (L-TAP) recapitulates earlier observations that despite the overwhelming evidence favoring intervention, lipid disorders are not treated as aggressively as they might be [8]. In L-TAP, investigators assessed the percentage of study patients receiving lipid-lowering therapy who achieved LDL-cholesterol goals as defined by US National Cholesterol Education Program (NCEP) guidelines. A total of 4,888 patients from five regions of the USA were studied. Of these, 23% had fewer than two CHD risk factors and no evidence of CHD (low-risk group), 47% had two or more risk factors and no evidence of CHD (high-risk group), and 30% had established CHD.

Overall, only 38% of patients achieved target levels of LDL cholesterol: success rates were 68% among low-risk patients, 37% among high-risk patents, and 18% among patients with CHD. Drug therapy was significantly (p ⩽ 0.01) more effective than nondrug therapy in all patient risk groups. However, in US guidelines, the target level for LDL cholesterol becomes more stringent as the risk increases (i.e., < 130 mg/dl (3.36 mmol/l) for high-risk primary prevention, but ⩽ 100 mg/dl (2.59 mmol/l) for CHD patients). Therefore, the lower success rate for the more ambitious target is somewhat unsurprising. Nevertheless, large proportions of patients receiving lipid-lowering therapy may require more aggressive treatment to attain goals.

Of the available lipid-altering drugs, the statins as a class have emerged as being the most prescribed and have driven the growth in this market.[9] A 4-year study in Ireland evaluated the impact of the landmark statin trials on local prescription practices and showed that statin use increased steadily after publication of the Scandinavian Simvastatin Survival Study (4S) in 1994 and the West of Scotland Coronary Prevention Study (WOSCOPS) in 1995, occurring to a greater extent in women than men [10]. More women than men older than 65 years are receiving statins. Compared with the landmark studies as the basis for prescription, the use of statins are generally not being used in the dosages demonstrated to be effective in trials.

Two considerations may help explain under-utilization of statins: i) uncertainty about whom should be treated, and ii) concerns about the cost-effectiveness and practicality of providing the broader population with drug therapy. The former consideration will yield as the diversity of clinical trials in progress in special populations like women, the elderly, or patients with diabetes come to fruition. Meanwhile, defining the boundaries of treatment represents a critical impasse in optimizing statin treatment, but "how should this question be decided? And who should decide: patients, physicians, or health maintenance organizations?" [10].

While there is little dissent that giving statins in secondary prevention is both worthwhile and cost-effective, making the case for primary prevention has proved to be far more contentious. Prosser et al. evaluated the cost-effectiveness ratios of cholesterol-lowering therapies according to NCEP risk categories [11]. Data were drawn from women and men aged 35–84 years with LDL-cholesterol levels of 160 mg/dl (4.1 mmol/l) or greater, who were divided into 240 risk subgroups according to age, sex, and the presence or absence of four CHD risk factors (smoking status, blood pressure, LDL-cholesterol level, and HDL-cholesterol level). The investigators considered Step I diet, statin therapy, and no preventive treatment for primary and secondary prevention. Incremental cost-effectiveness ratios for primary prevention with Step I diet ranged from US$1,900 per quality-adjusted life-year (QALY) gained for the highest-risk patient to US$500,000 per QALY for the lowest-risk patient. Primary prevention with a statin compared with diet therapy was US$54,000 per QALY to US$1,400,000 per QALY from highest risk to lowest risk. Secondary prevention with a statin cost less than US$50,000 per QALY for all risk subgroups. The authors conclude that primary prevention with a Step I diet seems to be cost-effective for most risk subgroups but may not be cost-effective for otherwise healthy young women. They also argue that primary prevention with a statin may not be cost-effective for younger men and women with few risk factors, "given the option of secondary prevention and of primary prevention in older age ranges." [11]

In a meta-analysis by LaRosa et al., the effects of statin therapy in the elderly and women in the landmark statin trials were evaluated. Overall, statin treatment reduced the risk by 31% for major coronary events (95% CI, 26–36%) and 21% for all-cause mortality (95% CI, 14–28%). The risk reduction in major coronary events was similar between women (29%; 95% CI, 13–42%) and men (31%; 95% CI, 26–35%), and between persons aged at least 65 years (32%; 95% CI, 23–39%) and persons younger than 65 years (31%; 95% CI, 24–36%).

In general, the absolute risk reduction for an event was greater in men than in women, except in the CARE trial, where women receiving pravastatin did significantly better than men. This effect was not replicated in the larger secondary prevention LIPID trial; therefore, the reason for the greater benefit in women in CARE remains to be elucidated. In the elderly, statin therapy was associated with the lowest number needed to treat in patients older than 65. On the one hand, this finding would seem to support the recommendation of Prosser et al. However, limiting treatment or delaying primary prevention until patients reach an older age discounts the lifelong pathology of atherosclerotic disease and presents important ethical concerns that should be addressed before excluding primary prevention on the basis of cost-effectiveness alone. Recent epidemiological data from three large cohorts affirm this critique: elevated cholesterol levels in younger men ($\leqslant 39$ years) were associated with an increased long-term risk for coronary, cardiovascular, and all-cause mortality. Conversely, more favorable cholesterol levels (< 200 mg/dl (5.17 mmol/l)) in this age range were associated with an estimated greater life expectancy of 3.8–8.7 years [13].

Identifying the effects of lipid modification in the acute coronary syndrome

As the number of statins has increased, an important controversy has arisen regarding whether the benefits of the statins are unique to each agent or whether there is a class effect dependent on the degree of LDL-cholesterol reduction achieved [14].

Adding to the controversy are data regarding the vascular effects of statins that may be independent of cholesterol modification, such as improvement of endothelial dysfunction, reduction of inflammatory parameters, and protection against lipoprotein oxidation [15]. For example, beneficial effects of simvastatin and lovastatin on nitric oxide synthase expression in a rat model have suggested a mechanism for the stroke protection observed in secondary prevention trials [16]. Also, differential effects on smooth muscle proliferation have been demonstrated ex vivo, with pravastatin having the least inhibitory effect on this mechanism [17].

Despite potential differences between statins in cardioprotective mechanisms additive to lipid control, a review of the major trial findings suggests a consistency of coronary benefit with the drugs lovastatin, pravastatin, and simvastatin. Data are fewer or unavailable so far for the so-called second generation statins (fluvastatin, atorvastatin, and cerivastatin) and newer agents. Nevertheless, lipid modification appears to be the primary mechanism for risk reduction in patients with or without stable coronary disease. Investigators are now examining the effects of statins in the acute coronary syndrome, where statin pleiotropy may be applicable to unstable atherosclerotic plaque in the acute phase of the disease. Until the results of such trials are known, the clinical significance of non-lipid-modifying effects remains speculative.

The Myocardial Ischemia Reduction with Aggressive Cholesterol Lowering (MIRACL) study has assessed the effects of atorvastatin therapy on early recurrent ischemic events in patients with either unstable angina or non-Q-wave acute MI [18]. Within 1—4 days of hospitalization for either of these conditions, patients in this double-blind study will be randomized to either atorvastatin 80 mg/day or placebo. Both treatment groups will receive dietary counseling.

A total of 3,000 patients were randomized and followed for 16 weeks. The primary outcome measure in MIRACL was the time to an ischemic event, defined as death, nonfatal acute MI, cardiac arrest with resuscitation, or recurrent symptomatic myocardial ischemia requiring emergency rehospitalization. With a sample size of approximately 1,500 per treatment group, the study has a 95% power to detect a 30% reduction in this endpoint at the 5% level of significance. The results of this study may provide important insights into the short-term effect of aggressive lipid-lowering as early intervention in acute coronary syndromes.

Two other investigations in this emerging area are being planned. The Aggrastat-to-Zocor (A-2-Z) study will randomize post-acute coronary patients to treatment first with tirofiban, unfractionated vs. low-molecular weight heparin, then re-randomize them to receive either simvastatin, 40—80 mg/day, vs. diet + simvastatin, 20 mg/day. The PRavastatin Or atorVastatin Evaluation and Infection Therapy (PROVE-IT) trial will compare pravastatin, 40 mg/day, with atorvastatin, 80 mg/day, in 4,000 post-acute coronary patients. This equivalency study will also have an antibiotic treatment arm, in order to evaluate the infection hypothesis in atherosclerosis.

Elucidating hypothetical applications and safety concerns of statin therapy

Another area that has seen some intriguing preliminary data relates to the hypothetical applications and safety concerns of statin therapy in hypertension, osteoporosis, cognitive function, and renal disease. It must be emphasized that the database for many of these effects is incomplete, and that the clinical implications of these findings remain speculative at the present time.

Statins in hypertension

Statins improve vasodilatation and endothelial dysfunction that frequently accompanies hypertension and hypercholesterolemia, possibly through their effects on nitric oxide synthesis. Glorioso et al. demonstrated a modest antihypertensive effect of pravastatin in a small study of patients with moderate hypercholesterolemia and untreated hypertension [19]. Borghi et al. observed a greater reduction of systolic and diastolic blood pressure values in patients taking antihypertensive drugs and treated for 3 months with statins when compared with other groups [20]. Furthermore, the combination of a statin with an ACE inhibitor or calcium channel blocker appeared to have a greater antihypertensive effect compared with control. The results of this study suggest that the use of statins in combination with antihypertensive drugs may improve blood pressure control in patients with uncontrolled hypertension and high serum cholesterol levels. The authors speculate that the additional blood pressure reduction observed in patients treated with statins is only partially related to the lipid-lowering effect.

Statins in osteoporosis

Osteoporosis and other diseases of bone loss are a serious public health problem. Mundy et al. demonstrated the osteogenic effect of statins in vitro and in rodents [21]. This effect was associated with increased expression of the bone morphogenetic protein-2 (BMP-2) gene in bone cells. Lovastatin and simvastatin increased bone formation when injected subcutaneously over the calvaria of mice and increased cancellous bone volume when orally administered to rats. These data suggest statins may have therapeutic applications for the treatment of osteoporosis.

Several studies have recently been published in support of this supposition. Chan et al. undertook a population-based case control study at six health maintenance organizations in the USA to investigate the relationship between statin use and fracture risk among women aged 60 years or more [22]. There were 928 cases and 2,747 controls. Compared with women who had no record of statin dispensing during the previous 2 years, women with 13 or more statin dispensings during this period had a decreased risk for nonpathological fracture (odds ratio 0.48 (95% CI 0.27—0.83)) after adjustment for age, number of hospital admissions during the previous year, chronic disease score, and use of nonstatin lipid-lowering drugs. No association was observed between fracture risk and fewer than 13 dispensings of statins or between fracture risk and use of nonstatin lipid-lowering drugs. Long-term exposure to statins therefore seemed to protect against nonpathological fracture among older women.

Meier et al. demonstrated similar effects based on data from the UK-based General Practice Research Database, comprising some 300 practices, with data collected from the late 1980s until September 1998 [23]. The investigators identified 3,940 case patients who had a bone fracture and 23,379 control patients matched for age, sex, general practice attended, calendar year, and years since enrollment in the database. After controlling for body mass index, smoking, number of physician visits, and corticosteroid and estrogen use, current use of statins was associated with a significantly reduced fracture risk (adjusted odds ratio (OR), 0.55; 95% CI, 0.44—0.69) compared with nonuse of lipid-lowering drugs. Current use of other lipid-lowering drugs was not related to a significantly decreased bone fracture risk.

These data, while promising, require confirmation in large-scale randomized trials. The Cerivastatin for Hyperlipidemia After Reaching Menopause (CHARM) study in a cohort of postmenopausal women will include the effects of this statin on osteoporosis as a study endpoint. Certainly any beneficial effect on bone formation should be considered supplementary to the primary indications of statins as anti-atherosclerotic agents or LDL-cholesterol-lowering drugs.

Statins and cognitive function

Animal research and cross-sectional studies suggest that serum lipid concentrations may influence cognitive function, mood, and behavior, and the potentially deleterious effects of cholesterol modification on psychological parameters have long been cited by critics of the lipid hypothesis. It is worth noting that none of the large statin trials have noted an appreciable difference in these kinds of endpoints (e.g., violent behavior, accidents, suicide) upon safety analysis.

However, data have been presented that suggest small but statistically significant detriments on attention and psychomotor speed tasks with lovastatin treatment [24]. In this double-blind investigation, 209 generally healthy adults with a serum LDL-cholesterol level of 160 mg/dl (4.14 mmol/l) or higher were randomly assigned to 6 months of treatment with lovastatin, 20 mg/day, or placebo. Measures of psychological well-being were not affected by lovastatin. In a study of 176 adults with elevated cholesterol (> 198 mg/dl (5.2 mmol/l)), treatment with either a low-fat or the Mediterranean diet similarly had no impact on mood or measures of cognitive function with the exception of poorer performance on a sustained attention task compared with a control group [25]. Additional studies will be required to determine the relevance of these findings.

One such trial will be the PROspective Study of Pravastatin in the Elderly at Risk (PROSPER), a randomized, double-blind, placebo-controlled trial designed to test the hypothesis that treatment with pravastatin will diminish the risk of subsequent major vascular events in a cohort of men and women (70—82 years old) with pre-existing vascular disease or significant risk of developing this condition [26]. In addition to receiving advice on diet and smoking, 5,804 men and women have been randomized equally to treatment with 40 mg pravastatin/day or a matching placebo. Following an average 3.5-year intervention period, a primary assessment will be made of the influence of this therapy on major vascular events (a combination of CHD, death, nonfatal MI, and fatal and nonfatal stroke). In addition to an assessment of disability, hospitalization or institutionalization, vascular mortality, and all-cause mortality, a key tertiary endpoint in the study will be the effects of treatment on cognitive function, which may be especially relevant for older patients.

Statins in renal disease

Ischemic heart disease is the major cause of death in dialysis patients, with 22% of cardiac deaths attributed to acute MI. In a meta-analysis of dialysis patients with acute MI, the in-hospital death rate was approximately 26% [27]. The all-cause mortality was 59% at 1 year and 73% at 2 years. The 1- and 2-year cardiac mortalities were 41 and 52%, respectively. Therefore, these patients represent an extremely high-risk group for complications of atherosclerotic disease.

Experimental and clinical studies have suggested a correlation between the progression of renal disease and dyslipidemia. Indeed, apolipoprotein-B-containing lipoproteins have been demonstrated to be an independent risk factor for the progression of renal disease in humans [28]. The effects of statins on inflammation may be relevant to treating the progression of renal disease. In addition, effects on fibrogenesis may influence not only the development of glomerulosclerosis, but also interstitial fibrosis. These potentially major effects of lipid-lowering agents appear to be related to the effects on intracellular synthesis of non-sterol isoprenoids, which are involved in prenylation of critical small molecular weight proteins involved in cell signal transduction.

The clinical impact of cerivastatin in this population will be assessed by the CHORUS trial. The objective of this study will be to determine if early intervention with cerivastatin, 0.4 mg, and usual care, or usual care alone, will reduce cardiovascular morbidity and mortality in patients with end-stage renal disease who are new to hemodialysis. The follow-up will be at least 24 months of treatment.

Conclusions: entering the 21st century

In the last 50 years, substantial progress has been made in understanding the relationship between lipid disorders and prevention of coronary disease. Clinical trials validate the modification of an unfavorable lipid profile, although implementing those findings in the clinical setting remains a challenge. Elucidating the applications of available drug therapies and expanding the groups to target for treatment is another critical goal for the future.

Also, the identification of new therapeutic targets and new lipid-modifying agents will expand treatment options. Newer statins are currently in clinical development and may prove valuable additions to the pharmacopeia [29]. Inhibitors of acyl-CoA:cholesterol acyltransferase (ACAT) might work against atherosclerosis in three different ways: first, inhibiting cholesteryl ester accumulation at arterial walls could be a direct antiatherosclerotic effect; while inhibiting cholesterol absorption inhibition at the intestine and accelerating cholesterol excretion acceleration at the liver would result in a reduction of blood cholesterol level [30]. Also, inhibitors of microsomal triglyceride transfer protein (MTP) may favorably impact blood lipid levels [31]. Finally, genetic agents, such as vascular endothelial growth factor (VEGF), that affect the vasculature or lesion directly are currently undergoing evaluation in humans [32].

While these new directions hold promise, they do not forecast a panacea, nor a replacement for the rationale that has informed clinical management of coronary risk for the last half century: namely, aggressive promotion of lifestyle therapy, risk factor modification, and reasonable application of drug therapy.

References

1. Bucher HC, Griffith LE, Guyatt GH. Systematic review on the risk and benefit of different cholesterol-lowering interventions. Arterioscl Thromb Vasc Biol 1999;19:187–195.
2. World Health Organization. WHO cooperative trial on primary prevention of ischemic heart disease with clofibrate to lower serum cholesterol: final mortality follow-up. Report of the Committee of Principal Investigators. Lancet 1984;2:600–604.
3. Huttunen JK, Heinonen OP, Manninen V, Koskinen P, Hakulinen T, Teppo L, Mänttäri M, Frick MH. The Helsinki Heart Study: an 8.5-year safety and mortality follow-up. J Intern Med 1994;235:31–39.
4. Rubins HB, Robins SJ, Collins D, Fye CL, Anderson JW, Elam MB, Faas FH, Linares E, Schaefer EJ, Schectman G, Wilt TJ, Wittes J, for the Veterans Affairs High-Density Lipoprotein Cholesterol Intervention Trial Study Group. Gemfibrozil for the secondary prevention of coronary heart disease in men with low levels of high-density lipoprotein cholesterol. N Engl J Med 1999;341:410–418.
5. The BIP Study Group. Secondary prevention by raising HDL cholesterol and reducing triglycerides in patients with coronary artery disease. The Bezafibrate Infarction Prevention (BIP) Study. Circulation 2000;102:21–27.
6. Downs JR, Clearfield M, Weis S, Whitney E, Shapiro DR, Beere PA, Langendorfer A, Stein EA, Kruyer W, Gotto AM Jr, for the AFCAPS/TexCAPS Research Group. Primary prevention of acute coronary events with lovastatin in men and women with average cholesterol levels. Results of AFCAPS/TexCAPS. JAMA 1998;279:1615–1622.
7. Pearson TA, Laurora I, Chu H, Kafonek S. The lipid treatment assessment project (L-TAP): a multicenter survey to evaluate the percentages of dyslipidemic patients receiving lipid-lowering therapy and achieving low-density lipoprotein cholesterol goals. Arch Intern Med 2000;160: 459–467.
8. Siegel D, Lopez J, Meier J. Use of cholesterol-lowering medications in the United States from 1991 to 1997. Am J Med 2000;108:496-499.
9. Feely J, McGettigan P, Kelly A. Increase in Statin Prescription Rates Following Landmark Trials. Growth in use of statins after trials is not targeted to most appropriate patients. Clin Pharmacol Ther 2000;67:438–441.
10. Sprecher DL. Where to draw the line using statins: lessons from 4S to AFCAPS/TexCAPS. Cleve Clin J Med 2000;67:169–171.
11. Prosser LA, Stinnett AA, Goldman PA, Williams LW, Hunink MG, Goldman L, Weinstein MC. Cost-effectiveness of cholesterol-lowering therapies according to selected patient characteristics. Ann Intern Med 2000;132:769–779.
12. La Rosa JC, He J, Vupputuri S. Effect of statins on risk of coronary disease: a meta-analysis of randomized controlled trials. JAMA 1999;282:2340–2346.
13. Stamler J, Daviglus ML, Garside DB, Dyer AR, Greenland P, Neaton JD. Relationship of baseline serum cholesterol levels in 3 large cohorts of younger men to long-term coronary, cardiovascular, and all-cause mortality and to longevity. JAMA 2000;284:311–318.
14. McAlister FA, Laupacis A, Wells GA, Sackett DL. Users' guides to the medical literature: XIX. Applying clinical trial results B. Guidelines for determining whether a drug is exerting (more than) a class effect. JAMA 1999;282(14):1371–1377.

15. Vaughan CJ, Gotto AM, Basson CT. The evolving role of statins in the management of atherosclerosis. J Am Coll Cardiol 2000;35:1—10.

16. Endres M, Laufs U, Huang Z, Nakamura T, Huang P, Moskowitz MA, Liao JK. Stroke protection by 3-hydroxy-3-methylglutaryl (HMG)-CoA reductase inhibitors mediated by endothelial nitric oxide synthase. Proc Natl Acad Sci USA 1998;95(15):8880—8885.

17. Negre-Aminou P, van Vliet AK, van Erck M, van Thiel GCF, van Leeuwen REW, Cohen LH. Inhibition of proliferation of human smooth muscle cells by various HMG-CoA reductase inhibitors; comparison with other human cell types. Biochim Biophys Acta 1997;1345:250—268.

18. Schwartz GC, Oliver MF, Ezekowitz MD, Ganz P, Waters D, Kane JP, Texter M, Pressler ML, Black D, Chaitman BR, Olsson AG. Rationale and design of the myocardial ischemia reduction with aggressive cholesterol lowering (MIRACL) study that evaluates atorvastatin in unstable angina pectoris and in non-Q-wave acute myocardial infarction. Am J Cardiol 1998;81:578—581.

19. Glorioso N, Troffa C, Filigheddu F, Dettori F, Soro A, Parpaglia PP, Collatina S, Pahor M. Effect of the HMG-CoA reductase inhibitors on blood pressure in patients with essential hypertension and primary hypercholesterolemia. Hypertension 1999;34:1281—1286.

20. Borghi C, Prandin MG, Costa FV, Bacchelli S, Degli Esposti D, Ambrosioni E. Effect of statins vs. diet in patients with HTN. Use of statins and blood pressure control in treated hypertensive patients with hypercholesterolemia. J Cardiovasc Pharmacol 2000;35:549—555.

21. Mundy G, Garrett R, Harris S, Chan J, Chen D, Rossini G, Boyce B, Zhao M, Gutierrez G. Simvastatin increases in vitro bone formation in mice murine calvaria. Science 1999;286:1946—1949.

22. Chan KA, Andrade SE, Boles M, Buist DS, Chase GA, Donahue JG, Goodman MJ, Gurwitz JH, La Croix AZ, Platt R. Inhibitors of hydroxymethylglutaryl-coenzyme A reductase and risk of fracture among older women. Lancet 2000;355:2185—2188.

23. Meier CR, Schlienger RG, Kraenzlin ME, Schlegel B, Jick H. HMG-CoA reductase inhibitors and the risk of fractures. JAMA 2000;283:3205—3210.

24. Muldoon MF, Barger SD, Ryan CM, Flory JD, Lehoczky JP, Matthews KA, Manuck SB. Effects of lovastatin on cognitive function and psychological well. Am J Med 2000;108:538—547.

25. Wardle J, Rogers P, Judd P, Taylor MA, Rapoport L, Green M, Nicholson Perry K. Randomized trial of the effects of cholesterol-lowering dietary treatment on psychological function. Am J Med 2000;108:547—553.

26. Shepherd J, Blauw GJ, Murphy MB, Cobbe SM, Bollen EL, Buckley BM, Ford I, Jukema JW, Hyland M, Gaw A, Lagaay AM, Perry IJ, Macfarlane PW, Meinders AE, Sweeney BJ, Packard CJ, Westendorp RG, Twomey C, Stott DJ. The design of a PROspective Study of Pravastatin in the Elderly at Risk (PROSPER). PROSPER Study Group. PROspective Study of Pravastatin in the Elderly at Risk. Am J Cardiol 1999;84:1192—1197.

27. Herzog CA. Acute myocardial infarction in patients with end-stage renal disease. Kidney Int 1999;56(Suppl 71):S130—S133.

28. Oda H, Keane WF. Recent advances in statins and the kidney. Kidney Int 1999;56(Suppl 71): S2—S5.

29. Suzuki H, Aoki T, Tamaki T, Sato F, Kitahara M, Saito Y. Hypolipidemic effect of NK-104, a potent HMG-CoA reductase inhibitor, in guinea pigs. Atherosclerosis 1999;146(2):259—270.

30. Lee HT, Roark WH, Picard JA, Sliskovic DR, Roth BD, Stanfield RL, Hamelehle KL, Bousley RF, Krause BR. Inhibitors of acyl-CoA:cholesterol O-acyltransferase (ACAT) as hypocholesterolemic agents: synthesis and structure-activity relationships of novel series of sulfonamides, acylphosphonamides and acylphosphoramidates. Bioorg Med Chem Lett 1998;8:289—294.

31. Pan M, Liang Js, Fisher EA, Ginsberg HN. Inhibition of translocation of nascent apolipoprotein B across the endoplasmic reticulum membrane is associated with selective inhibition of the synthesis of apolipoprotein B. J Biol Chem 2000;275:27399—27405.

32. Rosengart TK, Lee LY, Patel SR, Sanborn TA, Parikh M, Bergman GW, Hachamovitch R, Szulc M, Kligfield PD, Okin PM, Hahn RT, Devereux RB, Post MR, Hackett NR, Foster T, Grasso

TM, Lesser ML, Isom OW, Crystal RG. Angiogenesis gene therapy: phase I assessment of direct intramyocardial administration of an adenovirus vector expressing VEGF121 cDNA to individuals with clinically significant severe coronary artery disease. Circulation 1999;100(5):468–474.

© 2000 Elsevier Science B.V. All rights reserved.
Atherosclerosis XII.
S. Stemme and A.G. Olsson, editors.

Epidemiology and mechanisms of atherosclerosis: bringing the perspectives together

Michael Marmot
International Centre for Health and Society, University College London, UK

Keywords: coronary heart disease, mortality, pathophysiology, psychosocial, socioeconomic.

Research on the mechanisms of atherosclerosis and on the distribution of heart disease in populations has proceeded with little common regard. Atherosclerosis research has moved swiftly into the molecular age and advances in the understanding of pathogenetic mechanisms have been rapid and dramatic. If there has been any meeting at all between this research and epidemiology, it has been around risk factors. To put it simply, epidemiology has shown that plasma cholesterol is important as a risk factor for coronary heart disease; atherosclerosis research has suggested mechanisms to explain why it might be important.

It is important for a molecular approach to cardiovascular disease to attempt to understand why there have been major changes in the occurrence rate of coronary heart disease. Conversely, a population approach to cardiovascular disease would benefit greatly from understanding the pathogenetic mechanisms that underlie shifts in the rate of occurrence of disease. To be more specific we have been concerned both with socioeconomic differences in the rate of occurrence of cardiovascular disease within countries and contrasts between countries in time trends in cardiovascular disease.

In this lecture, I propose to focus on these two problems: the social gradient in cardiovascular mortality within countries and east-west differences across Europe in coronary heart disease; to present a simple model of how social and economic factors might be responsible for the occurrence of coronary heart disease; and to present a small amount of data on how these pathways might affect biological factors.

The social gradient

For more than 20 years, we have been reporting on the social distribution of deaths from cardiovascular and other diseases among British civil servants — the Whitehall study [1—5]. We first reported in the 1970s that coronary heart dis-

---

Address for correspondence: Prof Michael Marmot, International Centre for Health and Society, University College London, 1—19 Torrington Place, London WC1E 6BT, UK. Tel.: +44-207-679-1717. Fax: +44-207-813-0240. E-mail: M.Marmot@public-health.ucl.ac.uk

ease mortality followed an inverse social gradient: the lower the status in the employment grade hierarchy, the higher the mortality [1]. At that time, conventional wisdom had it that heart disease was a disease of affluence and that our finding that appeared to challenge the orthodoxy was either wrong or that British civil servants were somehow atypical. We showed that there had been a change in the social distribution of heart disease in England and Wales from being more common in higher social classes to being more common in lower [6]. Subsequently, heart disease mortality in England and Wales has declined to a greater extent in higher than in lower social classes, thus leading to a steepening of the social gradient [7,8]. Similar changes appear to have taken place in other countries [9,10].

The patterns we observed after 10 years of follow-up [2] have persisted after 25 years [4]. Table 1 shows mortality from all causes and from coronary heart disease according to employment grade at entry to the study [5]. It shows clearly that the slope of the gradient linking employment grade to coronary heart disease is in evidence after 25 years of follow-up and is similar for coronary heart disease and all-cause mortality. Not shown here is the fact that the social gradient is similar for many of the major causes of death [5]. This latter finding, the fact that the gradient cuts across major causes of death, suggests that we have to look beyond risk factors for specific diseases to understand causal processes.

This is illustrated further in the last column of Table 1. Here the rate ratios comparing the lowest with the highest grade have been adjusted for age, smoking, systolic blood pressure, plasma cholesterol concentration and glucose intolerance. For coronary heart disease, adjusting for these major risk factors has reduced the rate ratio in the lowest compared to the highest grade from 1.77 to 1.52; for all causes the reduction has been from 2.07 to 1.75. It may be objected that adjusting for risk factors measured at baseline is an inadequate way to summarise their effect over a 25-year period. We therefore examined the social gradient in mortality in the subgroup of the population (approximately 13%) who were nonsmokers with low plasma cholesterol, and low blood pressure. In this low risk group the rate ratios for lowest vs. highest employment grade was 2.3 for all causes and 2.61 for ischaemic heart disease. This makes it clear that factors other than these risk factors are responsible for the social gradient. It should be emphasised that this does not mean that these other risk factors are unimportant. The figures for lung cancer make this point clearly. The last column of Table 1 suggests that adjusting for smoking did not abolish the social gradient in lung cancer mortality. However, smoking was overwhelmingly the major risk factor for lung cancer, as only 5% of lung cancer deaths occurred in nonsmokers who had never smoked. The figures for ischaemic heart disease are less dramatic than for lung cancer. Nevertheless, the importance of these major risk factors in Whitehall is shown by the fact that only 6% of the ischaemic heart disease deaths occurred in the 13% of the population who were classified as low risk.

Table 1. Age-adjusted mortality rates by employment grade and mortality rate ratios for "other" grade vs. administrative[a] adjusted for age, and risk factors, for the whole population.

Causes of death (ICD-8)	Mortality rates (number of deaths)				Mortality rate ratio (95% CI), "other" grade vs. administrative[a]	Whole population (n = 18001) Mortality rate ratio (95% CI) adjusted for age and risk factors[b], "other" grade vs. administrative
	Administrative (n = 962)	Professional/ executive (n = 12269)	Clerical (n = 2981)	Other (n = 1789)		
All causes	16.76 (295)	20.74 (4733)	27.43 (1779)	30.91 (1246)	2.07 (1.90, 2.25)	1.75 (1.60, 1.91)
Malignant neoplasm of lung (162.1)	0.76 (16)	1.53 (358)	2.80 (181)	3.28 (147)	4.08 (3.10, 5.38)	2.75 (2.09, 3.63)
Other neoplasms (140—239 excl. 162.1)	4.00 (72)	4.57 (1088)	4.94 (313)	5.53 (207)	1.43 (1.17, 1.74)	1.36 (1.11, 1.66)
Ischaemic heart disease (410—414)	6.41 (105)	7.29 (1679)	9.10 (583)	10.07 (394)	1.77 (1.53, 2.06)	1.52 (1.24, 1.86)
Cerebrovascular disease (430—438)	1.43 (26)	1.79 (380)	2.12 (144)	1.81 (81)	1.35 (0.99, 1.85)	1.11 (0.81, 1.53)
Other cardiovascular (390—404,420—429,440—458)	1.18 (23)	1.73 (385)	2.42 (160)	2.38 (104)	2.13 (1.59, 2.86)	1.66 (1.23, 2.24)
Chronic bronchitis (491—492)	0.10 (2)	0.23 (44)	0.77 (51)	1.14 (48)	10.76 (5.96, 19.42)	6.53 (3.59, 11.87)
Other respiratory disease (460—490,493—519)	1.10 (20)	1.59 (337)	2.82 (192)	3.68 (155)	4.13 (3.15, 5.43)	2.98 (2.26, 3.93)
Gastrointestinal disease (520—577)	0.66 (8)	0.41 (94)	0.54 (37)	0.88 (30)	2.42 (1.35, 4.36)	1.93 (1.07, 3.49)
Genitourinary disease (580—607)	0.25 (4)	0.26 (53)	0.31 (20)	0.51 (25)	3.27 (1.59, 6.71)	2.61 (1.25, 5.46)
Accident and violence (800—949,960—978)	0.13 (3)	0.20 (51)	0.28 (16)	0.36 (11)	2.38 (0.98, 5.78)	2.47 (1.00, 6.10)
Suicide (950—958,980—989)	0.10 (2)	0.17 (45)	0.25 (15)	0.21 (6)	1.65 (0.60, 4.50)	1.20 (0.43, 3.37)
Other deaths	0.57 (11)	0.93 (207)	1.05 (63)	0.97 (36)	1.43 (0.91, 2.24)	1.24 (0.78, 1.97)

[a]Based on exponent of three times the coefficient of employment grade assessed with Cox proportional hazards models in which employment grade was added as a continuous variable (values 1,2,3,4). [b]Adjusted for age, smoking, systolic blood pressure, plasma cholesterol concentration and glucose intolerance.

East-west differences in heart disease: socioeconomic differences between countries

There has been much recent interest in the widening east-west gap in mortality across Europe. Cardiovascular disease is responsible for about one-half of the gap in mortality between the countries of central and eastern Europe and those of "the west" [11].

One way of illustrating these trends therefore is to look at life expectancy at age 15. This is shown in Fig. 1 for males and illustrates the increasing gap that developed over the 1970s and 1980s and, in the case of the former Soviet Union, widened in the early 1990s. In women, there was no decline in life expectancy, as was true in some countries among men, but there was, similarly, a widening east-west gap.

Given the social and economic differences between east and west before the cataclysmic political changes that began in 1989, and the diverging economic fortunes of central and eastern European countries after 1989, it is reasonable to wonder if these are important in generating the changes in coronary and other diseases. Figure 2 plots changes in mortality between 1989 and 1996 against changes in Gross Domestic Product (GDP) over the same period. In the Ukraine and Russia, where GDP in 1996 was 60% or less of the 1989 level, mortality rates among middle age men had increased by 60%. In Poland and the Czech Republic, two countries that had negligible change in their GDP, there was little overall change in mortality during this period. Hungary and Belarus, that had intermediate declines in GDP, had a clear rise in mortality, but not to the extent of Russia and Ukraine.

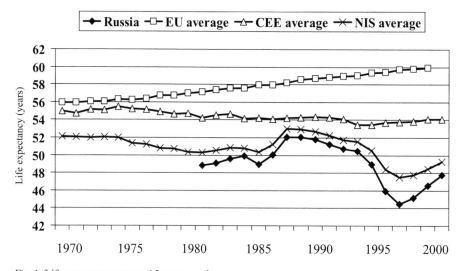

Fig. 1. Life expectancy at age 15 years, males.

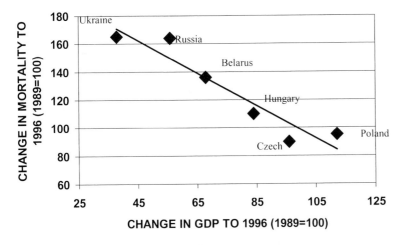

Fig. 2. Changes in mortality, men 40–49 years.

A model linking social and economic factors to pathogenesis and disease

The hypothesis developed from these two areas of research is that social and economic forces are crucial in determining the social gradient in disease within countries and the dramatic changes that have occurred among European countries. We have developed a simple model to guide the research which is illustrated in Fig. 3. It aims not to be comprehensive but to illustrate the pathways by which

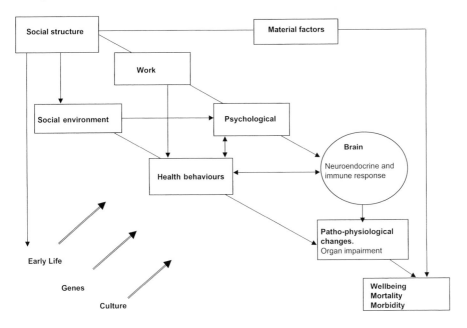

Fig. 3. Social determinants of health [28].

social and economic forces might operate to influence the occurrence of coronary heart disease, other diseases and general functioning.

Our research centre has been aiming to fill in pieces of this model, not in one grand research design but in targeted studies. There is a large body of work on the importance of behaviours to coronary heart disease occurrence. Patterns of diet, exercise, smoking and drinking may all be related to cardiovascular risk. What this model attempts to show is that these patterns of behaviour are affected by social and economic circumstances. Many of them now show a social gradient. In the Whitehall study, smoking, lack of physical activity in leisure time and moderate drinking were all socially patterned in a way that favoured people according to their place in the hierarchy: healthier patterns the higher the position. Interestingly, dietary fat intake did not differ by social position and there was no social gradient in plasma total cholesterol.

An important question therefore is the degree to which these behaviours account for the social gradient in disease. As shown in Table 1, they do make a contribution, but that contribution is limited.

The model shows that the social structure can, of course, begin to exert its effect from the earliest period of life. Barker's work has pointed to the possibility that the intrauterine environment can affect subsequent cardiovascular disease risk when the fetus becomes an adult. He has shown that low birth weight, or other features of the newborn, relate to risk of cardiovascular disease and diabetes during subsequent adult life [12]. Given the marked social distribution of infant mortality and low birth weight, it is possible that some of the effects of social position can originate early in life [13].

The genome does not make a strong appearance in this model, as it is not the primary focus of research that seeks to understand the reason behind rapidly changing patterns of distribution of disease. Nevertheless, environmental factors, including those with origin in the social environment, are likely to have differential impact on individuals according to their genetic make-up. Hence, exploration of gene environment interactions may be instructive.

It has been suggested that genetic differences may account for social position [14] and hence for social class differences in disease rates. Characteristics of individuals that lead to upward social mobility will, like most other human characteristics, be determined by a mixture of genes and environment. Many of the social changes in society, however, are determined by structural changes in our society. In Britain, for example, the huge decline in blue collar manufacturing jobs and more or less equal increase in white collar service jobs has had little to do with the changing characteristics of individuals. Were it the case that individuals' positions in the social hierarchy was strongly influenced by genetic endowment, it does not follow that this genetic endowment is responsible for the socioeconomic differences in disease rates. There is evidence that features of the environment in which people live and work may play an important role in generating observed social patterning of disease occurrence.

If the standard coronary risk factors account for a small part of the social gradient in cardiovascular disease, what accounts for the rest? There may be factors operating right through the lifecourse [15]. One set of hypotheses that we have been pursuing is that psychosocial factors, acting in adult life, are related to cardiovascular disease and may make important contributions both to the social gradient within countries and the east-west differences across Europe.

It is worth drawing attention to the fact that psychosocial factors, that are the result of the circumstances in which people live and work, may affect cardiovascular disease through the mechanism of health behaviours such as smoking, eating, physical activity and drinking, or directly through the brain and its effect on the neuroendocrine system.

We are in the process of summarising a full account of where we have reached in our understanding of these pathways but for the present purpose, I will illustrate with data on parts of the model.

Psychosocial work environment

A body of research has pointed to the importance of the psychosocial work environment in cardiovascular disease [16]. Early work in this area focussed on "stress" in the workplace. This had the disadvantage of difficulty in definition. Two dominant models have emerged from a large body of research in this area, the demand/control or job strain model, and the effort-reward imbalance model. The first posits that it is a combination of high psychological demand and low control in the workplace that leads to increased cardiovascular risk. Some studies show support for the full model; others support the importance of low control. This is the case for the Whitehall II study of civil servants.

Figure 4 shows the relationship between control and coronary heart disease incidence over a 5-year period in the Whitehall II study, and shows that the lower

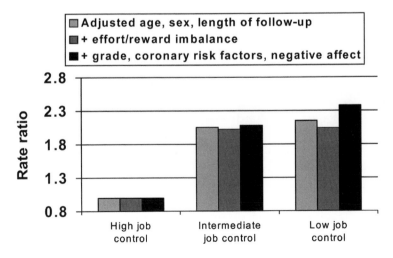

Fig. 4. Self-reported job control and CHD incidence — the Whitehall II study, men and women [18].

the degree of control the higher the subsequent incidence of coronary heart disease [17]. The second bar shows that the relationship between low control and coronary heart disease is independent of effort reward imbalance (see below). The third bar shows that the relationship is independent of the standard coronary risk factors and negative affect as a measure of general tendency to complain.

We have also shown that imbalance between efforts and rewards, i.e., high effort in the presence of inadequate reward, is associated with an increased risk of coronary heart disease independent of low control [18].

Figure 5 shows data from a case control study in a community sample in the Czech Republic [19]. For this study, we took the Whitehall questions on work and translated them into Czech. As in Whitehall II, high demand, here measured by high pace of work, was not associated with increased risk; the relationship may even have gone in the other direction. As in Whitehall II and most other studies, low control was associated with increased risk of myocardial infarction.

We have shown that a combination of low control in the workplace, high levels of smoking and some other coronary risk factors appear to account for a major part of the social gradient in coronary heart disease.

Social environment outside work

The Whitehall II study has been investigating social gradients in cardiovascular disease in a working population. As shown above, it has produced evidence on the importance of psychosocial work characteristics. Two comments are relevant here. First, although in Whitehall II social position is defined on the basis of position in the occupational hierarchy, factors other than those in the workplace may be important. Second, there is a social gradient in cardiovascular disease in people who are not working in the formal labour market: housewives, unem-

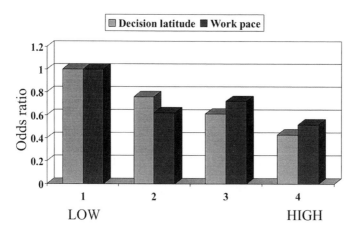

Fig. 5. Control, pace and MI in men — Czech case control study. Adjusted for age, district, education, smoking, waist/hip ratio, blood pressure, cholesterol, diabetes [19].

ployed and retired.

Wilkinson has argued that features of the social environment that correlate with income inequality are related to mortality rates [20]. This body of work will not be reviewed here. There is a separate corpus of research showing that low levels of social supports are, importantly, related to mortality rates [21]. It has long been recognised that single men have higher rates of morbidity and mortality than married men. Among the hypotheses that could account for this observation is that single men have less support. In several central and east European countries the disadvantage of higher mortality among single compared to married increased [22–24]. In Hungary for example, the increase in mortality that occurred in the 1980s was most marked in single men, thus increasing their health disadvantage. This apparent disadvantage of being single at a time of great social change requires explanation.

Pathophysiology

In searching for links between the social environment and risk of cardiovascular disease, the obvious avenues to explore first are those relating to established risk factors. As already indicated, in the Whitehall studies plasma cholesterol level offered little prospect for explaining the social gradient. In the first Whitehall study, plasma cholesterol levels were marginally higher in higher employment grades [1]. In the second Whitehall study, conducted 20 years after the first, there was no difference in plasma total cholesterol according to social position [25].

Many studies have shown a social gradient in blood pressure levels [26]. In Whitehall I, blood pressure levels were higher in low grades, although this was not the case in Whitehall II [25]. It may be that clinic blood pressure is too limited a way to examine blood pressures. Certainly there is evidence that blood pressure measured outside the clinical setting is related to psychosocial characteristics [27].

We have been particularly interested in three other biological measures: plasma fibrinogen level, the metabolic syndrome, and von Willebrand's factor. As shown in Fig. 6, plasma fibrinogen and the components of the metabolic syndrome all show a social gradient. For men, there is little exception to the pattern of lower status higher level of risk, and all the trends are statistically significant. Although the picture is similar in women, there is a suggestion that the highest grade women may be less protected than those immediately below them in the hierarchy. This requires further investigation. It is possible that both the hypothalamic pituitary adrenal axis and the sympathetic nervous system are involved in generating this social gradient in the metabolic syndrome [28].

The social gradient in plasma fibrinogen level may be important for different reasons. First, plasma fibrinogen is involved in the haemostatic system and has been shown to be a predictor of cardiovascular disease [29]. Second, plasma fibrinogen may be of interest because it is part of the acute phase reaction. Given the interest in infection and inflammation as possibly contributing to coronary

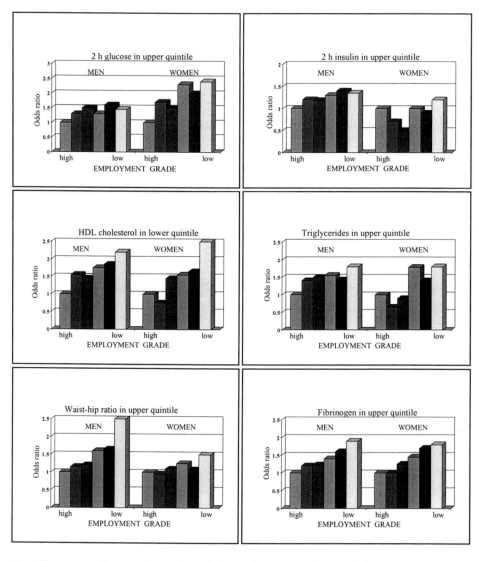

Fig. 6. Prevalence of adverse levels of metabolic syndrome variables and fibrinogen by employment grade in the Whitehall II study. Adjusted for age and, in women, menopausal status [28].

heart disease [30], the demonstration that an acute phase protein follows a social gradient and may be related both to psychosocial factors and influences from early life suggests that the link between social processes and inflammation needs to be explored. This has been done well for the common cold [31].

We examined von Willebrand's factor as a possible marker of endothelial dysfunction. It too showed a clear social gradient [32]. This suggests a further avenue for research: factors affecting endothelial dysfunction.

The focus of this lecture has been on social and economic factors in the occurrence of coronary heart disease. As the model presented in Fig. 3 allows, there may also be important cultural differences. We have also been interested in the observation that in Britain immigrants from the Indian subcontinent (South Asians) have higher mortality from coronary heart disease than the English average [33]. Immigrants from the Caribbean have lower than average ischaemic heart disease mortality. Figure 7 shows that South Asian men compared to white men have lower levels of hdl cholesterol and higher levels of glucose intolerance and fasting insulin [34,35]. By contrast, Afro-Caribbeans, although having a high prevalence of diabetes, do not have adverse patterns of these metabolic factors [35,36].

Avenues for research

I wish to finish with the same two problems with which I began. There is a need to adapt the understanding of pathophysiological processes in atherosclerosis to account for observed patterns of occurrence of cardiovascular disease in populations. How does new knowledge of atherosclerosis help us to understand variations in disease according to time, place, and person?

Conversely, those of us concerned with the population patterns of disease and, in particular, how social and economic factors influences its rate of occurrence, need to understand how these factors affect the biology of cardiovascular disease. This is part of a fuller aetiological understanding. We are pursuing a model that loosely relates psychosocial factors to the operation of the hypothalamic pituitary adrenal system and the sympathetic nervous system. These, in turn, may be related to metabolic changes and hence, through atherosclerosis and thrombosis, to disease. The evidence for this is suggestive rather than definitive. There may, of course, be other pathways involved.

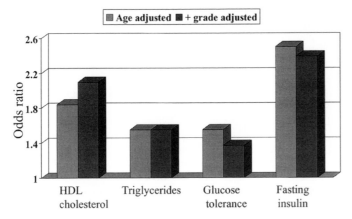

Fig. 7. Biochemical risk factors* for South Asian men (compared to white men) [35]. *Odds ratio of being in adverse quartile.

136

Acknowledgements

This work is supported by an MRC Research Professorship and by the John D. and Catherine T. Macarthur Foundation Research Network on Socioeconomic Status and Health.

References

1. Marmot MG, Rose G, Shipley M, Hamilton PJS. Employment grade and coronary heart disease in British civil servants. J Epidemiol Commun Health 1978;32:244–249.
2. Marmot MG, Shipley MJ, Rose G. Inequalities in death — specific explanations of a general pattern. Lancet 1984;1:1003–1006.
3. Marmot M, Davey Smith G. Socioeconomic differences in health: the contribution of the Whitehall studies. J Health Psychol 1997; 2(3):283–296.
4. Marmot MG, Shipley MJ. Do socioeconomic differences in mortality persist after retirement? 25-year follow-up of civil servants from the first Whitehall study. Br Med J 1996;313:1177–1180.
5. Van Rossum C, Shipley M, Van de Mheen H, Grobbee D, Marmot MG. Employment grade differences in cause specific mortality. 25-year follow-up of civil servants from the first Whitehall study. J Epidemiol Commun Health 2000;54:178–184.
6. Marmot MG, Adelstein AM, Robinson N, Rose G. The changing social class distribution of heart disease. Br Med J 1978;2:1109–1112.
7. Drever F, Whitehead M. Health Inequalities: Decennial Supplement. Series DS No.15, 1–257. London: The Stationery Office, Office for National Statistics, 1997.
8. Independent Inquiry into Inequalities in Health Report. 1–164. London: The Stationery Office, 1998.
9. Kunst AE, Looman CWN, Mackenbach JP. Socioeconomic mortality differences in the Netherlands in 1950–1984: a regional study of cause specific mortality. Soc Sci Med 1990;31:141–152.
10. Pappas G, Queen S, Hadden W, Fisher G. The increasing disparity in mortality between socioeconomic groups in the United States, 1960 and 1986. N Engl J Med 1993;329:103–109.
11. Bobak M, Marmot MG. East-West mortality divide and its potential explanations: proposed research agenda. Br Med J 1996;312:421–425.
12. Barker DJ. The Fetal and Infant Origins of Adult Disease. London: BMJ Books, 1992.
13. Davey Smith G, Hart CL, Blane D, Hole DJ. Adverse socioeconomic conditions in childhood and cause specific adult mortality: prospective observational study. Br Med J 1998;316:1631–1635.
14. Hernstein RJ, Murray C. The Bell Curve: Intelligence and Class Structure in American Life. New York: Simon & Shuster Inc., 1994.
15. Kuh D, Ben-Shlomo Y. A Life Course Approach to Chronic Disease Epidemiology. Oxford: Oxford University Press, 1997.
16. Hemingway H, Marmot M. Psychosocial factors in the aetiology and prognosis of coronary heart disease: systematic review of prospective cohort studies. BMJ 1999;318(7196):1460–1467.
17. Bosma H, Marmot MG, Hemingway H, Nicholson A, Brunner EJ, Stansfeld S. Low job control and risk of coronary heart disease in the Whitehall II (prospective cohort) study. Br Med J 1997;314:558–565.
18. Bosma H, Peter R, Siegrist J, Marmot MG. Alternative job stress models and the risk of coronary heart disease. Am J Public Health 1998;88:68–74.
19. Bobak M, Hertzman C, Skodova Z, Marmot M. Association between psychosocial factors at work and non-fatal myocardial infarction in a population based case-control study in Czech

men. Epidemiol 1998;9:43—47.

20. Wilkinson RG. Unhealthy Societies: The Afflictions of Inequality. London: Routledge, 1996.
21. Stansfeld SA. Social support and social cohesion. In: Marmot MG, Wilkinson R (eds) Social Determinants of Health. Oxford: Oxford University Press, 1999;155–178.
22. Watson P. Explaining rising mortality among men in Eastern Europe. Soc Sci Med 1995;41: 923—934.
23. Blazek J, Dzurowa D. The decline of mortality in the Czech Republic during the transition: a counterfactual case study. In: Cornia GA, Paniccia R (eds) The Mortality Crisis in Transitional Economies. Oxford: Oxford University Press, 2000;303–327.
24. Hajdu P, McKee M, Bojan F. Changes in premature mortality differentials by marital status in Hungary and in England and Wales. Eur J Pub Health 1995;5:259—264.
25. Marmot MG, Davey Smith G, Stansfeld SA, Patel C, North F, Head J et al. Health inequalities among British civil servants: the Whitehall II study. Lancet 1991;337:1387—1393.
26. Colhoun H, Hemingway H, Poulter NR. Socioeconomic status and blood pressure: an overview analysis. J Hum Hypertens 1998;12:91—110.
27. Steptoe A, Cropley M, Griffith J, Joekes K. The influence of abdominal obesity and chronic work stress on ambulatory blood pressure in men and women. Int J Obes 1999;23:1184—1191.
28. Brunner EJ, Marmot MG. Social organisation, stress and health. In: Marmot MG, Wilkinson RG (eds) Social Determinants of Health. Oxford: Oxford University Press, 1999;17–43.
29. Meade TW, Ruddock V, Stirling Y, Chakrabarti R, Miller GJ. Fibrinolytic activity, clotting factors, and long-term incidence of ischaemic heart disease in the Northwick Park Heart Study. Lancet 1993;342:1076—1079.
30. Danesh J, Whincup P, Walker M, Lennon L, Thomson A, Appleby P et al. Low grade inflammation and coronary heart disease: prospective study and updated meta-analyses. Br Med J 2000;321:199—204.
31. Cohen S, Doyle WJ, Skoner DP, Rabin BS, Gwaltney JM. Social ties and susceptibility to the common cold. J Am Med Ass 1997;277:1940—1944.
32. Kumari M, Marmot M, Brunner E. Social determinants of von Willebrand factor. Arterioscl Thromb Vasc Biol (In press).
33. Marmot MG, Adelstein AM, Bulusu L. Lessons from the study of immigrant mortality. Lancet 1984;1:1455—1458.
34. McKeigue PM, Pierpoint T, Ferrie JE, Marmot MG. Relationship of glucose intolerance and hyperinsulinaemia to body fat pattern in South Asians and Europeans. Diabetologia 1992;35: 785—791.
35. Whitty CJM, Brunner EJ, Shipley MJ, Hemingway H, Marmot MG. Differences in biological risk factors for cardiovascular disease between three ethnic groups in the Whitehall II study. Atherosclerosis 1999;142(2):279—286.
36. Chaturvedi N, McKeigue PM, Marmot MG. Relationship of glucose intolerance to coronary risk in Afro-Caribbeans compared with Europeans. Diabetologia 1994;37:765—772.

Workshop abstracts

Diabetes

Why is the protection provided by female gender wiped out in diabetes

B.V. Howard. *MedStar Research Institute, Wash., DC, USA*

Diabetes has been shown to be a significant independent risk factor for cardiovascular disease (CVD), especially in women. Review of population data reveals that the prevalence of type 2 diabetes is higher in women and it increases the risk of CVD in women to a greater extent than in men. The dyslipidemia characteristic of diabetes, hypertension and other adverse changes in CVD risk factors have been shown to play a major role in the development of CVD in individuals with diabetes. More adverse changes in several CVD risk factor occur in diabetic women; mechanisms for this may include the insulin resistance that accompanies type 2 diabetes, and diabetes-associated changes in sex hormones. These findings highlight the need for increased attention to CVD risk factors in the care of diabetic women and for further research into the mechanisms of the accelerated atherosclerosis in diabetes.

Vascular effects of insulin

Hannele Yki-Järvinen. *Department of Medicine, University of Helsinki, Helsinki, Finland*

Insulin resistance has been associated with the development of cardiovascular disease and hypertension but the mechanisms are poorly understood. In vivo in normal subjects, insulin regulates vascular function at multiple sites. In peripheral resistance vessels, insulin acts as a slow vasodilatator via a mechanism, which can be abolished by inhibiting nitric oxide synthesis, and is masked by sympathetic vasoconstrictor tone. Defects in insulin action on peripheral vasodilatation have been described in various insulin resistant states. These defects have, however, been observed at supra- rather than physiological insulin concentrations or after prolonged infusions of insulin, which make them unlikely to contribute to hemodynamic alterations such as increased peripheral vascular resistance and diastolic blood pressure in insulin resistant individuals. Another recently described action of insulin involves acute insulin induced decreases in arterial stiffness in pre-resistance vessels in normal subjects. This action of insulin is observed at physiological insulin concentrations within 30 min. A defect in insulin regulation of arterial stiffness characterizes insulin resistant individuals including those with insulin resistance secondary to obesity or chronic hyperglycemia. The ability of insulin to diminish stiffness is also blunted in insulin resistant subjects with untreated essential hypertension. The inability of insulin to decrease stiffness increases augmentation i.e. the pressure difference between the second and first systolic peak of the aortic pressure wave and thereby increases pre-load and decreases diastolic filling of the left ventricle. The mechanisms underlying these changes in humans remain unknown due to the inaccessibility of pre-resistance arteries. Taken together these data demonstrate the existence of resistance to insulin's antiatherogenic actions in arteries greater than those controlling peripheral vascular resistance.

Plasminogen activator inhibitor type 1: Influence of metabolic factors and pharmacological control

E. Tremoli, C. Banfi, L. Sironi, L. Mussoni. *Institute of Pharmacological Sciences, University of Milan, Milan, Italy*

PAI-1 is a glycoprotein synthesized by cells of the vessel wall, adipose tissue and hepatocytes. Both environmental and genetic factors are involved in the biosynthesis of this glycoprotein. Recent data have demonstrated a crucial role of metabolic variables such as insulin and/or insulin resistance, obesity, triglycerides and blood pressure as determinants of circulating PAI-1 in healthy and diseased subjects, thus suggesting a link between the insulin resistance syndrome and fibrinolytic system. In support of this, in vitro studies have demonstrated that insulin and triglycerides stimulate PAI-1 biosynthesis by cultured endothelial and hepatic cells. Moreover, insulin and triglycerides, either directly or through an effect mediated by long-chain fatty acids act synergistically in inducing PAI-1 synthesis in these cells. Angiotensin II has also been shown to upregulate PAI-1 biosynthesis in human endothelial and smooth muscle cells. The mechanisms by which these metabolic factors influence PAI-1 have been recently elucidated and involve the activation of a complex network of signalling pathways leading to the activation of the MAP kinase cascade. The knowledge of the mechanisms involved in PAI-1 biosynthesis is of particular importance for the development of specific therapeutic strategies to decrease the cardiovascular risk in these patients. At present, triglyceride lowering drugs, statins, angiotensin converting enzyme inhibitors and/or angiotensin receptor type 1 inhibitors are under evaluation also for their potential effects in controlling PAI-1 biosynthesis.

The atherogenic dyslipidemia of visceral obesity

J.P. Després. *Québec Heart Institute, Lipid Research Center, Laval University, Sainte-Foy, Canada*

Studies published over the last 20 years have emphasized the role of body fat distribution, especially of visceral adipose tissue accumulation as a critical correlate of metabolic abnormalities that were in the past associated with excess fatness per se. Thus, excess visceral adipose tissue accumulation, which can be assessed by imaging techniques such as computed tomography, has been associated with hyperinsulinemia, insulin resistance, glucose intolerance which may lead to NIDDM among genetically susceptible individuals, hypertriglyceridemia, elevated LDL particle concentration, increased proportion of small-dense LDL and HDL particles and reduced plasma HDL cholesterol concentrations leading to a substantial increase in the cholesterol/HDL-cholesterol ratio. Results of the prospective Québec Cardiovascular Study have emphasized that this cluster of metabolic abnormalities is associated with a substantial increase in the risk of coronary heart disease (CHD). As most visceral obese patients have rather "normal" cholesterol levels, it is suggested that CHD risk in these individuals should be assessed, in addition to conventional risk variables, by a triad of metabolic abnormalities which include hyperinsulinemia, hyperapo B and small-dense LDL particles. We have also developed a low cost screening approach where a high proportion of visceral obese individuals with the insulin resistance dyslipidemic syndrome could be identified. We have reported that more than 80% of men with waist circumference values above 90 cm and with fasting triglyceride levels above 2.0 mmol/l were characterized by the atherogenic metabolic triad (hyperinsulinemia, elevated apo B and small dense LDL phenotype). It is proposed that simple and inexpensive variables such as the waist circumference and fasting triglyceride levels may be helpful markers for the screening of high risk patients.

Postprandial hyperglycemia is a risk factor for cardiovascular death in newly diagnosed type 2 diabetes: The Diabetes Intervention Study (DIS)

M. Hanefeld[1], U. Julius[1], H. Schmechel[2], U. Schwanebeck[1]. *[1]Medical Faculty C.G. Carus Dresden; [2]Weimar, Germany*

Objective: Prospective studies have consistently shown that the risk of myocardial infarction (MI) and cardiovascular death (CD) in type 2 diabetes is 2–4 fold higher than in non-diabetic subjects matched for major risk factors. We therefore analysed the importance of fasting and postprandial blood glucose (ppBG) on the incidence of MI and CD.

Methods: 1139 newly diagnosed type 2 diabetics classified as diet controlled without other severe diseases. Follow-up time $\geqslant 11$ years. BG was measured after 4 weeks on diet before and one hour after breakfast, major risk factors were recorded under standard conditions. Statistics: Cox regression analysis and cumulative incidence stratified by gender and categories of quality of risk factor control according to NIDDM Policy criteria.

Results: 11 year follow-up data were available for 828 patients of which 71 (8.6%) died from CD. In multivariate analysis age, blood pressure, triglycerides and smoking were independent risk factors for MI and age, male sex, ppBG, triglycerides and blood pressure for CD resp. In Cox regression analysis comparing categories of quality control of risk factors smoking (relative risk (RR) vs. non-smokers 1.51), ppBG (RR poor vs. good control 2.09) and blood pressure (RR poor vs. good control 2.2) for subsequent MI and smoking (RR 1.65) poor ppBG (RR 2.24), poor blood pressure (RR 3.23) and poor triglycerides (RR 2.18) for CD resp. were of significant importance. PpBG was a stronger predictor in females than males.

Conclusions: Our data show that pp hyperglycemia is an independent risk factor for coronary heart disease in type 2 diabetes which could substantially add to the excessive cardiovascular mortality in these patients.

Chylomicron remnant kinetics in post-menopausal women with and without diabetes

P.H.R. Barrett[1], D. Chan[1], C. Dane-Stewart[1], B. Stuckey[2], J.C.L. Mamo[4], T.G. Redgrave[3], G.F. Watts[1] *Departments of [1]Medicine; [3]Physiology; [2]Keogh Institute for Medical Research, University of Western Australia; [4]Department of Nutrition, Dietetics and Food Science, Curtin University, Perth, Western Australia*

Objective: To examine the kinetics of chylomicron remnants (CR) in post-menopausal women with and without diabetes.

Methods: 12 post-menopausal (PM) women with non-insulin dependent diabetes mellitus (NIDDM) and 23 PM women without NIDDM of similar age, BMI and waist-hip ratio were studied. CR metabolism was measured using an intravenous bolus injection of CR-like particles labelled with cholesteryl ^{13}C-oleate, with subsequent measurement $^{13}CO_2$ in the breath over 10 hours by isotope ratio mass spectrometry. The fractional clearance rate (FCR) of the CR-like particles was derived from the appearance of $^{13}CO_2$ in breath using a multi-compartmental model (SAAM-II). Fasting lipid and lipoproteins including apolipoprotein B-48 (apoB-48) and remnant-like particle cholesterol (RLP-C) were also measured.

Results:

	Without NIDDM	With NIDDM	p value
Triglyceride, mmol/l	1.02 ± 0.41	1.95 ± 1.02	*0.010*
Cholesterol, mmol/l	5.86 ± 0.78	5.50 ± 0.79	0.204
HDL-C, mmol/l	1.60 ± 0.37	1.28 ± 0.23	*0.004*
Non-HDL-C, mmol/l	4.26 ± 0.83	4.22 ± 0.87	0.897
Glucose, mmol/l	4.90 ± 0.56	8.62 ± 3.82	*0.001*
RLP-C, mmol/l	0.24 ± 0.11	0.27 ± 0.08	0.462
ApoB-48, µg/ml	13.14 ± 4.46	12.56 ± 3.92	0.716
FCR of CR, pools/hr	0.15 ± 0.12	0.07 ± 0.03	*0.006*

In a pooled analysis, the fractional clearance rate of CR was correlated with cholesterol (r = –0.46, p = 0.006), HDL-C (r = 0.36, p = 0.035) and glucose (r = –0.31, p = 0.07).

Conclusions: The findings suggest that CR clearance is impaired in PM diabetic women in the absence of elevated post-absorptive plasma concentrations of RLP-C or apoB48. This kinetic defect may contribute independently to the increased risk of cardiovascular disease in NIDDM and requires further investigation.

Plasma cholesteryl ester transfer and hepatic lipase activity are determinants of low high density lipoprotein cholesterol associated with insulin resistance in type 2 Diabetic and non-diabetic subjects

A. Van Tol[1], S.C. Riemens[2], L.M. Scheek[1], R.P.F. Dullaart[2] *[1]Erasmus University Rotterdam; [2]University Hospital Groningen, The Netherlands*

Objectives: To evaluate the hypothesis that rates of plasma cholesteryl ester transfer (CET) and lipase activities are influenced by insulin sensitivity (IS) and contribute to the low high density lipoprotein cholesterol (HDL-C) levels observed in type 2 diabetic (DM) and insulin resistant non-DM subjects.

Methods: IS was measured as the glucose infusion rate (M-value) during the last h of a 3 h euglycaemic hyperinsulinaemic clamp (150 mU/kg/h, blood glucose target 4.6 mM) in 16 DM and 16 non-DM men. DM and non-DM subjects were divided in equal groups with low or high IS. Post-heparin plasma lipoprotein lipase (LPL) and hepatic lipase (HL) activities were measured in plasma samples obtained 1-2 weeks before the clamp. CET was measured using a radioisotope method.

Results: In non-DM with high IS, plasma CET was lower than in the other groups (p < 0.05 for all). Plasma CET (R_s = –0.62, p < 0.001 in all subjects combined, n = 32) and HL activity (R_s = –0.49, p < 0.01, n = 32) but not LPL activity (R_s = 0.01, n = 32) were inversely correlated with the M-value. HDL-C was also inversely correlated with plasma CET (R_s = –0.48, p < 0.01, n = 32) and with HL activity (Rs = –0.47, p < 0.01, n = 32).

Conclusions: Both high plasma CET and high HL activity may be determinants of low HDL-C associated with insulin resistance in type 2 DM patients and in non-DM subjects.

Thrombosis and fibrinolysis

Thrombosis and fibrinolysis: lessons from clinical trials

T.W. Meade. *MRC Epidemiology and Medical Care Unit, Wolfson Institute for Preventive Medicine, London, UK*

Clinical trials nearly always have their origin in observational studies showing associations between a medicine or a putative risk factor that it appears valuable to modify and the occurrence of clinical events such as myocardial infarction and coronary death. However, confounding and selection biases can never be excluded as explanations for the results of observational studies. A randomised controlled trial ensures that the groups under comparison are identical in all respects. A difference in outcome following an intervention can then confidently be attributed to the intervention. One objective of a randomised trial may be to try to confirm or refute the causal contribution of a risk factor. Most trials are of course undertaken to evaluate the place of treatments in preventive and clinical practice. Platelet-active agents and anticoagulants are of proven worth in primary prevention, the clinical management of acute events and in secondary prevention. The remarkable success of thrombolytic therapy in early suspected myocardial infarction adds to the evidence that the level of fibrinolytic activity is also involved. There is increasing interest in the potential value of combination therapy, either with platelet-active agents and anticoagulants or with platelet-active agents with different actions — provided there is no unacceptable increase in the risk of bleeding. Many newer agents are under consideration, a major contrast compared with older treatments being that it will still be some years before their full safety profiles have been established. An important outstanding question is the value of lowering raised fibrinogen levels. Nearly all trials throw up unexpected findings. Whether these are chance observations or suggest true effects (e.g., greater benefit in one group than another) is difficult to judge but since there is a limit to the number of trials that can be carried out, the clinical significance or otherwise of results that were not anticipated has to be considered.

Functional mutations predisposing to arterial thrombosis

C. Kluft. *Gaubius Laboratory, TNO-PG, Leiden, The Netherlands*

The human genome shows in individuals on average in one in 500 nucleotides a sequence variation some of which may be of significance for developing arterial disease or for the response to intervention or prevention. In addition to silent mutations, mutations in protein sequence with consequences for the function and mutations in the regulatory sequences for protein production do occur. Haemostatic factors are important in arterial thrombosis. In these factors genetic variation in function and regulation has been observed. They concern amongst others fibrinogen, factor VII, GP IIIA, t-PA, PAI-1, factor XIII, factor XII. What has been observed is that some of the genetic variations concern variations in response to internal or external stimuli. Thus it has been shown for fibrinogen that the response in the acute phase reaction is modulated by a genetic variation in the promotor region involved in interleukin-6 stimulation. It has been shown for PAI-1 that a 4G/5G length polymorphism in the promotor region is involved in chronic (lipids, glucose) and acute differences (infection) in blood level of PAI-1. Such variations in response may be of particular importance in chronic disease and acute situations and a particular example of disease-dedicated gene environment interaction. The distinction between genetic variations that act as a marker and genetic variations that are functional in disease is important for the application of the genetic variation in individual counselling. It requires at least the demonstration of functional, biological consequences of the genetic variation. However, the demonstration of functional/biological consequences is not sufficient as theoretically such variations may also serve as a marker of another genetic variability that really matters.

The endogenous fibrinolytic enzyme system: regulation and significance for cardiovascular disease

A. Hamsten. *King Gustaf V Research Institute, Karolinska Institute, Stockholm, Sweden*

Impaired fibrinolytic function secondary to elevated plasma plasminogen activator inhibitor-1 (PAI-1) activity is associated with precocious coronary heart disease (CHD) and with recurrent cardiovascular events in subjects with manifest CHD. Molecular explanations of clinically important gene-environment interactions that determine the regulation of PAI-1 are now emerging. From a clinical perspective elevated plasma PAI-1 activity can be considered as a component of the insulin resistance syndrome. A common 4/5 guanosine (4G/5G) polymorphism in the promoter region of the PAI-1 gene has been indicated to influence plasma PAI-1 activity and to be involved in an allele-specific response to triglycerides. Very low density lipoproteins (VLDLs) induce transciption of the human PAI-1 promoter in endothelial cells, and promoter activity is influenced by the 4G/5G polymorphic site which is located adjacent to and upstream of the binding site of a VLDL/fatty acid-inducible transcription factor. A blunting effect of PAI-1 on intravascular fibrinolytic function is generally considered to be the principal mechanism by which PAI-1 enhances the risk of thromboembolic events. However, other mechanisms have also been suggested since increased PAI-1 expression has been detected in atherosclerotic plaques. Regulation of plasmin generation by PAI-1 in the vessel wall might play an important role in the regulation of smooth muscle cell proliferation and activation of matrix metalloproteinases, two processes considered to be important for plaque growth and plaque rupture.

Tissue factor in atherothrombosis and the acute coronary syndromes

L. Badimon. *Cardiovascular Research Center, IIBB/CSIC-HSCSP-UAB, Barcelona, Spain*

Atherosclerotic plaque rupture and superimposed thrombosis is the underlying cause of acute coronary syndromes (ACS) in 75—80% of cases, the remanding being associated to plaque erosion. Thrombosis on atherosclerotic plaques seems to be triggered by tissue factor (TF) present in the boundary layer of the ruptured plaque. Indeed local treatment of human atherosclerotic plaques with recombinant tissue factor pathway inhibitor (rTFPI) or with antibodies against TF has shown to significantly reduce the thrombotic mass triggered by the plaque when perfused at characterized hemodynamic conditions in the Badimon perfusion chamber. Intravenous treatment with rFVIIai has also shown to significantly inhibit thrombosis triggered by severe arterial injury. Interestingly we have recently found that TF expression is absent in arterial intimal thickenings of the human coronary arteries, but it is already found in human coronary atherosclerotic plaques of type II and III (following the AHA classification), plaques that are not very stenotic and that contain intracellular lipid. Therefore, TF is already expressed in the vessel wall of mildly stenotic coronaries. Upon exposure to circulating blood TF can trigger the initiation of the coagulation cascade and locally generate thrombin that by a feedback activation mechanism increases its production.

New functions for TF are being uncovered; as such, the knock out of the TF gene in mice has been found incompatible with embryonic survival. TF function in angiogenesis seems fundamental for embryonic development.

Modulation of monocyte atherosclerotic and thrombotic antigen expression by platelets

D.J. Lamb, J. Wright, S. Kharodia, H. Sandhu, A.H. Goodall. *University of Leicester, Leicester, UK*

Objective: It has been shown that monocyte-platelet aggregates form spontaneously in the circulation. There is growing evidence that this is mediated by P-selectin tethering and alters monocyte tissue factor (TF) expression. The aim of this study is to determine whether platelets modify monocyte expression of CD11b, ICAM-1 and tissue factor expression.

Methods: Monocyte antigen expression was determined on free and platelet-bound monocytes (PBMs) using a novel 3-colour whole blood flow cytometric technique. Briefly, monocytes were identified using a CD14-RPE/Cy5 monoclonal antibody and the PBMs were then differentiated using a CD42b-RPE monoclonal antibody. Surface expression of CD11b, ICAM-1 and TF was determined on monocytes and PBMs using specific FITC-labelled monoclonal antibodies.

Results: Compared to platelet-free monocytes, resting PBMs expressed markedly higher levels of TF (70.8 ± 33.9 vs. 2.9 ± 1.3) and CD11b (195.8 ± 21.6 vs. 112.3 ± 15.9), but not of ICAM-1 (6.2 ± 0.9 vs. 4.7 ± 0.8). Furthermore, lipopolysaccharide induced a more rapid expression of TF and ICAM-1, but not CD11b, in PBMs compared to platelet-free monocytes. Additionally, the platelets adherent to monocytes bound more fibrinogen (6076 ± 3109 vs. 159 ± 110), expressed higher levels of P-selectin (590.5 ± 312.8 vs. 4.1 ± 2.6) and exhibited greater phosphatidylserine exposure (34.1 ± 27.1 vs. 0.9 ± 0.1) than free platelets.

Conclusion: Monocytes with adherent platelets exhibit increased expression of the procoagulant tissue factor and to a lesser extent the adhesion molecules CD11b and ICAM-1. These data suggest that activated platelets may increase the thrombogenic and atherogenic potential of monocytes in the circulation.

DNA-protein interactions at the t-PA promotor shear stress responsive element in intact human conduit vessels exposed to high shear stress

L. Selin Sjögren, L. Rasmussen, U. Hägg, L.-M. Gan, S. Jern. *Clinical Experimental Research Laboratory, Göteborg University, Göteborg, Sweden*

Objective: We recently showed that shear stress increases tissue-type plasminogen activator (t-PA) gene expression and protein synthesis in endothelial cells of intact human conduit vessels. We tested the hypothesis that this effect is mediated by interaction of NF-KB with the shear stress responsive element (SSRE) of the t-PA promotor, as shown for PDGF-B.

Methods: Human umbilical veins were perfused at high or low laminar shear stress (25 vs. < 4 dyn/cm^2) and identical intraluminal pressure (20 mmHg) for 1.5, 3, and 6 h in a computerized bio-mechanical perfusion system. Total RNA or nuclear proteins were extracted from explanted endothelial cells. t-PA mRNA was quantified after reverse-transcription with TaqMan real-time PCR using GAPDH as endogenous control. DNA-protein interactions were studied by electrophoretic mobility shift assay (EMSA).

Results: t-PA mRNA increased by $54 \pm 14\%$ (p = 0.002) relative to control after 6 h of high-shear perfusion. A distinct, transient SSRE interaction peaking after 1.5 h was observed with no difference in band shifts between high and low sheared vessels. Competition experiments indicated that NF1 but not NF-KB was involved in this interaction. With labelled consensus sequences, NF1-binding showed a shear-independent up-regulation with a similar time course as the SSRE interaction, whereas NF-KB complex formation was shear-dependently upregulated after 1.5 and 3 h.

Conclusion: Induction of t-PA gene expression by shear stress in intact pressurized vessels appears to be independent of interactions with its promotor SSRE. Since two binding sites for NF1 are present within and close to the t-PA SSRE, it is possible that the interaction of an NF1-like protein with this region may sterically hinder shear-induced NF-KB to interact with SSRE in this particular gene.

A new mechanism for platelet formation

J. Pedreño, M. Moncusí, A. Cabré, Ll. Masana. *School of Medicine, Rovira; Virgili University of Reus, Spain*

The site and mechanism of platelet formation by fragmentation of the bone marrow megakaryocytes (MKs) are still a matter of controversy. Nevertheless, platelet shedding has never been observed. In this study, we show for the first time that the ultrastructural subcellular events of platelet production take place into the blood stream. Using a new isolation method we have demonstrated the presence of MK processes in whole blood and platelet-rich plasma (PRP). Morphology and ultrastructure were analyzed by transmission and scanning electron microscopy (TEM, SEM). A high number of MK processes with different forms and sizes was found. The long axis ranged from 10 µm to 1,000 µm and the short from 2.5 µm to 8 µm. According to the size MK processes were classified into the four categories. Small (long axis < 10 µm), intermediate (10—100 µm), big (100—500 µm) and giant (> 500 µm). Small and intermediate were slender and beaded and they always showed the presence of constriction points. In contrast, big and giant MK processes were bulky or slender but beads were never present. TEM experiments showed that MK processes contain mature platelets in a resting state. Small and intermediate MK processes contained one large (> 2.5 µm) mature platelet per constriction point. However, big and giant MK processes contained a lot of small (< 2.5 µm) mature platelets. The specificity of MK processes was demonstrated by immunofluorescence microscopy and immunogold labeling techniques combined with TEM (IG-TEM) using a wide panel of monoclonal antibodies (anti-actin, anti-actinin, anti-CD36, anti-GPIIIa and anti-CD34). Finally, thrombin was able to cause the rupture of MK processes, leading to the release of mature platelet in an activated state. Our results demonstrate that MK processes containing mature resting platelets are present in human blood and that platelet shedding takes place after thrombin-induced activation.

Dr. Pedreño was the recipient of The Daria Haust Award 1996 of IAS.

Imaging of atherosclerosis

Quantitative angiography and intravascular ultrasound as research tools for the imaging of atherosclerosis

P.J. de Feyter. *Thoraxcentre, Rotterdam, The Netherlands*

Quantitative coronary angiography (QCA) has been used as a surrogate endpoint to study progression/regression of coronary atherosclerosis in several (MARS, CCAIT, MAAS, REGRESS, HARP, PLACI) intervention studies using cholesterol lowering treatment. Indeed progression of disease could be retarded but not stopped and occasionally a lesion regressed. However, QCA is lumenography so that only the "fingerprints" of atherosclerosis can be detected if the disease is progressed so far that it encroaches upon the lumen. During the development of early lesions the coronary lumen is preserved due to remodelling of the coronary artery and thus is angiographically unnoticed. This is the main reason that angiography seriously underestimates the extent of CAD.

Intracoronary ultrasound (IVUS) is a tomographic technique which allows to study the coronary wall and the lumen.

User interactive border detection algorithms allow precise quantification of coronary plaque and lumen, whereas sequential measurements of a coronary vessel segment provide volumetric quantification of the plaque and permits investigations of the remodelling process. Various long-term randomized interventional studies are now being conducted which use both QCA and IVUS techniques to provide further insights into the mechanisms of plaque progression/regression and coronary artery remodelling.

The results of these studies will become available within a few years.

Extravascular ultrasound and CT measures of coronary calcium as research tools to better understand early atherosclerosis/subclinical disease

G. Burke. *Wake Forest University, Winston-Salem, North Carolina, USA*

Objective: To describe the importance of different diagnostic tools used to evaluate atherosclerosis and subclinical disease.

Methods/Results: Noninvasive imaging of atherosclerosis/subclinical disease is essential to facilitate further reductions in cardiovascular disease (CVD) morbid and mortal events. Carotid ultrasound is a proven strategy for evaluation of intimal medial thickness and stenosis. Intimal medial thickness has been shown to be related to traditional CVD risk factors and is an independent predictor of CVD outcomes. Brachial artery ultrasound assessment of flow-mediated vasodilatation has been linked to CVD risk factors, however, less data is available on the association with CVD outcomes. CT Coronary artery calcium (CAC) correlates highly with coronary angiography findings and is associated with CVD risk factors and outcomes. CAC measures have the distinct advantage of evaluating atherosclerotic burden in the coronary bed. Conversely, much less is known about the importance of change in CAC (i.e., does it reflect true atherosclerotic progression or plaque stabilization?). Future opportunities include using MRI to evaluate plaque characteristics in the carotid and coronary beds.

Conclusions: The different subclinical disease measures may individually provide valuable information for the earlier detection of higher risk populations to facilitate more effective interventions for reduction of future CVD burden. Opportunities may exist to use a combination of these different subclinical measurements to better understand the etiology of early subclinical disease. New research studies are currently underway to better determine the incremental gain of using these subclinical measures in prediction of CVD outcomes beyond traditional CVD risk factors.

Low dose metoprolol and fluvastatin slow progression of atherosclerosis. Main results from BCAPS

G. Berglund, J. Wikstrand, L. Janzon, H. Wedel, B. Hedblad. *For the BCAP study group; University Hospital, Malmö, Sweden*

Background/Objectives: Several trials have shown that statins can slow the progression of atherosclerosis. Betablockers are known to reduce cardiovascular events, sudden deaths and death from heart failure, but antiatherosclerotic effects have not been shown in humans. The Betablocker Cholesterol-lowering Asymptomatic Plaque Study (BCAPS) aimed at assessing the effects of low-dose metoprolol and fluvastatin alone and in combination on carotid atherosclerosis.

Methods: Degree of atherosclerosis was determined with B-mode ultrasound. Asymptomatic subjects with an atherosclerotic plaque in the right carotid bifurcation (n = 793) were randomly allocated to fluvastatin 40 mg once daily, metoprolol 25 mg once daily, the combination or placebo for 36 months. Subjects were seen every sixth month and ultrasound of the right carotid artery was performed initially and after 18 and 36 months. Mean intima media thickness (IMTmean) over 10 mm in the common carotid artery and maximal intima-media thickness in the bifurcation (IMTmax), were the main effect variables. Death and cardiovascular events were monitored, although insufficient statistical power was foreseen.

Results: Fluvastatin significantly reduced the rate of progression of the IMTmean (p < 0.001) compared to placebo. Metoprolol significantly reduced the progression of IMTmax (p < 0.003). The combination of the two drugs reduced both measures of progression compared to placebo. First cardiovascular event tended to be lower in the metoprolol (n = 6) than in the placebo group (n = 13), although not significant, p = 0.055.

Conclusion: This is the first evidence in humans that a betablocker can slow progression of carotid atherosclerosis. As previously shown the statin also slowed progression of carotid atherosclerosis. Further studies are of interest to clarify the different effect of the two drugs on signs of atheroscloross in the common carotid and in the bifurcation.

Coronary calcification score and predicted risk of coronary heart disease

G.R. Thompson[1], R.S. Elkeles[2], K. Gibson[3], M. Rubens[4], R. Underwood[4]. *[1] Hammersmith; [2] St. Mary's; [4] Royal Brompton; Hospitals; and [3] BUPA Medical Centre, London, UK*

Objective: Lipid-lowering therapy is less cost effective in the primary prevention of coronary heart disease (CHD) than in secondary prevention because only a minority of those at high risk will sustain an event if left untreated. This study assesses quantification of coronary calcification by electron beam computed tomography (EBCT) as a means of discriminating between hypercholesterolaemic subjects with and without preclinical CHD.

Methods: Asymptomatic men aged 45–64 years with a plasma cholesterol $\geqslant 6.5$ mmol/l were further selected according to whether their absolute risk of CHD was low $\leqslant 10\%/10$ years) or high $\geqslant 20\%/10$ years), computed with the Framingham Equation. Of 286 eligible subjects, 223 underwent EBCT scanning.

Results: The mean log coronary calcification score was significantly higher in the 97 high risk men than in the 189 low risk men (1.58 ± 0.84 vs. 1.00 ± 0.85, $p < 0.001$), arithmetic means 158 vs. 55, and the proportion
with a high coronary calcification score (> 400) was greater (11 vs. 2%, $p < 0.01$). However, 27% of the high risk group had a low coronary calcification score $\leqslant 10$), which is known to be associated with minimal angiographic abnormalities.

Conclusion: The observation that over a quarter of hypercholesterolaemic men with an absolute risk of CHD of $\geqslant 20\%/10$ years had a coronary calcification score indicative of a low likelihood of significant coronary artery disease is novel. However, uncertainties about the predictive power of coronary calcification for clinical events must be resolved before EBCT scanning can be validated as a means of screening asymptomatic subjects at high risk of CHD.

Noninvasive imaging and quantitation of atherosclerosis with radiolabeled oxidation-specific antibodies

S. Tsimikas, W. Palinski, P.X. Shaw, J.L. Witztum. *University of California San Diego, La Jolla California, USA*

Methods to detect preclinical, "high risk" atherosclerotic lesions are urgently needed. Current noninvasive methods do not directly assess the presence of oxidized LDL (OxLDL) which is enriched in vulnerable plaques. We have developed murine monoclonal antibodies that bind to epitopes of OxLDL. Intravenous injection of 125I-MDA2, a prototype oxidation-specific antibody that binds to malondialdehyde-lysine epitopes on LDL (MDA-LDL), resulted in 8–10-fold higher uptake in plaque vs. normal tissue within the same aortas in Watanabe rabbits and mice with atherosclerosis. Autoradiography showed that 125I-MDA2 accurately reflected the lipid-strained lesions whereas no signal was seen in areas with normal tissue. Aortic 125I-MDA2 uptake showed a linear correlation with traditional lesion parameters (% surface area covered by lipid strained lesions and aortic weight). In a dietary regression study in LDLρ-/- mice, in vivo uptake of 125I-MDA2 correlated well with the percent surface area and aortic weight in progressing atherosclerosis but was more sensitive in detecting the depletion of OxLDL following a regression diet with or without antioxidants. Autoantibody titers (IgM and IgG) to Cu-OxLDL and MDA-LDL increased up to 80% with the high fat diet but decreased with the regression diet (chow or chow + vitamins E and C) and also correlated well with 125I-MDA2 uptake. 99mTc-MDA2 imaging of live Watanabe rabbits showed accurate detection of atherosclerotic lesions. Because murine antibodies have several disadvantages in human applications, we have cloned a human antibody to OxLDL, IK17, which binds to both the oxidized lipid and protein moiety of OxLDL and shows similar in vivo aortic uptake patterns. These studies describe a novel approach that could lead to noninvasive imaging, quantitation and surveillance of OxLDL-rich lesions in humans.

Are small lesions in atherosclerotic rabbit aorta shown by histology visible on magnetic resonance images?

L. Hegyi[1], P.D. Hockings[4], J.N. Skepper[2], T.A. Carpenter[3], G.A. Whelan[4], D.C. Grimsditch[4], G.M. Benson[4], K.E. Suckling[4], P.L. Weissberg[1]. *[1]Dept Medicine; [2]Multi-Imaging Centre; [3]Wolfson Brain Imaging Centre, Cambridge University; and [4]SmithKline Beecham Pharmaceuticals, Harlow, UK*

Objective: Our objective is to develop MRI methods to image the detailed structure of atherosclerotic lesions using a rabbit model of atherosclerosis.

Methods: 18 New Zealand White (NZW) rabbits were fed a diet supplemented with 0.2% cholesterol. The abdominal aortas of the rabbits were injured using a 4F Fogarty embolectomy catheter at a balloon pressure of 1 atmosphere. MRIs were acquired with a fast spin-echo technique either with or without fat suppression on a 2T Bruker Medspec at 20–30 weeks after injury. Image resolution was $250 \times 250 \times 2000$ micrometer. After imaging the rabbits were culled and their aortas were examined by histology. MRI images were compared with histological sections.

Results: All 18 rabbits used in the study developed atherosclerosis shown by MRI and histology. The thickness of the lesions produced by balloon injury in 0.2% cholesterol fed NZW rabbits was variable. It was up to 1 mm, well within the resolution of MRI. MRI images showed marked thickening of the aorta wall. Histology confirmed the presence of extensive intimal remodelling and enlargement in the same regions. We found that not only large but as small as 300-μm thick lesions are visible on MRI.

Conclusion: Small atherosclerotic lesions of 300 micrometer can be readily imaged by MRI in NZW rabbits.

Infections, CHD, and atherosclerosis

Consistence between infection and atherosclerosis

P. Saikku. *Department of Microbiology, University of Oulu, KTL, Oulu, Finland*

Already in 19th century inflammation caused by infection was proposed to be behind atherosclerosis and septic bacterial infections in experimental animals caused lesions resembling atherosclerosis. The idea was revived when herpes viruses were found to cause atherosclerosis in animals. Human herpes viruses, HSV– 1 and CMV have been associated with atherosclerosis and restenosis, and enteroviruses have been mentioned. Also bacteria, like *Helicobacter pylori* and dental pathogens, are suspected, but the most compelling evidence is from *Chlamydia pneumoniae*, a small gram-negative intracellular bacterium, which is a common cause of respiratory tract infections worldwide. Its association with atherosclerosis was found with seroepidemiology in 1988 and now nearly 30 studies have confirmed the original observations. Moreover, the presence of the agent in the lesions, discovered in 1992, has been verified in over 30 studies. Successful animal experiments have been reported from 1997 onwards and two out of the three preliminary intervention studies with antibiotics were positive. The presence of an infectious agent in the atherosclerotic lesions could easily explain their inflammatory nature, and in vitro several mechanisms how *C. pneumoniae* could cause these alterations have been demonstrated. When waiting the results of larger intervention trials we should find out in animal and in vitro experiments the pathogenetic mechanisms of chronic *C. pneumoniae* infections, how the diagnose them in patients, and what type of treatment is effective in eradicating them.

Infections and athero-thrombotic risk: The role of sero-epidemiology

D. Siscovick. *University of Washington, Seattle, Washington, USA*

The possible role of infection in the etiology of atherosclerosis has long been of investigative interest. However, the contribution of sero-epidemiologic studies of infection and atherosclerotic risk remains a source of controversy, in part because the findings from prior studies appear inconsistent. While cross-sectional sero-epidemiologic studies have suggested possible associations of prior infection with atherosclerotic risk, recent reports from several prospective studies have failed to demonstrate associations between the presence of IgG antibodies to *Chlamydia pneumoniae*, herpes simplex virus, type 1 (HSV-1), and cytomegalovirus (CMV) and incident myocardial infarction. In general, evidence from pathologic, animal-experimental, and molecular studies support a possible etiologic role of infection in atherosclerosis. For these reasons, some have questioned the contribution of sero-epidemiologic studies. In this presentation, we review the major findings from sero-epidemiologic studies in the context of other research paradigms, explore alternative explanations for the inconsistent findings, and suggest a further role for sero-epidemiologic studies of infection and athero-thrombotic risk.

Identifying and treating patients in the framework of infection and atherosclerosis

Enrique P. Gurfinkel. *Coronary Unit, Favaloro Foundation, Buenos Aires, Argentina*

The occurrence of inflammation in atherosclerotic lesions, which is mediated at least to some extent by cellular immune mechanisms, is now recognized. There are serological, pathological evidences that show an association between Chlamydial infection and acute myocardial infarction. These findings suggested a potential contribution of the cytopathologic effects of infection, including the inflammatory response of the endothelium to atherosclerosis. In addition, new data suggest that the HLA system and HSP-60 may be implicated in this process.

The ROXIS Pilot Study was the first clinical trial with a primary clinical endpoint to prove the benefit of antibiotics in coronary artery disease. Patients treated with roxithromycin had a significantly lower rate of combined clinical endpoints. These early results need confirmation by large-scale studies not only to prove the efficacy of antibiotic treatment, but also to define the potential population to be treated and how long should be the optimal treatment period.

Folate deficiency, hyperhomocyst(e)inemia and *Chlamydia pneumoniae*, — who came first?

O. Stanger[1], B. Tiran[2], H. Semmelrock[2], B. Rigler[1], A. Tiran[2]. *[1] University Hospital Graz, Div. of Cardiac Surgery; and [2] Div. of Laboratory Medicine, Graz, Austria*

Objective: We investigated a hypothesized interference of plasma homocyst(e)ine (Hcy) concentrations and *Chlamydia pneumoniae* infection in patients with coronary artery disease (CAD).

Methods: Fasting plasma homocyst(e)ine and IgG antibody titers against Chlamydia pneumoniae (C. p.) were measured in 184 male CAD patients under 60 years of age.

Results: 35 patients were hyperhomocysteinemic (Hcy > 14 µmol/l group A) vs. 149 patients with Hcy levels < 14 µmol/l (group B). Prevalence of IgG seropositivity against C. p. was significantly higher in patients of group A (66% vs. 41%, p = 0.007), as were also mean antibody titers (p = 0.026). Hcy was significantly associated with folate levels (p = 0.018) and hypertension (p = 0.007). Age, smoking, body mass index, vitamin B_6 and B_{12}, diabetes and lipids were not associated with either hyperhomocyst(e)inemia or IgG seropositivity.

Conclusions: Elevated plasma Hcy levels are associated with chlamydial IgG seropositivity in patients with CAD. Causality remains elusive at present. Explanations for our findings include damage of vascular cells through high Hcy concentrations and/or cell lysis after replication of C. p. with increased mutual susceptibility. Folate deficiency increases Hcy, but may also impair cell-mediated immunity with higher rates of intracellular infections.

Leucocytes count and fibrinogen level are associated with carotid and femoral intima-media thickness

T. Temelkova-Kurktschiev, E. Henkel, S. Fischer, F. Schaper, M. Hanefeld. *Institute of Clinical Metabolic Research, University Clinic Dresden, Germany*

Objective: Inflammatory processes are supposed to play a role in atherogenesis. The intima-media thickness (IMT) of the carotid and femoral artery is an accepted marker of atherosclerosis. The aim of this study was to examine the relationship of leucocytes count and fibrinogen level to carotid and femoral IMT, as well as to known risk factors for atherosclerosis.

Methods: A total of 597 subjects, aged 40–70 years, were analysed from the Risk factors in IGT for Atherosclerosis and Diabetes (RIAD) Study. Carotid and femoral IMT was determined by B-mode ultrasound. A variety of cardiovascular risk factors were measured by established methods.

Results: In univariate analysis carotid and femoral IMT was significantly correlated to leucocytes count and fibrinogen level. Leucocytes count significantly correlated to blood pressure, body mass index, waist to hip ratio, triglycerides, high-density lipoprotein cholesterol, insulin resistance (HOMA), fibrinogen, plasminogen activator inhibitor, tissue plasminogen activator, microalbuminuria, smoking and low physical activity, as well as to fasting and postprandial levels of plasma glucose, proinsulin and specific insulin. Fibrinogen was significantly related to blood pressure, body mass index, total cholesterol, triglycerides, insulin resistance (HOMA), plasma glucose, von Willebrandt factor, plasminogen activator inhibitor, tissue plasminogen activator, alcohol consumption and low physical activity. In multivariate analysis leucocytes count was an independent determinant of the maximal carotid IMT and fibrinogen level — of carotid and femoral IMT.

Conclusions: Our data support the hypothesis that inflammatory processes could contribute to carotid and femoral atherosclerosis.

Antibodies to *Chlamydia pneumoniae* react non-specifically with lipid in macrophages in human atherosclerotic arteries

S. Sriskandarajah, N. Singh, R.N. Poston. *Centre for Cardiovascular Biology and Medicine, King's College London; Guy's Hospital Campus, London, UK*

Objective: To detect *Chlamydia pueumoniae* in the human atherosclerotic arterial wall by immunohistochemistry.

Methods: Avidin-biotin complex immunohistochemistry on 30 paraffin embedded carotid artery endarterectomy specimens with antigen retrieval by microwaving. *Chlamydia pneumoniae* antigens were recognised by antibodies to HSP60, MOMP, LPS, and MOMP/LPS. Controls were 5 mouse plasmacytoma immunoglobulins of the same Ig classes.

Results: Surprisingly, all Chlamydia antibodies gave extensive staining of lipid-laden macrophages in the atherosclerotic plaques of every specimen. The reactivity was too extensive to be explained by Chlamydial infection. A lysosomal granular pattern was obtained, similar to that produced by a CD68 antibody. It was also similar to the distribution of lipofuscin, an insoluble advanced oxidation product of lipoprotein. Four of five control mouse immunoglobulins used at the same concentrations gave little or no reactivity, but one gave similar but weaker staining.

An ELISA assay for reactivity against human LDL showed increased binding by the Chlamydia antibodies compared to the control mouse immunoglobulins.

Conclusion: Paraffin section immunohistology can show a novel ability of immunoglobulins to react with LDL in atheroma macrophages. The panel of Chlamydia antibodies all showed this reactivity. It can give false positive results in the detection of arterial wall Chlamydiae by immunohistochemistry.

Antibodies to *Chlamydia pneumoniae* are related to the intima-media thickness in the carotid artery and to an atherogenic fatty acid profile

A. Holmlund[1], B. Wessby[2], J. Gnarpe[3], H. Gnarpe[3], T. Kahan[4], L. Lind[1]. *Depts of [1]Internal Medicine; and [2]Geriatrics, University Hospital, Uppsala; [3]Microbiology, Gävle Hospital; and [4]Medicine, Danderyds Hospital, Sweden*

Objective: To investigate the impact of IgA antibodies to *Chlamydia pneumoniae* on the intima-media thickness in the carotid artery and the lipid profile.

Methods: IgA antibodies to *Chlamydia pneumoniae*, the intima-media thickness in the carotid artery (far wall in the common artery), lipoproteins and the free fatty acid composition in cholesterol esters and phospholipids were investigated in a population sample of 56 healthy middle-aged subjects.

Results: Eight of the subjects showed detectable IgA antibodies to *Chlamydia pneumoniae*. These subjects showed an increased intima-media thickness in the carotid artery compared to the others (0.85 ± 0.15 SD vs. 0.75 ± 0.17 mm, $p < 0.05$). Neither age, nor the lipoprotein pattern differed, but the subjets with antibodies showed an increased proportion of dihomogammalinoleic acid and a reduced arachidonic to dihomogammalinoleic acid ratio (both $p < 0.05$) when compared to those without.

Conclusions: The occurance of IgA antibodies to *Chlamydia pneumoniae* is related to the intima-media thickness in the carotid artery and to an atherogenic fatty acid profile in appearently healthy individiuals.

Growth factors, cytokines, and atherosclerosis

Regulation of signal transduction in endothelial cells

L. Claesson-Welsh. *Department of Genetics and Pathology, Uppsala, Sweden*

Objective: To define molecular mechanisms in positive and negative regulation of endothelial cells.

Methods: Endothelial cells in culture are analyzed with respect to proliferation, migration and tubular morphogenesis in three-dimensional collagen gels. Angiogenesis in vivo is studied using the chicken chorioallantoic membrane assay and using different tumor models in mice.

Results: Endothelial cell morphogenesis induced by growth factors such as fibroblast growth factor (FGF) and vascular endothelial growth factor (VEGF) involves the Ras pathway and members of the Src family of cytoplasmic tyrosine kinases. In contrast, phospholipases A2, C and D are not required. Phosphatidyl inositol 3' kinase (PI3-kinase) is critical in regulation of endothelial cell survival and therefore contributes to the morphogenic response. Endostatin and latent antithrombin inhibits angiogenesis by counteracting the effects of FGF and VEGF. The mechanism of action of endostatin involves induction of an as yet unidentified tyrosine kinase. As a consequence, endothelial cells undergo apoptosis. Induction of tyrosine kinase activity and apoptosis by endostatin is dependent on its heparin-binding ability. Latent antithrombin also induces apoptosis, but does not induce tyrosine kinase activity.

Conclusions: Positive regulation of endothelial cell function by FGF and VEGF is dependent on specific signal transduction pathways, such as the Ras, Src and PI3-kinase pathways. Angiogensis inhibitors may act by subversion of those pathways.

Chemokines, monocytes, T cells, and the adaptive immune response in atherosclerosis

L. Gu, S. Tseng, P. Libby, B.J. Rollins. *Dept. of Adult Oncology, Dana-Farber Cancer Institute, Dept. of Medicine, Brigham & Women's Hosptial, Harvard Medical School, Boston, Massachusetts, USA*

In the inflammatory model of atherosclerosis, endothelial damage is thought to elicit emigration of circulating monocytes into the arterial wall where they ingest lipid and become the foam cells of the fatty streak. Chemokines have been thought to play a part in this process because of their ability to attract leukocytes. Monocyte chemoattractant protein-1 (MCP-1) is a particularly attractive candidate because of its expression in diseased vessels. Experiments using mice deficient for MCP-1 or its receptor, CCR2, have confirmed an important role for this chemokine in LDL-R-deficient, apoE-deficient, and apoB transgenic models of atherosclerosis. In the absence of MCP-1, fatty streak formation is reduced 60–80% for extended periods of time with no effect on plasma lipoprotein levels. Decreased fatty streak formation in MCP−/− and CCR−/− mice is associated with decreased numbers of arterial wall macrophages.

While these results fit a straightforward model of chemokine-induced monocyte infiltration, recent observations demonstrate that MCP-1 can also have an important effect on adaptive immunity. In response to immunological challenge, MCP—/− mice produce almost no IL-4, IL-5, or IL-10, but normal amounts of IFN-γ and IL-2. They cannot achieve the Ig subclass switching characteristic of T helper type 2 responses, and are less susceptible to L. major. Thus, MCP-1 may contribute to atherosclerosis not only by directly recruiting foam cell precursors, but also by enhancing the Th2 character of T lymphocyte-dependent aspects of lesion formation, a process that has been associated with lesion progression.

Role of shear and pressure in regulation of PDGF-B in intact human conduit vessels

L. Gan, M. Miocic, A. Johansson, U. Hägg, R. Doroudi, S. Jern. *Clinical Experimental Research Laboratory, Sahlgren's University Hospital/Östra, Göteborg, Sweden*

Objectives: PDGF-B is a potent vascular growth factor involved in the vascular remodelling process. In the present study, we investigated the possible roles of combined shear and pressure on PDGF-B expression at a whole-vessel level.

Methods: Human umbilical veins were exposed to high vs. low shear stress (25 vs. < 4 dyn/cm^2) at identical intraluminal pressure (20 mmHg) or high vs. low pressure (40 vs. 20 mmHg) at identical shear stress (10 dyn/cm^2) for 1.5, 3 or 6 h in a new computerized perfusion system. Endothelial cells were eluated with collagenase treatment and total RNA was extracted. After reverse transcription, PDGF-B gene expression was quantified by real-time RT-PCR using Taqman probe and primers (reverse primer spanning exon junction). GAPDH was used as endogenous control. Localization and semi-quantification of PDGF-B protein expression was achieved by computer-aided semi-quantitative immunohistochemistry.

Results: PDGF-B protein expression was localized mainly in the vascular endothelium. Shear stress and pressure induced significantly different temporal regulation patterns of PDGF-B gene expression (ANOVA, $p = 0.006$). After an initial transient upregulation, the PDGF-B gene expression was significantly down-regulated by 39% after 6 h shear perfusion, while in pressure stimulated vessels an 89% upregulation was detected (contrast analysis, $p = 0.01$).

Conclusions: Shear stress and pressure exerts differential regulating effects on PDGF-B gene expression. The results emphasize the importance of studying the vascular function in a complex hemodynamic environment.

Elimination of PDGF-B from only the circulating cells of APOE−/− mice significantly impacts atherosclerotic lesion formation

E.W. Raines[1], K. Kozaki[1], J. Tang[1], W.E. Kaminski[1], P. Lindahl[3], P. Martin[2], R. Ross[1], C. Betsholtz[3]. *[1]University of Washington; [2]Fred-Hutchinson Cancer Research Center, Seattle, Washington, USA; and [3]University of Göteborg, Sweden*

Platelet-derived growth factor (PDGF) is a potent stimulant of smooth muscle (SMC) migration and proliferation in culture. To test the role of PDGF in the accumulation of SMC in vivo, we evaluated ApoE−/− mice that develop complex lesions of atherosclerosis. Although targeted deletion of the PDGF genes is embryonic lethal, we have developed chimeric mice in which fetal liver cells from PDGF-B-deficient embryos were used to replace the circulating cells of lethally irradiated ApoE−/− mice. One month after transplant, all monocytes in PDGF-B−/− chimeras are of donor origin (lack PDGF), and no PDGF-BB is detected in circulating platelets, primary sources of PDGF in lesions.

Although lesion volumes are comparable in the PDGF-B+/+ and –/– chimeras at 35 weeks, lesions in PDGF-B –/– chimeras contain mostly macrophages, appear less mature and have a marked reduction in fibrous cap formation as compared with PDGF-B+/+ chimeras. Data from 45-week animals are being evaluated for the extent of SMC accumulation in lesions at a very late time point. Gene array analysis of peritoneal macrophages from PDGF-B+/+ and –/– chimeras suggests that the absence of PDGF alters macrophage gene products that may contribute to modified lesion formation in PDGF-B–/– chimeras. Thus, elimination of PDGF-B from circulating cells in ApoE–/– mice is sufficient to significantly reduce SMC infiltration into lesions and delay lesion progression.

(Supported in part by NIH grant HL 18645 to EWR and RR and by grant Ka 1078/1 from the Deutsche Forschungsgemeinschaft to WEK.)

Proto-oncogene product Crk differentially interacts with PDGF α- and β-receptors

K. Yokote, S. Mori, T. Matsumoto, M. Takemoto, Y. Saito. *Second Department of Internal Medicine, Chiba University School of Medicine, Chiba, Japan*

Objective: To identify intracellular proteins which are involved in signal transduction pathway specific for the PDGF α-receptor.

Methods: Affinity purification using an immobilized synthetic peptide containing phosphorylated Tyr-762 in the PDGF α-receptor was performed. Wild-type or tyrosine-residue mutated PDGF α-receptors were stably transfected into porcine endothelial (PAE) cells. The cells were treated with PDGF-BB, lysed and subjected to immunoprecipitation followed by Western blotting. Tyrosine phosphorylated GST fusion protein of CrkII was produced in *E. coli* encoding inducible tyrosine kinase gene.

Results: Proteins in HeLa cell lysate of molecular sizes 27, 38 and 40 kDa bound to the phosphorylated but not to the unphosphorylated peptide. Partial amino acid sequences of the purified proteins indicated that they were identical to SH2-containing proto-oncogene products CrkI, CrkII and CrkL, respectively. CrkII bound to wild-type but not to Y762F PDGF α-receptor upon ligand-stimulation of PAE cells. In contrast, association between CrkII and PDGF β-receptor was negligible, whereas CrkII became prominently phosphorylated by the β-receptor. GST-CrkII fusion protein could bind activated PDGF β-receptor in vitro, and the association was diminished by tyrosine phosphorylation of the fusion protein.

Conclusion: Tyr-762 in the PDGF α-receptor serves as the binding site for CrkII. CrkII can also bind to PDGF β-receptor in vitro. However, CrkII can hardly associate with the b-receptor in vivo, because internal tyrosine phosphrylation of CrkII negatively regulate its binding to the target molecules. Differential binding of CrkII to the PDGF α- and β-receptors may be a rationale for functional diversity of the two receptors.

Cytokine regulation of endothelial cell function: new molecules in an old paradigm

Alberto Mantovani, Cecilia Garlanda. *Istituto di Ricerche Farmacologiche Mario Negri, Milan, Italy*

IL-1 is a prototypic activator of endothelial cells which induces expression of a set of prothrombotic/proinflammatory functions. We found that vascular cells, as well as cells of other origin, respond to IL-1 exclusively via the type I IL-1 receptor (R). The type II R acts as a decoy for IL-1, regulated by anti-inflammatory signals. Recent evidence, including gene transfer and identification of a novel rapid pathway of release is consistent with the decoy R concept. The IL-1 receptor family includes the various Toll, some of which are expressed in endothelium. Their signaling pathway will be discussed. Among IL-1 inducible genes, we identified a new molecule related to pentraxins (PTX3). The sequence, genomic organization, predicted structure and in vitro and in vivo expression of mouse and human PTX3 will be discussed. Evidence will be presented of restricted expression of PTX3 in certain vascular beds. The ligand binding properties of PTX3 suggest that it may represent a mechanism of local resistance. Initial results on PTX3 in human diseases, including acute myocardial infarction, will be discussed.

References

1. Mantovani A, Bussolino F, Introna M. (1997) Cytokine regulation of endothelial cell function: from molecular level to the bed side. Immunol Today 18:231–239.
2. Romano M, Sironi M, Toniatti C et al. (1997) Role of IL-6 and its soluble receptor in induction of chemokines and leukocyte recruitment. Immunity 6:315–325.
3. Muzio M, Natoli G, Saccani S et al. (1998) The human Toll signaling pathway: divergence of Nuclear Factor kB and JNK/SAPK activation upstream of tumor necrosis factor receptor-associated factor 5 (TRAF6). J Exp Med 187:2097–2101.

New aspects of statin treatment

Statins and the atherogenic process

J. Davignon, R. Laaksonen. *Hyperlipidemia and Atherosclerosis Research Group; Clinical Research Institute of Montreal, Montreal, Quebec, Canada*

Statins, like most biologically active molecules, have multiple actions. Reduction in cardiovascular events following sustained statin therapy results from a combination of beneficial effects. Separating the relative contributions of these effects is as complex as determining causality in a multifactorial disease such as atherosclerosis. The complex etiology of atherosclerosis and recognition of the contribution of a wide spectrum of risk determinants in a given individual is readily accepted. In contrast, the notion that the effect of a drug is the algebraic sum of its many positive and negative effects is not given the attention it deserves in current practice. Many properties of statins could directly influence lesion formation. Statins have antioxidant effects that can be demonstrated both in vitro and in vivo. They take place at therapeutic plasma concentrations. They differ among statins, may characterize the parent compound or a metabolite, influence both LDL and HDL oxidation, impart a paraoxonase-sparing effect or be modified by a slight change in the molecular structure. Statins' anti-inflammatory properties confirmed in clinical trials complement their plaque stabilizing effects. They inhibit inflammatory cytokines as well as proliferation of inflammatory cells. There is evidence that adhesion molecules may be reduced by statins. The effect on cell proliferation is a key feature of lipophilic statins. The significance of their ability to or not to inhibit smooth muscle cell proliferation is still a matter of controversy. Macrophages may be affected by statins so as to reduce foam cell formation. Statins inhibit the ability of macrophages to oxidize LDL, and reduce the expression of scavenger receptors including CD36, and LOX-1 on their surface. The effect of statins on apolipoprotein E production by macrophages is currently being investigated. A better understanding of the pleiotropic effects influencing the atherogenic process could eventually allow for the refining of indications of the various statins and help in the appraisal of their individuality.

Statins and C-reactive protein (CRP)

T.E. Strandberg. *Department of Medicine, University of Helsinki, Helsinki, Finland*

C-reactive protein (CRP) was first found in the 1930s in plasma of patients with pneumococcal pneumonia. Nowadays CRP is a widely used measure to evaluate the activity of inflammation and diagnose bacterial infections. CRP belongs to acute phase proteins, the concentrations of which in serum are increased by inflammatory cytokines (for example interleukin-6) up to 1,000-fold. Conventionally, CRP concentrations below 10 mg/l have been intrepreted as normal, and CRP of healthy individuals is generally below 2 mg/l. Results from several follow-up studies have revealed that CRP concentrations over 2 mg/l — but below 10 mg/l — predict future coronary heart disease events. This suggests that silent inflammation, either in the coronary arteries or elsewhere in the body, could play a role in the development of atherosclerosis. CRP may also have pathogenetic significance, because CRP has been found in atherosclerotic arteries. Interesting new findings of CRP and coronary prevention are the following:
1. Pravastatin seemed to prevent coronary events more effectively in those patients whose

CRP was increased at baseline;

2. In coronary patients with hyperlipidemia both short-term and long-term statin treatment is associated with decreased CRP levels; and

3. CRP change is not associated with LDL reduction during statin treatment, but at least in short-term inversely with change in HDL cholesterol.

Practical consequencies of the statin effects on CRP are currently obscure, but reduction of CRP and inflammation may play a role in the early stabilization of the atherosclerotic plaque.

Effect of statins on the synthesis of lipoprotein containing apo B-100

A.L. Catapano. *Institute of Pharmacological Sciences University of Milan, Italy*

Statins effectively lower plasma LDL cholesterol. Their action takes place through the inhibition of the HMG CoA Reductase, a key step in the cholesterol biosynthetic pathway. By inhibiting cholesterol synthesis statins induce an up regulation of LDL receptors, thus leading to a sharp decrease of plasma LDL levels. Recent data, however, suggest that statins may lower plasma lipids also by different mechanisms. In the liver the secretion of LDL depends on a finely tuned balance between synthesis and intracellular degradation of apoB-100. In the poorly lipidated form apo B is readily degraded intracellularly and this mechanism, rather than apolipoprotein synthesis, appears to be the mayor determinant of apolipoprotein B-100 secretion. Statins by lowering cholesterol availability (both free and esterified) may decrease apolipoprotein B-100 secretion. To address this question we studied the effects of NK-104, a competitive inhibitor of HMGCoA-Reductase on apoB-100 synthesis and secretion from the human hepatoma cell line HepG2. Cells were preincubated with NK-104 (0.01–5 µM) for 24 h. The incubation with the drug continued for further 4 h in the presence of absence of oleate (0.8 mM). ApoB-100 in the medium was determined by an ELISA assay. Incubation of HepG2 with NK-104 resulted in a marked inhibition of cholesterologenesis, determined as incorporation of 14 C-acetate into sterol, and decreased apoB-100 secretion in a dose-dependent manner (about –20% vs control, both in basal conditions and after incubation with oleate). Evaluation of the distribution of apoB-100 among different lipoprotein secreted showed a reduction of apoB-100 associated with lipoproteins in the LDL density range. Pulse-chase experiments demonstrated that NK-104 did not affect the synthetic rate of apoB-100 but increased intracellular degradation of newly synthesised protein; apoB-100 mRNA levels were not affected. These data, together with other in vitro and in vivo findings, suggest that statins may decrease lipoproteins secretion especially in patients with LDL overproduction.

Atorvastatin increases the catabolism of chylomicron remnants in normolipidemic subjects

K.G. Parhofer[1], P.H.R. Barrett[2], P. Schwandt[1]. *[1]Med. Dept. II, Klinikum Grosshadern, University Munich, Germany; and [2]Dept. Medicine, University Western Australia, Perth, Australia*

Objective: Atorvastatin (atorva) is a potent HMG-CoA reductase inhibitor that also decreases fasting triglyceride concentrations. Because of the positive association between elevated triglycerides and CAD we investigated the effect of atorva on postprandial lipoprotein metabolism.

Methods: We evaluated the effect of 4 weeks of atorva (10 mg.d^{-1}) on postprandial lipoprotein metabolism in 10 normolipidemic men (30 ± 2 years, 22 ± 3 kg.m^{-2}, cholesterol (chol) 187 ± 21, triglyceride (TG) 130 ± 44, HDL-chol 45 ± 7, LDL-chol 116 ± 19 mg.dl^{-1}). Postprandial lipoprotein metabolism was evaluated with a standardized fat load (1300 kcal, 87% fat, 7% carbohydrates, 6% protein, 80,000 IU Vitamin A) given after 12 h fast. Plasma was obtained every 2 h for 14 h. Chylomicrons (C) and chylomicron-remnants (CR) were isolated by ultracentrifugation and chol, TG, apoB, apoB-48 and vitamin A (vitA) was determined.

Results: Atorva significantly (p < 0.001) decreased fasting chol (–28%), TG (–30%), LDL-chol (–41%) and apoB (–39%), while HDL-chol increased (4%, NS). The area under the curve for plasma-TG (–27%) and CR-TG (–40%), CR-Chol (–49%), CR-apoB-48 (–43%) decreased significantly (p < 0.05), while CR-vitA decreased slightly (–34%, p = 0.08). In contrast, none of the C-parameters changed with atorva therapy.

Conclusions: Atorva decreases postprandial CR but not C. This indicates, that atorva has no effect on hydrolysis, but induces an increase in CR clearance, presumably due to decreased competition for receptors and/or because of an increased receptor activity or number. Thus, atorva does not affect C formation, secretion or catabolism, but increases CR catabolism.

Pravastatin reduces mortality: The Prospective Pravastatin Pooling Project

J. Simes[1], A. Tonkin[2], E. Braunwald[3], J. Shepherd[4], T. Craven[5], B.R. Davis[6], C. Furberg[5]. [1] *NHMRC Clinical Trials Centre, Sydney;* [2] *National Heart Foundation, Melbourne, Australia;* [3] *Brigham and Women's Hospital, Boston, Massachusetts, USA;* [4] *University of Glasgow, UK;* [5] *Bowman Gray School of Medicine, Winston-Salem, NC;* [6] *University of Texas, Houston, Texas, USA*

Objective: To definitely address the effects of pravastatin 40 mg daily on total mortality, CHD morbidity, and specific non-CHD events within important subgroups.

Methods: The Prospective Pravastatin Pooling Project was designed to address the effects of pravastatin 40 mg/day on all-cause and cause-specific mortality by combining data from three large prevention trials, the West of Scotland Coronary Prevention Study (WOSCOPS), Cholesterol And Recurrent Events (CARE), and Long-term Intervention with Pravastatin in Ischaemic Disease (LIPID), according to objectives specified before the results of any trail were known. Combining these three 5-year trials yielded a database that included 19,768 patients and 112,330 person years of follow-up. In addition to all these trials, the combined results for the two trials in patients with prior CHD (CARE and LIPID) were compared to those of the trial in patients without prior CHD (WOS-COPS).

Results: Patients taking pravastatin (vs. placebo) had significantly lower all-cause mortality (relative risk reduction [RRR] 20%, 95% confidence interval [CI] (12–27%; p < 0.0001), due largely to significantly reduced CHD mortality (RRR 24%, 95%CI 14–33%). Differences in other vascular deaths and noncardiovascular deaths were insignificant. The greatest reductions in absolute risk were estimated, however, in patients with a history of CHD.

Conclusions: Pravastatin is effective in the prevention of (CHD) mortality across a broad range of cholesterol levels, with the absolute benefit of treatment related principally to the baseline risk of CHD death.

A large, 36 week study of the HDL-C raising effects and safety of simvastatin versus atorvastatin

J.R. Crouse[1], J. Kastelein[2], J. Isaacsohn[3], L. Corsetti[4], M. Liu[4], M. Melino[4], L.M. Mercuri[4], O'Grady[4], L. Ose[5]. [1]Wake Forest University, Winston-Salem; [3]Metabolic and Atherosclerosis Research Center, Cincinnati; [4]Merck & Co., Inc., Rahway, New Jersey, USA; [2]Academic Medical Center, Amsterdam, The Netherlands; and [5]Lipid Clinic, Rikshospitalet, Oslo, Norway

Objective: This study evaluated the HDL-C, apo A-I raising effects and safety of simvastatin (S) and atorvastatin (A) at their upper dosage ranges.

Methods: In a double-blind, parallel, 36 week dose escalation study, 826 hypercholesterolemic patients (LDL-C > 4.14 mmol/l) were randomized to S (40 mg 6 weeks, 80 mg 6 weeks, 80 mg 24 weeks) or A (20 mg 6 weeks, 40 mg 6 weeks, 80 mg 24 weeks).

Results: S was superior to A at raising HDL-C (primary endpoint) and apo A-I at each dose comparison.

Treatment		HDL-C (mean%)			Apo A-I (mean%)		
	N	Change		Diff	Change		Diff
		A	S	S vs. A	A	S	S vs. A
		412	414				
W06	A 20 vs. S 40	6.1	7.4	1.3	3.2	4.8*	1.6
W12	A 40 vs. S 80	5.1	8.2**	3.2**	0.2	4.6**	4.5**
W12–36	A 80 vs. S 80	2.1	6.5**	4.4**	–4.3	1.7**	6.0**

Change = from baseline; Diff = between treatment; *p = 0.051, **p < 0.001

Both A and S lowered mean LDL-C substantially by 46—55% and 43—49%, respectively (p < 0.001 in favor of A at each dose comparison). During the 24 week A 80 versus S 80 mg period, a significantly larger number of patients (p = 0.004) were discontinued because of clinically meaningful (> 3 × upper limit of normal) consecutive increases in hepatic transaminases with A (14/392; 3.6%) than with S (2/384; 0.5%).

Conclusions: S had superior HDL-C and apo A-I raising effects across the doses studied, which was more prominent at the highest doses. At the 80 mg dose of each drug, S also had a better hepatic safety and tolerability profile.

Cholesterol-lowering therapy with pravastatin in older patients (aged 65—75 years) in the lipid study

D. Hunt[1], P. Young[2], J. Simes[2], D. Colquhoun[3], W. Hague[2], A. Tonkin[4]. [1]University of Melbourne; [2]NHMRC Clinical Trials Centre, Sydney; [3]Core Research Group, University of Queensland, Brisbane; [4]National Heart Foundation, Melbourne, Australia

The LIPID (Long-Term Intervention with Pravastatin in Ischaemic Disease) study found that, for patients with coronary heart disease (CHD) (prior myocardial infarction (MI) or unstable angina) and cholesterol levels of 4—7 mmol/l, therapy with pravastatin reduced total and CHD mortality. Of the 9014 patients, 3514 were in prespecified older age group (aged 65—75 years). We aimed to ascertain the effects of pravastatin on total mortality and on CHD death or nonfatal MI in the older patients.

The older patients had a higher risk for the prespecified outcomes than the younger patients (both $p < 0.001$). The risk of an MI or fatal stroke was also higher for older patients (both $p < 0.001$), but they were less likely to undergo revascularization ($p = 0.035$). Pravastatin reduced the relative risk of the prespecified outcomes to a similar extent in the older and younger group; as the absolute risk of events was higher in the older age group, the absolute benefit of therapy was larger for them.

Prespecified event	Age group (years)	Risk of event	Relative risk reduction (%)	Absolute risk reduction (%)	NNT*
CHD death or nonfatal MI	31–64	13.4	22	3.0	33
	65–75	19.7	21	4.2	24
Total mortality	31–64	9.8	22	2.2	43
	65–75	20.6	20	4.1	25

*Numbers needed to treat over 6 years per 1000 patients

Conclusion: Treatment with pravastatin appears useful and effective in this older age group of patients with previous MI or unstable angina.

Fatty acids: the link between insulin resistance and dyslipidaemia

Pathogenesis of fatty acid induced atherogenic dyslipoproteinemia

Allan D. Sniderman. *McGill University, Montreal, Quebec, Canada*

Hypertriglyceridemic hyperapoB is the most common atherogenic dyslipoproteinemia. It has four major features: hypertriglyceridemia; increased numbers of small dense LDL particles; low HDL cholesterol; and delayed postprandial triglyceride (TG) clearance. Inappropriate diversion of fatty acids (FA) to the liver due to reduced FA trapping by adipose tissue appear to be the most common pathogenetic mechanism underlying hypertriglyceridemic hyperapoB and the objective of this presentation will be to explicate what is known of the molecular mechanisms responsible for this phenomenon.

Our attention has focused on the regulation of the rate at which FA can be taken up by adipocytes and converted to TG. That effort has led to the description of the Acylation Stimulating Protein (ASP) pathway which regulates the rate adipocyte TG synthesis and influences FA release. The proportion of FA which are released from chylomicrons that enter the nearby adipocytes is variable and is determined by the ability of the adipocyte to incorporate these newly released FA into TG. Diminish FA trapping by adipocytes and necessarily, FA delivery to the liver will increase and so will hepatic apoB secretion and plasma apoB.

We have recently completed an initial series of experiments in ASP knockout mice. The results support an important physiologic role for the ASP pathway but indicate that the phenotypic consequences of dysfunction of the ASP pathway are critically modulated by gender and insulin sensitivity. These studies point to a model of linked, but distinguishable, steps in peripheral clearance of TG rich lipoproteins and their interaction will have to be appreciated if the pathogenesis of familial combined hyperlipidemia is to be explicated.

Insulin resistance and postprandial lipid metabolism

D.W. Erkelens. *Utrecht, Netherlands*

Insulin resistance is at the origin of the syndrome X, encompassing among many risk factors hypertriglyceridemia. It may however well be that the second is operative in enhancing the first or that both are the consequence of one causative mechanism.

Artificial hypertriglyceridemia, with free fatty acid (FFA) increase, strongly reduces insulin mediated glucose uptake during clamping. Postprandial suppression of free fatty acid levels is reduced or even reversed in both insulin resistant type 2 DM patients and familial combined hyperlipidemia (FCH) patients. Growth hormone deficiency is among others characterized by a delayed postprandial clearance of triglyceride rich remnant particles. Spontaneous daily triglyceride profiles (day-trip's) show even in normal males a substantial dependance on insulin resistance (assessed as HOMA ratio).

These and other data suggest that insulin resistance and disturbed postprandial lipid metabolism are closely linked, mutually dependant and possibly caused by insufficient suppression of free fatty acid flux from lipolysis.

Fatty acids and insulin resistance: A genetic and physiological perspective

Timothy J. Aitman. *MRC Clinical Sciences Centre and Imperial College School of Medicine, Hammersmith Hospital, London, UK*

Glucose and fatty acids are major cellular energy substrates. In many states of insulin resistance, excess availability of fatty acids co-exists with decreased insulin-mediated glucose uptake and utilisation. We have studied the genetics of glucose and fatty acid metabolism in adipocytes from the spontaneously hypertensive rat (SHR). In this model, defects in adipocyte fatty acid metabolism and insulin action associate with insulin resistance and dyslipidaemia at the whole body level. In a genome-wide linkage scan, a major SHR quantitative trait locus (QTL) for defective insulin action shared coincident peak linkage to the telomere of rat chromosome 4 with defective fatty acid metabolism. Previously mapped SHR QTLs for dyslipidaemia and hypertension also map to the same chromosome 4 locus. Using cDNA microarrays and radiation hybrid mapping, we identified a defective SHR gene, Cd36, that resides at the peak of linkage to these QTLs. *Cd36* is a transmembrane transporter of long-chain fatty acids and receptor for oxidised low density lipoproteins, and is proposed to play a key part in foam cell formation. *Cd36* is directly induced by PPApg, the target of the thiazolidinedione insulin-sensitising drugs and *Cd36* knockout and transgenic mice display marked abnormalities of lipid and carbohydrate metabolism. These observations indicate that Cd36 plays a key role in regulation of cellular and whole body metabolism of carbohydrates and lipids.

Fatty acid binding proteins in different human adipose tissue depots: Relationships to serum insulin concentrations

R.M. Fisher[1], P. Eriksson[1], J. Hoffstedt[2], A. Hamsten[1], P. Arner[2]. *[1]King Gustaf V Research Institute; [2]Department of Medicine, Huddinge Hospital, Karolinska Institute, Stockholm, Sweden*

Objective: To investigate the fatty acid binding proteins (FABPs) adipocyte lipid binding protein (ALBP) and epidermal fatty acid binding protein (EFABP) expressed in different human adipose tissue depots.

Methods: Omental (om) and subcutaneous (sc) adipose tissue samples were obtained from 19 obese individuals (10 female, 9 male, age 41.1 ± 2.4 years, BMI 42.8 ± 1.2 kg/m^2). ALBP and EFABP RNA levels were quantified by northern blot analysis (expressed relative to the ribosomal 18S subunit), ALBP protein levels by Western blot analysis (expressed relative to actin).

Results: In sc compared to om adipose tissue, ALBP RNA and protein levels were 37% ($p < 0.02$) and 11% (not significant) higher respectively. There were no significant differences in EFABP RNA levels. The ALBP:EFABP RNA ratio was 23% higher in sc compared to om adipose tissue ($p < 0.03$). ALBP:EFABP RNA ratios were inversely related to serum insulin concentrations in both sc and om adipose tissue ($r = -0.618$ and $r = -0.577$ respectively, both $p \leqslant 0.02$). ALBP protein and serum insulin levels were inversely correlated in om ($r = -0.475$, $p < 0.04$), but not in sc adipose tissue.

Conclusions: Differences in ALBP and EFABP expression in sc and om adipose tissue might be related to the metabolic differences observed between these two depots. Adipose tissue FABPs may be important in man in the link between obesity and insulin resistance.

Changes in matrix proteoglycans induced by fatty acids in hepatic cells; effects on lipoprotein binding

U. Olsson[1], A.-C. Egnell[1,2], M. Rodríguez Lee[1], G. Bondjers[1], G. Camejo[1,2].
[1]Wallenberg Laboratory, Göteborg, AstraZeneca; [2]Mölndal, Sweden

Objective: The dyslipidemia of insulin resistance and type 2 diabetes is characterized by elevated circulating non-esterified fatty acids (NEFA) and lipoprotein remnants. Microvascular and macrovascular complications of type 2 diabetes are characterized by changes in extracellular matrix proteoglycans (PG). Excess exposure to NEFA in vitro alters the amount and composition of extracellular PG in endothelial cells and arterial smooth muscle cells [1,2]. In liver extracellular PG contribute to the uptake of triglyceride (TG)-rich lipoprotein remnants [3]. We explored if NEFA can also alter the extracellular PG of hepatic cells and if this could change their affinity for remnant lipoproteins, a hypothetical mechanism that could contribute to the dyslipidemia of insulin resistance and type 2 diabetes.

Methods: Cultured HepG2 cells and livers from obese rats were used as in vitro and ex vivo models to study PG synthesis and binding of lipoproteins.

Results: HepG2 cells cultured in medium with 300 μM albumin-bound linoleic acid increased markedly their PG secretion. The glycosaminoglycans of the secreted proteoglycans where enriched in chondroitin sulfate proteoglycans (CS) at the expense of heparan sulfate. Livers of obese Zucker fa/fa rats that are insulin resistant and have high circulating levels of NEFA and TG-rich remnants showed also an increased expression of CS-proteoglycans when compared to lean littermates. The changed proteoglycan composition decreased the affinity of remnant bVLDL particles to PG isolated from HepG2 cells and Zucker obese rat livers.

Conclusions: Elevated fatty acid levels modulate PG in hepatic cells. If present in vivo, this could affect the clearance rate of remnant particles in insulin resistance and type 2 diabetes and contribute to its dyslipidemia.

References

1. Hennig, B. et al. (1995) Prostagl. Leukot. Essent. Fatty Acids 53, 315—24
2. Olsson, U., Bondjers, G., and Camejo, G. (1999) Diabetes 48, 616—22
3. Reference: Mahley, R.W., and Ji, Z. (1999) J. Lipid Res. 40, 1—16

Adipose tissue insulin resistance in familial combined hyperlipidemia (FCH), but not type 2 diabetes mellitus (DM2)

C.J.H. van der Kallen, F.G. Bouwman, R.W.J. van de Hulst, W.D. Boeckx, T.W.A. de Bruin. Lab. Molecular Metabolism and Endocrinology, Maastricht University, Maastricht, The Netherlands

Objective: To test in both DM2 and FCH the hypothesis that in both DM2 and FCH insulin induced suppression of hormone sensitive lipase (HSL) activity is reduced as consequence of insulin resistance.

Methods: Subcutaneous adipose tissue biopsies were obtained from healthy controls (C, n = 11), DM2 (n = 12) and FCH (n = 10) subjects. Immediately following isolation, mature adipocytes were incubated with isoprenaline or insulin for 2 hours. Both glycerol and free fatty acids (FFA) levels were measured in the incubation media.

Results: Isoprenaline stimulated the release of glycerol as well as FFA in all groups, with the highest release in DM2 ($p < 0.05$ vs. C and FCH). Insulin decreased FFA release in C and DM2, but not in FCH, indicating impaired insulin sensitivity towards fractional FFA re-esterification in the adipocytes. Data in table represent nmol/40,000 cells/2 h (mean ± sd).

		Controls	DM2	FCH
FFA	Basal	26.6 ± 10.8	56.2 ± 48.9	25.8 ± 9.8
	Isoprenaline	137.9 ± 83.6*	332.7 ± 176.8	94.0 ± 57.4*
	Insulin	18.8 ± 8.6*	32.6 ± 17.8	27.3 ± 7.3
Glycerol	Basal	11.1 ± 5.3	34.0 ± 43.1	9.6 ± 3.1
	Isoprenaline	61.6 ± 45.9*	136.8 ± 95.8*	33.7 ± 17.7*
	Insulin	11.2 ± 5.6	17.1 ± 10.8	11.0 ± 3.9

Conclusions: In DM2 maximum lipolysis activity is high, probably due to larger adipocytes (data not shown). In FCH adipocytes, FFA release did not change under the influence of insulin. This suggests that in FCH the FFA metabolism is disturbed. This may be due to impaired acylation, or TG synthesis, or oxidation, eventually resulting to a higher FFA flux to the liver, contributing to the hyperlipidemia.

Spectrum of nuclear lamin A/C mutations and metabolic phenotypes in familial partial lipodystrophy

Robert A. Hegele, Carol M. Anderson, Jian Wang, Henian Cao. *The John P. Robarts Research Institute, London, Canada*

We were the first to report that Dunnigan-type familial partial lipodystrophy (FPLD) with insulin resistance, diabetes, hyperlipidemia, hypertension and early atherosclerosis results from a mutation, namely R482Q, in *LMNA*, the gene that encodes nuclear lamins A and C. We have since identified three novel and extremely rare missense mutations in *LMNA*, namely V440M, R482W and R584H. Examination of the clinical and biochemical phenotypes in carriers of mutant *LMNA* revealed that hyperinsulinemia and perturbations in plasma lipids preceded the development of plasma glucose abnormalities and hypertension. Our findings indicate that: 1) a spectrum of *LMNA* mutations underlies FPLD; 2) aberrant lamin A, and not lamin C, underlies FPLD, since R584H occurs within *LMNA* sequence that is specific for lamin A; 3) compound heterozygosity for mutant *LMNA* is associated with a relatively more severe FPLD phenotype, but not with complete lipodystrophy; and 4) environmental factors appeared to be partially related to the variation in phenotype severity in *LMNA* mutation carriers. Thus, rare mutations in a nuclear structural protein are associated with markedly abnormal qualitative and quantitative metabolic phenotypes. The precise mechanism by which mutant *LMNA* causes fat-wasting in specific anatomical sites is unknown. It is also not clear whether the metabolic disturbances in FPLD are a direct result of deficient or defective intracellular function due to the mutant *LMNA* or are merely secondary to the abnormal distribution of adipose tissue. In either event, our genetic analysis has implicated an etiologic role for aberrant nuclear lamin A in FPLD. These naturally occurring *LMNA* mutations can now be evaluated with in vitro molecular and cellular analyses in order to understand why specific cell types and tissues are selectively affected.

Gene therapy and other new treatments

VEGF gene transfer in the treatment of coronary heart disease and peripheral vascular disease

S. Ylä-Herttuala. *A.I. Virtanen Institute and Department of Medicine, University of Kuopio, Kuopio, Finland*

Vascular gene therapy is a new area where only a few preliminary results from human trials are available [1]. Most of the clinical trials are centered around therapeutic angiogenesis, treatment of restenosis, arterial cytoprotection or a combination of these effects. Intravascular adenoviral gene transfer in human peripheral arteries in the leg has been proved feasible with infusion-perfusion catheters [2]. Detectable transgene expression was achieved in a maximum of 5% of arterial cells. Beneficial effects have been reported after intramuscular VEGF gene transfer into the muscle or artery of an ischaemic limb or myocardium [3—6]. Several gene therapy trials with various types of VEGF are currently ongoing [1]. Results are expected within 1–2 years.

Based on current information, gene therapy in the cardiovascular system seems to be safe and well tolerated, although edema has been seen in legs treated with intramuscular VEGF gene therapy and hypertension has been reported in some patients. Even though gene therapy has shown promising results in some areas of cardiovascular diseases, further developments in gene transfer vectors, gene delivery techniques and identification of effective treatment genes will be required before the full therapeutic potential of gene therapy can be assessed.

References

1. Ylä-Herttuala S, Martin JF. Cardiovascular gene therapy. Lancet 2000;355:213—222.
2. Laitinen M et al. Hum. Gene Ther. 1998;9:1481—1486.
3. Baumgartner I et al. Circulation 1998;97:1114—23.
4. Losordo DW et al. Circulation 1998;98:2800-804.
5. Rosengart TK et al. Circulation 1999;100:468-74.
6. Laitinen M et al. Hum. Gene Ther. 2000;11:263-270.

Gene therapy for dyslipidemias

Lawrence Chan. *Departments of Molecular & Cellular Biology and Medicine Baylor College of Medicine, Houston, Texas 77030, USA*

Elevation of atherogenic plasma lipoproteins is a major risk factor for atherosclerosis development. Somatic gene therapy is a novel experimental approach for the treatment of hyperlipoproteinemia and dyslipidemia. Successful gene therapy requires the availability of safe and efficient gene-delivery vectors. Although first and second-generation adenoviral vectors are highly efficient in delivering transgenes to the liver, they exhibit substantial toxicity and have been associated with significant morbidity and mortality in clinical trials. A helper-dependent adenovrial vector (HD-Ad) deleted of all viral protein genes was developed at Baylor College of Medicine, and an efficient production system for this vector was developed by Dr. Frank Graham at McMaster University. In collaboration with Dr. Arthur Beaudet in the Department of Molecular & Human Genetics at Baylor, we used HD-Ad to deliver lipid-lowering genes to the liver of mouse and nonhuman primate models of hyperlipidemia. A single injection of HD-Ads for LDL receptor, VLDL receptor, apoA-I or apoE produced long-term (6 months to >1 yr) hepatic transgene expression with negligible toxicity, reversed dyslipidemia and prevented atherosclerosis development. The data support the feasibility and safety of using HD-Ad vectors for the treatment of lipid disorders in clinical trials.

Gene therapy for proliferative vascular disease

K. Walsh. *Division of Cardiovascular Research, St. Elizabeth's Medical Center, and Program in Cell, Molecular, and Developmental Biology, Sackler School of Biomedical Sciences, Tufts University, Boston, MA, USA*

I will provide an overview of the candidate genes and delivery systems that we are evaluating for the therapy of proliferative vascular disorders. The promise of gene therapy for post-angioplasty restenosis is that one has the opportunity to deliver genetic material to the site of balloon inflation at the time of intervention. The delivery of genetic material to these sites creates a depot for recombinant protein expression, thereby avoiding limitations imposed on other therapies by the short retention periods experienced with small molecules and macromolecules delivered to the vessel wall. The altered expression of genes within the targeted cells will, in theory, alter the course of the wound healing process to minimize reocclusion of the vessel. I will discuss treatment strategies that have been shown to be efficacious in limiting post-angioplasty restenosis through evaluation with in vivo model systems. Candidate strategies that we have investigated utilize genes encoding factors that are either cytotoxic (Fas ligand and hammerhead ribozyme to Bcl-2) or cytostatic (Rb and p21). We have also investigated the therapeutic utility of a transcriptional regulator of integrin expression that was isolated from smooth muscle cells (Gax). I will also briefly discuss critical issues of delivery with devices and gene control that must be considered for successful application of this therapy.

VEGF-C adenovirus gene transfer reduces intima formation in rabbits

Mikko O. Hiltunen[1], Marja Laitinen[1], Mikko P. Turunen[1], Michael Jeltsch[2], Juha Hartikainen[1], Tuomas T. Rissanen[1], Johanna Laukkanen[1], Mari Niemi[1], Maija Kossila[1], Tomi P. Häkkinen[1], Antti Kivelä[1], Berndt Enholm[2], Hannu Mansukoski[1], Anna-Mari Turunen[1], Kari Alitalo[2], Seppo Yl ä-Herttuala[1]. *[1]A.I. Virtanen Institute, University of Kuopio, Kuopio; 2 Molecular Cancer Biology Laboratory, Haartman Institute, University of Helsinki, Helsinki, Finland*

Background: Gene transfer may provide new possibilities for the treatment of postangioplasty restenosis. In this study we analyzed the effects of adenovirus-mediated VEGF-C gene transfer on neointima formation after endothelial denudation in rabbits. For comparison, a second group was treated with VEGF-A adenovirus and a third group with *lacZ* adenovirus.

Methods and Results: Aortas of cholesterol-fed New Zealand White rabbits were balloon denuded and gene transfer was performed three days later. Animals were sacrificed 2 and 4 weeks after the gene transfer and intima/media ratio (I/M), histology and cell proliferation were analyzed. Two weeks after the gene transfer I/M in the *lacZ*-transfected control group was 0.57 ± 0.04. VEGF-C gene transfer reduced I/M to 0.38 ± 0.02 ($p < 0.05$ vs. *lacZ* group). I/M in VEGF-A treated animals was 0.49 ± 0.17 (ns). Expression of VEGF receptors 1, 2 and 3 were detected in the vessel wall by using immunocytochemistry and in situ hybridization.

Conclusions: VEGF-C adenovirus gene transfer is effective in reducing intimal thickening. VEGF-C may be useful for the treatment of postangioplasty restenosis and vessel wall thickening after vascular manipulations.

Feasibility of gene transfer through bone marrow cells using lentiviral vector

S. Jovinge[1,3], A. Harpf[2], L. Branén[3], P.K. Shah[1], T. Rajavashisth[1]. *[1]Atheroscl. Res. Center, Cedars-Sinai MC, UCLA, Los Angeles, CA; [2]UCLA CVRL, Los Angeles, CA, USA; [3]Dept. of Med, Univ. Hospital MAS, University of Lund, Malmö, Sweden*

Objective: To establish a feasible model for gene-transfer for vascular disease using bone-marrow cell transduction.

Methods: We investigated the hypothesis that lentiviral vectors transduce bone-marrow cells (BMC) which, when injected to totally body irradiated (TBI) C57Bl/6 mice, result in successful engraftment. A shuttle expression plasmid encoding the enhanced green fluorescent protein (EGFP) under the cytomegalovirus major immediate early promoter/enhancer (CMV) was packaged into lentiviral particles. For, comparison a CD11b controlled expression system was used.

Results: Transduced bone-marrow cells showed EGFP expression on flow-cytometry. EGFP expression was also detected in peripheral blood cells (PBC). The EGFP expression in PBC was detected up to six months after bone marrow transplantation. To increase the specificity of gene-transfer to the vessel wall, the same vector-system was used substituting the CMV-promoter with the monocyte/macrophage specific CD11b-promoter. The relative strength of this promoter was similar to the CMV-promoter in flow-cytometry based assay systems. This later system was used in bone marrow transplantation of apo E deficient mice and EGFP-expression in the atherosclerotic plaques was established demonstrated.

Conclusion: We have demonstrated the successful transduction of murine bone marrow cells using lentiviral vectors encoding EGFP. Furthermore, transplantation of bone-marrow transduced with lentiviral vectors driven by CD11b promoter, we have also demonstrated successful EGFP expression in atherosclerotic plaques in apo E deficient mice. These findings thus demonstrate the feasibility of bone marrow selective gene transfer with lentiviral vectors targeting the vasculature.

Therapeutic angiogenesis induced by HGF: Potential gene therapy for ischemic diseases

Motokuni Aoki[1], Ryuichi Morishita[2], Yoshiaki Taniyama[1], Keita Yamasaki[1], Yasufumi Kaneda[2], Toshio Ogihara[1]. *[1]Department of Geriatric Medicine; [2]Division of Gene Therapy Science, Osaka University Medical School, Suita, Japan*

Objectives: The feasibility of a novel therapeutic strategy using angiogenic growth factors by expediting collateral artery development has recently entered the realm of treatment of ischemic diseases. In USA, human gene therapy for angina and ASO has already begun and it gives a surprising effect. We already reported that HGF has a powerful effect on the proliferation of endothelial cells in vitro. In this study, we hypothesized the transfection of HGF gene into ischemic hindlimbs and infarcted hearts could induce angiogenesis, potentially resulting in a beneficial response to ischemia.

Methods & Results: Human HGF gene or control vector were transfected into ischemic limbs and myocardium by HVJ-liposome method. Although the concentration of endogenous HGF in ischemic hindlimbs and infarcted hearts were siginificantly decreased, this transfection showed a marked increase in rat immunoreactive HGF, accompanied by the over-expression of human HGF. In the myocardium transfected with HGF gene, a significant increase in PCNA-positive endothelial cells and the number of vessels could be observed at 14 days after transfection. Angiogenic activity was also confirmed by the activation of a transcription factor, ets, which is essential for angiogenesis, assessed by immunohistochemistry and electrophoretic mobility shift assay. Also, the complimented HGF by the transfection into the ischemic hindlimbs showed a significant increase in the number of vessels, resulting in a significant increase in blood flow assessed by Laser Doppler Image.

Conclusion: The constant production of the local HGF will be considered as an innovative therapeutic angiogenesis strategy for ischemic diseases.

Optimisation of in vivo arterial transfection

E. O'Brien, X. Ma, C. Glover, H. Miller. *Ottawa Heart Institute, Canada*

Objective: Gene therapy for the treatment of vascular disease is limited by low transfection efficiency and/or undesired biological responses (e.g., with viral vectors). The purpose of this study was to determine an efficient method of delivering liposome/DNA complexes into balloon-injured rabbit iliac arteries using a delivery catheter.

Methods: Cationic liposomes were made from a 1:1 (wt/wt) mixture of DOTAP and DOPE. The plasmid pCMV-AP containing the human placenta alkaline phosphatase (AP) reporter gene was used as a marker gene for these experiments. Prior to initiating the in vivo experiments, the optimal ratio of liposome to DNA complex, as well as the persistence of transgene expression were determined in vitro using cultured vascular SMCs. The liposome/DNA complex was then delivered under pressure using a Dispatch catheter to rabbit iliac arteries that were balloon injured 5 days prior gene delivery. Transfection efficiency was defined as the percentage of transfected cells/total cells per high power field.

Results: The optimal ratio of liposome to DNA was 8:1 (wt/wt). AP expression in transfected SMCs persisted for 28 days, although the percentage of transfected cells declined with time (e.g., at 24 hours: 27.3% ± 2.9%; at 28 days: 0.4% ± 0.1%). The peak transfection efficiency in cultured smooth muscle cells was seen at 24 hours post-transfection. As well, smooth muscle cell proliferation in vitro enhanced the transfection efficiency (e.g., 12.6 fold higher than quiescent cells). In vivo experiments were performed on 9 balloon injured rabbit iliac arteries, with half of the arteries receiving the pCMV-AP plasmid and the other half receiving the liposome only (no plasmid). Low levels of transfection were observed in arteries harvested 1 day post delivery. However, 6/7 arteries harvested 3 days post-delivery had multiple regions of focal transgene expression involving all 3 arterial layers. No gene expression was found in the uninjured aorta.

Conclusion: Liposome mediated gene transfection to all vessel layers can successfully be performed in vivo using local delivery, and may provide an ideal means of targeting vascular disease processes.

174

Geographic epidemiology of atherosclerosis

CHD risk factors in indians: A global comparison

K.S. Reddy. *All India Institute of Medical Sciences, New Delhi, India*

As the engines of health transition gather pace, the epidemic of coronary heart disease (CHD) is accelerating in India, with rise in CHD burdens reported especially in urban settings. Excess mortality due to CHD reported in migrant Indians in several countries, is also a portent of increased risk for Indians. Studies in migrants have been unable to explain the excess risk on the basis of conventional risk factors. High frequency of the metabolic syndrome, elevated lipoprotein 'a' levels and plasma homocysteine have been incriminated in migrant studies. Comparative studies of urban and rural populations in India and migrant-nonmigrant comparisons, however, reveal a gradient of CHD risk best explained by rising levels of conventional risk factors (body mass index, plasma cholesterol and blood pressure). For any level of total cholesterol, Indians appear to have a higher total cholesterol to HDL cholesterol ratio and for any level of LDL cholesterol, the small dense LDL fraction appears to be higher. Thus the lipid Pool is more atherogenic at each level of cholesterol, indicating the need for different guidelines for dyslipidemia. Increments of body mass index even within the "normal" range, are associated with a marked rise in CHD risk factors, in urban-rural comparisons. The migrant studies, comparing different gene pools in a similar environment, identify the non-conventional risk factors as explanatory. The urban-rural and migrant-nonmigrant comparisons, contrasting the same gene pool in different environments, identify the conventional risk factors as explanatory. The excess CHD risk of Indians seems to be related to a confluence of both sets of risk factors and warrants investigation and intervention at both levels.

Globalisation and coronary heart disease

R. Beaglehole. *Health and Sustainable Development, WHO, Geneva, Switzerland*

Objective: To explore the relationship between globalisation and the emerging epidemics of coronary heart disease (CHD) in developing countries.

Methods: The first part of this presentation analyses the critical elements of the modern phase of globalisation and their theoretical impacts on the occurrence of CHD. The second part describes recent trends in CHD in developing countries and assesses the actual impact of globalisation on the epidemics.

Results: The core of modern globalisation is economic interconnectedness and the associated policy regimes. The two facilitating domains are technological, especially of information and communication technologies, and cultural. The specific health risks of globalisation include: the spread of smoking-caused diseases as the tobacco industry rapidly globalises its marketing and promotion strategies; the diseases of dietary excesses, as food production and food processing becomes intensified and as urban consumer preferences are shaped by globally promoted images; the diverse public health consequences of the proliferation of private car ownership; and the resulting rise of obesity. These risks are likely to exacerbate the effects of ageing on the population risk for CHD. The burden of CHD is clearly increasing in developing countries. The age specific effects of the globalisation of risk on CHD rates are not yet so obvious, although the available evidence is limited.

Conclusion: The prevention and control of the emerging CHD epidemics will require a global policy response, not just national initiatives. Sustainable surveillance systems are required to monitor the epidemics and the effects of the prevention policies.

Males with mild and severe coronary atherosclerosis in five European populations over a 25 year period

N.H. Sternby[1], V.S. Zhdanov[2], A.M. Vikhert[2], J. Duskova[3]. *[1]Malmo University Hospital, Malmo, Sweden. [2]Russian Cardiology Complex, Moscow, Russia. [3]Charles University, Prague, Czech Republic*

Objective: To study atherosclerotic (Ath) changes over 25 years in subjects belonging to groups with mild or low atherosclerosis (LAth) and severe or high atherosclerosis (HAth).

Methods: Ath in the coronary arteries was studied on autopsy material during the early 1960s (1st study) and the late 1980s (2nd study) in males, 20—59 years of age, from Malmo, Sweden; Prague, the former Czechoslovakia; and Riga, Tallinn and Yalta, the former Soviet Union. During the 1st study 3597 and during the 2nd study 3456 cases were included. The HAth group included subjects who had died from manifestations of Ath, hypertensives and/or diabetics excluded. The LAth group included mainly subjects who had died from violence or suicide.

Results: The number in the HAth group was 911 and 1218, resp. in the 1st and 2nd study, in the LAth group 1146 and 665, resp. The proportion of males belonging to the HAth group increased in all populations except in Prague. The proportion of males belonging to the LAth group decreased in Riga, Tallinn and Yalta but showed no change in Malmo and Prague. In the HAth group Ath of coronary arteries expressed as extent of raised lesions, was of significantly greater severity in the 2nd study in Riga, Tallinn and Yalta but significantly less severe in Malmo; in Prague no difference was observed. The same pattern was found in the LAth group: Ath decreased in Malmo, did not change in Prague but increased in Riga, Tallinn and Yalta.

Conclusions: Differences in the development of Ath in males of five European populations over a 25-year period were expressed in changing proportions of subjects with mild and severe Ath, as well as changing level of Ath in these groups.

The second nation-wide study of atherosclerosis in infants, children and young adults in Japan

C. Yutani. *Japanese Pathological Study Group of Atherosclerosis in Youth; Department of Pathology, National Cardiovascular Center, Osaka, Japan*

Objective: This paper reports the results of the second nation-wide cooperative study of atherosclerosis in young Japanese with ages ranging from 1 month to 339 years, who were autopsied between 1991 and 1995 in 67 hospitals in Japan.

Methods: Atherosclerotic lesions in 1066 aortas and 974 coronary arteries from 1253 autopsied patients were classified into fatty streaks, fibrous plaques and complicated lesions and were then quantificated with the point-counting method. The definition and the method of the quantification of the atherosclerotic lesions most identical to those of the previous study which was performed 13 years ago and the results of the current study were compared with those of the previous study.

Results: Atherosclerosis of aorta, determined by surface involvement (SI) of atherosclerotic lesions and atherosclerotic index (AI), increased with age in both sexes of the former and the current studies and their tendency for the progression of the extent of atherosclerotic lesions appeared to be similar. Among the three segments of the aorta, the percent intimal surface involved with all lesions was greatest in the abdominal aorta for every age except less than 1 year and the proportion of raised lesions (the sum of the fibrous plaque and complicated lesion) to total lesions was greatest in the abdominal aorta. Fatty streaks preceded the other lesions and accounted for the largest portion of the lesions. Fibrous plaque and complicated lesions developed in the later decades of life. In the aortic segments no significant changes were detected between the two nation-wide studies. In the coronary arteries, the mean values of SI and AI in the males of the current study were significantly greater than those in the male of the former studies and in the female of the both studies in the 3rd and 4th decades.

Correlation of some risk factors with SI and AI of aorta and coronary arteries were analyzed. Age, serum total cholesterol, blood pressure, body mass index and heart weight were significantly correlated with SI and AI of aorta and coronary arteries.

Conclusion: Serum total cholesterol appeared to be more strongly correlated with the extent of fatty streaks than was systolic blood pressure and vice versa with that of fibrous plaques.

A pathologic survey of atherosclerotic lesions in chinese youth

Hai-Lu Zhao[1,2], Hong-Fen Li[1], Li-Bi You[1], Julian A.J.H. Critchley[2]. *[1]Department of Pathology, Chinese PLA General Hospital, Beijing; [2]Division of Clinical Pharmacology, Department of Medicine & Therapeutics, Prince of Wales Hospital, Hong Kong, China*

Objective: In order to provide justification about prevention of atherosclerosis, a pathologic survey was conducted to study the pathogenesis and prevalence of premature atherosclerosis in Chinese youth.

Methods: One-hundred and fifty-seven aortae and ninety-one hearts of autopsy were collected from Chinese youth who died of accident, with age ranging from 15 to 39 years. Both macroscopic and microscopic examinations were taken. Primary antibodies such as CD31, CD45RO, CD3, CD68, α-smooth muscle specific actin, and desmin were employed in the immunohistochemical technique.

Results: Types I, II lesion was found in all the aortae, and most of coronary arteries. The prevalence of type III lesion was 34% in aortae, 27% in coronary arteries, and significantly higher in smokers. Only one case with familial hypercholesterolemia showed severe and diffuse atherosclerotic lesions. Cubic structure change of endothelial cells, CD68-positive macrophage-derived foam cells and activated T lymphocytes (CD45RO and CD3 positive) underlying endothelial cells and predominant desmin negative smooth muscle cells were found in atherosclerotic lesions.

Conclusions: Early atherosclerotic lesions are common within arterial intima of Chinese youths and smoking is an important risk factor. Endothelial dysfunction, macrophage and T lymphocyte activation, and smooth muscle cell dedifferentiation are the major pathologic findings in early atherogenesis.

Hypercholesterolaemia as a risk factor for coronary heart disease in the Asia-Pacific region: The ASPAC study

A. Keech, R. Zambahari, G. Ritchie, V. Thongtang, H. White, A. Carruthers, H. Kalim. *For the Asia-Pacific CHD Risk Factor Collaborative Group; NHMRC Clinical Trials Centre, Sydney, Australia*

Objective: To determine the prevalence of hypercholesterolaemia and rates of dietary advice and drug treatment in CHD patients in more than 180 randomly selected hospitals in the Asia-Pacific region.

Methods: Medical records were reviewed over 6 months follow-up among 4,112 patients admitted with myocardial infarction or unstable angina. Hypercholesterolaemia was defined as documented history, blood level $\geq$ 5.5 mmol/l or use of lipid-lowering therapy at any time.

Results: Cholesterol measurement rates after CHD ranged from 42% (Thailand) to 99% (Japan) of patients. Mean cholesterol levels in Asian countries ranged from 4.9 to 5.9 mmol/l (190 to 229 mg/dl) with 33% (Taiwan) to 63% (Malaysia) of measured patients having blood levels of $\geq$ 5.5 mmol/l compared with 54% in Australia and 72% in New Zealand. Formal dietary advice appeared not to be given or documented in most countries. From 16% to 52% of hypercholesterolaemic patients received drug therapy, with HMG CoA reductase inhibitors most common. Follow-up measures were infrequent, but with 74% of elevated levels failing to fall below 5.5 mmol/l. Rates of use of cholesterol-lowering drugs correlated strongly with Gross National Product per capita.

Conclusions: The prevalence of hypercholesterolaemia in CHD varies more than two-fold in the region. Measurement and treatment rates also vary widely. A "treatment gap" exists between the recent evidence of benefit from cholesterol lowering treatment and our recent practice patterns. A coordinated approach to cholesterol management is needed.

Transplantation atherosclerosis

Renal transplantation arteriosclerosis is a cell-mediated intimal immune response

Hai-Lu Zhao[1,2], Hong-Fen Li[1], Li-Bi You[1], Julian A.J.H. Critchley[2]. *[1]Department of Pathology, Chinese PLA General Hospital, Beijing; [2]Division of Clinical Pharmacology, Prince of Wales Hospital, Hong Kong, China*

Objective: To study the pathogenesis of renal transplantation arteriosclerosis.

Methods: One-hundred and two human renal allografts were removed surgically due to function failure, examined pathologically. Cases with arteriosclerosis were studied using immunohistochemical technique. Antibodies specifically for T lymphocytes, B lymphocytes, macrophages, endothelial cells, smooth muscle cells, cytomegalovirus (CMV), bcl-2 protein, transforming growth factor (TGF-β_1) were employed.

Results: Thirty-eight renal allografts developed arteriosclerosis, which accounted for 93% of the failed allografts survived for more than 1 year. in CMV-infected renal transplants, the incidence of definite arteriosclerosis with intimal extensive lymphocyte and macrophage/foam cell infiltration is 82%, compared with 23% of those without CMV viral inclusions ($p < 0.001$). Immunostains showed that more than 80% of the intimal infiltrated inflammatory cells were activated T lymphocytes. The other infiltrates beneath endothelial cells were mainly macrophages and lipid-loaded foam cells. Endothelial cells appeared degeneration and proliferation changes, mitosis was occasionally found, a-Actin-positive smooth muscle cells predominated over desmin-positive ones. Aberrant bcl-2 and TGF-β_1 were also observed.

Conclusions: Transplantation arteriosclerosis is indicated the major limit for long-term renal allograft survival. It may be resulted from T lymphocyte-mediated arterial intimal immune injury with subsequent smooth muscle proliferation.

Expression of thrombospondin-1 (TSP-1) in human cardiac allografts

X.M. Zhao, Y. Hu, R. Michell, G. Miller, P. Libby. *Brigham and Women's Hospital, Boston, MA; Vanderbilt Medical Center, Nashville, TN, USA*

Expression of endogenous angiogenic growth factors is significantly elevated while angiogenesis is not present in cardiac allografts. We hypothesize that other factors expressed in allografts may alter vascular response to angiogenic growth factors. TSP-1 is a matrix glycoprotein that inhibits angiogenesis and facilitates the proliferation and migration of smooth muscle cells (SMC) by growth factors.

Methods: Quantitative RT-PCR and immunohistology were used to analyze expression of TSP-1 and its receptors in endomyocardial biopsies from human cardiac allografts and normal human hearts. In vitro experiments were used to investigate regulation of TSP-1 by cytokines and allostimulation.

Results: Expression of TSP-1 mRNA was significantly increased in human cardiac allografts compared to normal hearts. TSP/GAPDH ratio was 1.26 ± 0.21 in cardiac allografts vs. 0.26 ± 0.03 ($p = 0.005$) in normal hearts. Persistent elevation of TSP-1 was strongly associated with the severity of CAV. CD36 and CD47 were also elevated in allografts. Immunohistochemistry demonstrated intense expression of TSP-1 in cardiac allografts, predominantly in intimal SMC from arteries with severe CAV. In vitro experiments demonstrated that TSP-1 was induced in mixed lymphocyte cultures. IL-1 beta, IFN-gamma, and TNF alpha strongly induced TSP-1 expression in SMC.

Conclusions: Expression of TSP-1 and its receptors is significantly increased in human cardiac allografts and is associated with the severity of CAV. Cytokines and allostimulation regulate TSP-1 expression in SMC and T cells. Augmented levels of TSP-1 and its receptors in human cardiac allografts may alter vascular response to angiogenic growth factors by inhibiting angiogenesis and promoting SMC proliferation characteristic of CAV.

Transplant vascular disease: Potential sites of intervention

P. Häyry. *Transplantation Laboratory, University of Helsinki and Helsinki University Central Hospital, Helsinki, Finland*

Three separate target sites have so far been discovered to present fibrointimal dysplasia in chronic rejection after the process has become autonomous of the triggenring event. Interference with receptors, particularly with their early signaling events, regulating smooth muscle cell migration and replication and targeting to two sepatare sets of vasculo-protective gene products: somatostatin receptor subtypes 1, 4 and estrogen receptor beta. For rational drug design, aiming specifically to agonize or antagonize a given receptor, ligand or enzyme, the following four modalities exist. Gene therapy, monoclonal antibodies, chimeric or humanized, non-degradable peptides based on D- rather than L-amino acids and peptidomimetics, which are organic compounds lacking the peptide bond. Only the last approach will generate credible orally available drug candidates. This approach will need reliable modeling of the target receptor, combinatorial chemistry and high throughput screens using cell lines permanently overexpressing the desired genes. In regard to receptor protein tyrosine kinases, the crystal stucture of the phosphorylation sites of at least EGF, PDGF, FGF anf IGF-1 receptors are known and they are sufficiently different to generate receptor-specific drugs. In regard to 7-transmembrane G-protein coupled receptors, the modeling of SSTR subtypes will be a particularly demanding task, as the receptor cannot be crystallized. In regard to estrogen receptor subtypes, the ligand-binding domains have already been crystallized. Indications for these drugs would not be limited to transplantation but will also include other forms of fibroproliferative vasculopaties, such as complications of bypass surgery, PTCA procedures, autoimmune and diabetic vasculopathies and possibly variations of the common form of atherosclerosis.

Endothelial cell changes in microvessels of organ allografts

Z. Jurukova[1], H.J. Knieriem[2], V. Minkova[1]. *[1] Dept. of Pathology, Med. Faculty Sofia, Bulgaria, [2] Dept. of Pathology, Bethesda Hospital, Duisburg, Germany*

Objective of the study was to evaluate the micro- and ultrastructure of microvessels in long term heart- and kidney allotransplants.

Methods: Histologic and electronmicroscopic investigations were performed on: a) endomyocardial biopsies from 16 long-term heart-transplant recipients, 2 of whom died 13, resp. 15 months after transplantation on cardiac failure; b) renal biopsies from 12 long-term kidney-transplant recipients, 2 of them died 11, resp. 25 months after transplantation on renal failure.

Results: In all of the 4 deceased patients consecutive biopsies from the organ allograft revealed during the entire post-transplant period only transitional signs of mild cellular rejection. By light microscopy some swelling or proliferation of microvessel endothelial cells were observed. Electronmicroscopy demonstrated however severe endothelial altera-tions in capillaries, arterioles and even venules, manifested by prominent swelling of endothelial cells with loss of subcellular organelles and severe narrowing of the vessel lumina. At autopsy the pattern of severe graft vasculopathy could be detected throughout the allograft.

Conclusion: Our findings in organ allograft biopsies suggest that microvascular endothelial damage could represent a marker for evolving transplant vasculopathy and chronic vascular rejection.

Lipoprotein(a) inhibits proliferation of human umbilical venous endothelial cells (HUVEC) in vitro

F. Wahn[1], D. Michalk[2], U. Querfeld[1]. *[1]Department for Pediatric Nephrology, University of Berlin Charité, Schumannstr. 20/21, 10117 Berlin; [2]Children's Hospital, University of Cologne, Germany*

Objective: We have previously shown that Lipoprotein(a) [Lp(a)] is a risk factor for chronic renal transplant rejection. Histologically, the affected vessels show a significant intima proliferation. To investigate if Lp(a) is a growth factor for endothelial cells we have studied the effect of Lp(a) on the proliferation of human umbilical venous endothe-lial cells (HUVEC) in a cell culture model.

Methods: HUVECs were activated by a 24-h incubation with interferon γ (IFvγ). After-wards, the cells were incubated with different concentrations of Lp(a) or low density lipo-proteins (LDL) for another 24 h in the presence of IFvγ. The proliferation of the cells was measured by the uptake of bromodesoxyuridyl (BrdU) of the cells as an expression for DNA-synthesis.

Results: While LDL-incubation stimulated the proliferation of endothelial cells in vitro, the incubation of HUVECs with Lp(a) inhibited proliferation. This effect was significant and dependent on the concentration (10—200 µg/ml) and time of incubation (4—48 h). The activation of the cells with IFvγ had no influence on these effects.

Conclusions: Against our expectations, Lp(a) seems to have an inhibitory effect on pro-liferation of HUVECs. To study this effect more closely further experiments are necessary.

Restenosis

The role of vascular smooth muscle cell apoptosis in atherosclerosis and restenosis

Martin R. Bennett. *Addenbrooke's Centre for Clinical Investigation, Addenbrooke's Hospital, Cambridge, UK*

The orthodox view holds that vascular smooth muscle cell (VSMC) proliferation is a major contributor to disease states such as atherosclerosis or restenosis after angioplasty, arguing that deregulated cell proliferation and phenotypic differences in VSMCs in these processes generate the disease. As a consequence, major efforts have been made to inhibit VSMC proliferation, which have been unsuccessful in inhibiting clinical events in either disease. More recently, it has been recognised that VSMCs and their products, extracellular matrix and collagen, comprise the major structural components of the atherosclerotic plaque, and a reduction in cell numbers, either by inhibition of cell proliferation or increased apoptosis may be detrimental. VSMC accumulation in atherosclerosis is now viewed as a repair process, and failure of repair may lead to plaque rupture. In fact, plaque VSMCs from advanced human plaques show poor proliferation, early senescence and increased apoptosis, and are thus a "senescent" phenotype, incapable of effective repair. Plaque VSMCs show intrinsic defects in both mitogenic and survival signalling, and activation of cell cycle machinery in plaque VSMCs induces apoptosis, not cell proliferation. Thus, although plaque VSMCs are surrounded by mitogens, they cannot repair a damaged plaque effectively. In addition, plaque VSMCs show increased sensitivity to agents that induce DNA damage and p53 activation, such as free radicals and nitric oxide.

In restenosis after angioplasty, the major determinant of restenosis is the extent of negative remodelling of the vessel, not the degree of neointimal accumulation. However, both VSMC proliferation and apoptosis regulate vessel calibre in remodelling, so that cell cycle inhibition may inhibit negative remodelling. In contrast to VSMCs from primary plaques, VSMCs from human restenosis lesions show increased cell proliferation and delayed senescence, but retain high rates of apoptosis, and the sensitivity to DNA-damage induced apoptosis. This appears to be a true "repair" phenotype. Examination of cell cycle machinery reveals stable differences in expression of cyclins, cdks, and cdk inhibitors that underlie this difference. Such differences may account for the failure of conventional antiproliferatives to inhibit neointimal accumulation in restenosis.

Inhibition of angioplasty restenosis by vascular brachytherapy: mechanisms of action and role of the adventitia

Josiah N. Wilcox. *Emory University, Atlanta, Georgia, USA*

Post-angioplasty restenosis is a major problem confronting cardiology today. While most studies have focused on neointimal development after angioplasty, recent data indicates that negative vascular remodeling, seen as constriction of the external elastic lamina, may contribute to lumen loss. Intravascular brachytherapy has been shown to be effective in blocking post-angioplasty restenosis and vascular remodeling in experimental animal models. Early results from clinical trials suggest that restenosis rates with brachytherapy are < 15%. Previously we have described the proliferation of myofibroblasts in the adventitia surrounding porcine coronary arteries after angioplasty. Tracing studies indicate that these cells migrate from the adventitia and contribute to the cellular mass of the neointima. Experimental studies from our laboratory suggest that adventitial myofibroblasts may be one of the most important targets of brachytherapy. Radiation treatment of porcine coronary arteries after angioplasty reduces proliferation of adventitial myofibroblasts, inhibits the expression of PDGF by these cells, prevents formation of a myofibroblast scar at the angioplasty site and improves vascular remodeling. One of the mechanisms by which radiation appears to work is by increasing the expression of p21 in adventitial cells. These studies support the hypothesis that adventitial myofibroblasts contribute to vascular remodeling associated with angioplasty and emphasize the potential of radiation therapy in the control of restenosis.

Construction and characterization of an HBGAM/FGF-1 chimera for vascular tissue engineering

L. Xue[1], S. Woloson[1], B. Hampton[3], W. Burgess[3], H. Greisler[1,2]. *[1]Department of Surgery; [2]Cell Biology, Maywood, Illinois; [3] Department of Tissue Biology, Holland Laboratories of the American Red Cross, Rockville, Maryland, USA*

Objective: Cardiovascular tissue engineering approaches to vessel wall restoration have focused on the potent but relatively nonspecific and heparin-dependent mesenchymal cell mitogen FGF-1. We constructed an heparin-binding growth-associated molecule (HBGAM)/FGF-1 chimera by linking full length human HBGAM to the amino-terminus of human FGF-1b (21-154) and tested it's activities on SMCs and ECs.

Methods: SMCs and ECs proliferations in response to the HBGAM/FGF-1 chimera and FGF-1 were measured by 3H-thymidine incorporation.

Results: In the presence of heparin the HBGAM/FGF-1 chimera stimulated less SMC proliferation ($p < 0.000001$ at 0.15 pmol) than did the wild-type FGF-1 with an ED50 of ~ 0.15 pmol vs. ~ 0.05 pmol. By contrast the chimera retained full stimulating activity on EC proliferation with an ED50 of 0.03 pmol for the both cytokines. Unlike the wild type protein, the chimera possessed heparin-independent activity and less synergistic response by the addition of heparin with no synergism at concentrations > 0.3 pmol. In the absence of heparin the chimera induced dose-dependent EC and SMC proliferation at 30.03 pmol compared to the wild-type FGF-1 which stimulated minimal DNA synthesis at 3.0 pmol concentrations.

Conclusions: The HBGAM/FGF-1 chimera displays significantly greater land uniquely heparin-independent mitogenic activity for both cell types and in the presence of heparin a significantly greater EC specificity.

This chimeric construct may provide a novel approach to engineering endothelialized surfaces without the concurrent fibroplastic reaction elicited by wild type FGF-1.

Relationship between monocyte chemoattractant protein-1 and restenosis after coronary angioplasty

F. Cipollone[1], M. Marini[1], M. Fazia[1], M. Torello[1], L. Paloscia[2], G. Materazzo[2], E. D'Annunzio[2], F. Chiarelli[1], F. Cuccurullo[1], A. Mezzetti[1]. *[1]Department of Medicine and Aging, University of Chieti "G D'Annunzio" School of Medicine, Chieti; [2]The Division of Cardiology, Spirito Santo Hospital, Pescara, Italy*

Objective: Inflammation appears to play a pivotal role in the development of restenosis after coronary angioplasty (PTCA). Activation of leucocytes to areas of vessel injury is an important factor in this inflammatory response. The monocytes chemoattractant protein-1 (MCP-1) is a specific chemoattractant of leucocytes and can modulate other functions of these cells e.g., generation of reactive oxygen species such as superoxide anion (O_2^-). The purpose of our study is to investigate the role of this chemokine in the restenosis.

Methods: We measured circulating levels of MCP-1 and vitamin C before and 1, 5, 15, 180 days after PTCA in 50 patients (30 M; 20 F; aged 62 ± 5 years) who underwent PTCA and who had repeat angiograms at 6-month follow-up. Restenosis occurred in 14 (28%) patients. Levels of MCP-1 were meausured by ELISA assay (values as pg/ml) and vitamin C was measured by a spectrophotometric assay (values as µmol/l).

Results: As shown in table, there were no differences before PTCA between the two groups. However, after PTCA, patients with restenosis showed significantly elevated levels of MCP-1 and significantly reduced plasma concentration of vitamin C.

Variables	Pre PTCA	1 day post	5 days post	15 days post	180 days post
MCP-1 restenosis	480 ± 42	$816 \pm 17^*$	$755 \pm 158^*$	$712 \pm 54^*$	$715 \pm 80^*$
no restenosis	470 ± 69	618 ± 102	594 ± 111	450 ± 72	445 ± 49
VIT. C restenosis	39 ± 3	$25 \pm 5^{**}$	23 ± 4	$24 \pm 5^{\#}$	$25 \pm 6^{\#}$
no restenosis	40 ± 4	35 ± 3	38 ± 3	40 ± 3	42 ± 5

$^*p < 0.0001$; $^{**}p = 0.007$; $^{\#}p < 0.0001$

Moreover, MCP-1 levels were significantly correlated ($p < 0.0001$) with monocyte activity, measured as O_2^- production from healthy subjects monocytes incubated with serum of patients, both before and 24 hours after PTCA $\rho = 0.87$ and $\rho = 0.528$, respectively).

Conclusion: This study suggests that: a) MCP-1 may play a key role in the pathophysiology of restenosis after PTCA; b) this effect is mediated, at least in part, by an increased monocyte O_2^- production and consequent circulating vitamin C consumption.

A novel model for restenosis in the carotid arteries of APOE−/− and LDLR−/− mice

J.H. von der Thüsen, Th.J.C. van Berkel, E.A.L. Biessen. *Division of Biopharmaceutics, Leiden/Amsterdam Center for Drug Research, Leiden University, The Netherlands*

Objective: Effective treatment of restenosis in existing animal models does frequently not translate into effectivity of these approaches in a clinical setting. This indicates the need for a more representative animal model, and we have therefore developed an advanced two-step model of restenosis in two atherosclerosis-prone mouse strains.

Methods: A silastic collar was placed around the carotid arteries of ApoE−/− and LDLR−/− mice, which has previously been shown to induce localised atherogenesis proximal to the collar. The thus obtained carotid lesions were angioplastied with a rigid balloon catheter and cross-sections of the artery were analysed morphometrically and histologically 3 weeks after the procedure.

Results: Post-angioplasty neointima enlargement was observed in both ApoE−/− and LDLR−/− animals. The respective cross-sectional plaque areas after treatment were 9.96×10^4 µm^2 (n = 8) and 2.31×10^4 µm^2 (n = 5) on a western-type diet. Immunohistochemical staining revealed a complex neointimal composition with large smooth muscle cell-rich areas in addition to moderate intimal macrophage accumulation. Omission of the high-cholesterol diet after angioplasty reduced these values to 4.59×10^4 μm^2 (n = 6) and 1.45×10^4 μm^2 (n = 4), resp., while increasing the relative smooth muscle cell content of the neointima.

Conclusions: This murine model closely resembles human post-angioplasty restenosis in aetiology and neointima composition, and we therefore believe it to be a valuable new tool in the study of restenosis. Evaluation of new treatment strategies for the prevention of restenosis in this model may also allow a more accurate prediction of the effectivity of these therapeutic entities in clinical practice.

Polylysine as a vehicle for extracellular matrix-targeted intravascular drug delivery, providing high accumulation and long-term retention within the vessel wall

D.V. Sakharov, J.J. Emeis, D.C. Rijken. *Gaubius Laboratory, TNO Prevention and Health, Leiden, The Netherlands*

Background: Catheter-based delivery methods are currently being elaborated for local intravascular delivery of concentrated drugs, particularly for treatment of restenosis after coronary angioplasty. Short retention time of the delivered drugs in the vessel wall critically reduces the efficacy of this technique. We propose an approach of extracellular matrix (ECM)-directed drug targeting. The approach is based on a concept of a bifunctional drug consisting of an anti-restenotic effector moiety and an "affinity vehicle" capable of delivering and retaining the drug within the ECM of the vessel wall. The "affinity vehicle" should bind to an abundant component of the vessel wall, in order to provide a high concentration and ubiquitous distribution of the bound drug within the vessel wall.

Objective: As a first step in the elaboration of this approach, we studied polylysine as one of potential "affinity vehicles", which might bind to negatively charged glycosaminoglycan components of the vascular ECM.

Methods and Results: Fluorescence-labelled poly-L-lysine was shown to bind abundantly to all layers of cross-sections of human vessels in a plasma environment. After delivery under pressure into a segment of
a human umbilical artery, polylysine was concentrated throughout a luminal layer (50—100 μm) of the vessel wall, and was retained therein after 72 h of perfusion without noticeable losses. Also after in vivo delivery into a segment of a rat carotid artery, polylysine was still present in the vessel wall after 72 h, whereas control FITC-albumin was washed out in 1—2 hours. No major thrombotic or inflammatory complications were documented.

Conclusions: Polylysine can be considered as a potential "affinity vehicle" within the proposed approach of ECM-targeted local drug delivery. Testing of antirestenotic drugs potentially usable within this approach is currently underway.

Diet and bioactive components of food

A locus conferring resistance to diet-induced hypercholesterolemia and atherosclerosis on mouse chromosome 2

A.J. Lusis[1], A. Mouzeyan[1], J. Choi[2], H. Allayee[1], X. Wang[1], J. Sinsheimer[1], J. Phan[3], L.W. Castellani[1], K. Reue[1,3], R.C. Davis[1]. [1]University of California, Los Angeles; [3]VA West Los Angeles Healthcare Center, USA; and [2]Seoul National University, Seoul, Korea

Dietary cholesterol is known to raise total and low density lipoprotein cholesterol concentrations in humans and experimental animals, but the response among individuals varies greatly. We identified a mouse strain, C57BL/6ByJ (B6By), that is resistant to diet-induced hyper-cholesterolemia, in contrast to m phenotype seen in other common strains of mice including the closely related C57BL/6J (B6J) strain. Compared to B6J, B6By mice exhibit somewhat lower basal cholesterol levels on a chow diet, and show a relatively modest increase in absolute levels of total and LDL/VLDL cholesterol in response to an atherogenic diet containing 15% fat, 1.25% cholesterol and 0.5% cholate. Correspondingly, B6By mice are also resistant to diet-induced aortic lesions, with less than 15% as many lesions as B6J. Food intake and cholesterol absorption are similar between B6By and B6J mice.

To investigate the gene(s) underlying the resistant B6By phenotype, we performed genetic crosses with the unrelated mouse strain, A/J. A genome-wide scan revealed a locus, designated Diet1, on chromosome 2 showing highly significant linkage (lod = 9.6) between B6By alleles and hypo-response to diet. Examination of known genes in this region suggested that this locus represents a novel gene affecting plasma lipids and atherogenesis in response to diet.

We have now isolated this locus by constructing congenic strains in which the Diet1 gene from B6By has been placed on other genetic backgrounds. Using these congenics, fine structure mapping of the gene has been initiated. We are also utilizing chip technologies to test for variations in gene expression to aid in the identification of candidate genes.

PPARS: Fatty acid-activated receptors controlling lipid metabolism and inflammation

B. Staels. U.325 INSERM, Dépt. D'Athérosclérose, Institut Pasteur, Lille, France

Peroxisome proliferator-activated receptors (PPARs) are ligand-activated transcription factors belonging to the nuclear receptor family. The hypolipidemic fibrates and the antidiabetic glitazones are synthetic ligands for PPARα and PPARγ, respectively. Furthermore, fatty acids and eicosanoids are natural PPAR ligands. PPARs function as regulators of lipid and lipoprotein metabolism and glucose homeostasis and influence cellular proliferation, differentiation and apoptosis. PPARα is highly expressed in tissues such as liver, muscle, kidney and heart, where it stimulates the b-oxydative degradation of fatty acids. PPARα furthermore mediates the action of the hypolipidemic drugs of the fibrate class on plasma lipoprotein metabolism. PPARγ is predominantly expressed in intestine and adipose tissue. PPARγ triggers adipocyte differentiation and promotes lipid storage. In addition, PPARs play a role in inflammation control. PPAR activators inhibit the activation of inflammatory response genes by negatively interfering with the NF-kB and AP-1 signalling pathways. PPAR activators exert these anti-inflammatory activities in different immunological and vascular wall cell types such as monocyte/macrophages, endothelial, epithelial and smooth muscle cells in which PPARs are expressed. These findings indicate a modulatory role for PPARs in the control of lipid and glucose metabolism, as well as in the inflammatory response with potential therapeutic applications in inflammation-related diseases, such as atherosclerosis.

Obesity and diabetes gene loci in genetically obese mice

Alan D. Attie, Jonathan Stoehr, Samuel Nadler, Mary Rabaglia, Brian Yandell, Kathryn Schueler, Stewart Metz. *Department of Biochemistry, University of Wisconsin-Madison, Madison, Wisconsin, USA*

While obesity is an important risk factor for Type-II Diabetes, background genetic factors substantially modify an individual's risk for developing the disease. We sought to identify modifier alleles present within a murine model of insulin resistance developed by our laboratory – the BTBR x C57BL6/J F1 mouse. In lean F1 mice, these alleles result in impaired glucose tolerance and impaired glucose uptake into muscle and adipose tissue. We hypothesized that these alleles might also lead to severe diabetes in ob/ob animals. If obese BTBR and B6 mice differed in their susceptibility to diabetes, we could identify the loci responsible for the modification of the diabetes syndrome. We introgressed the ob allele into the BTBR strain using marker-assisted backcrossing for 6 generations, and intercrossed to produce ob/ob mice. These N6F1 mice (BTBR. ob/ob) have markedly higher fasting levels of plasma glucose compared to B6- ob/ob at 10 weeks (females: 360 vs. 170 mg/dl, $p < 10$-7; males: 460 vs. 250 mg/dl, $p < 10$-4). BTBR. ob/ob mice also have significantly lower fasting plasma insulin levels at 8 and 10 weeks. We generated 250 F2 ob/ob mice. These F2 mice exhibit a 5-fold range in fasting plasma glucose at 10 weeks of age (150–750 mg/dl) and a 60-fold range in fasting plasma insulin (2–120 ng/ml). The F2 mice show great variability in pathophysiology of b-cells. We genotyped the F2 panel at 120 polymorphic markers and used composite interval mapping techniques to detect segregating QTL. We report two highly significant linkages to the plasma glucose trait. One of the two loci also shows highly significant linkage to the plasma insulin trait. Surprisingly, although all of the F2 animals were ob/ob, their body weight showed a large range – 40–75 g. We therefore mapped two gene loci that together control 30% of the variance in body weight. In conclusion, we have shown that alleles within the BTBR strain exacerbate the obesity/diabetes syndrome in ob/ob mice, and we have detected two such modifier loci with highly significant linkages. In addition, we have mapped two body weight loci that do not involve the leptin pathway.

Consumption of plant stanol esters increase LDL receptor expression in mononuclear cells from non-hypercholesterolemic subjects

J. Plat, R.P. Mensink. *Department of Human Biology, Maastricht University, Maastricht, The Netherlands*

Introduction: Plant stanol esters lower serum LDL cholesterol by reducing intestinal cholesterol absorption. This causes a compensatory increase in cholesterol synthesis. Whether LDL receptor expression is also changed, is not known. We therefore decided to analyze effects of stanol ester consumption on LDL receptor expression on three subpopulations of human mononuclear cells.

Methods: 112 men and women consumed for a four week run-in period a low erucic acid rapeseed (LEAR) oil based margarine and shortening, followed by an 8 week test period of the same rapeseed oil based products enriched with wood (n = 34) or vegetable oil (n = 36) based plant stanol ester mixtures. Daily stanol intake was 3.8—4.0 g. A control group consumed no plant stanol esters (n = 42). LDL receptor expression was measured in a subset of 36 subjects (n = 12 of each group) by flow cytometry using FITC labeled MABs against the LDL receptor. Monocytes, T-and B-lymphocytes were identified by PE-conjugated MABs.

Results: Consumption of plant stanol esters significantly (p < 0.001) lowered LDL cholesterol with 13—15%. LDL receptor expression on monocytes increased by 50% (p = 0.011) and 13% (p = 0.039) in the wood based and the vegetable oil based group respectively. Compared to the control group, T-lymphocyte LDL receptor expression was 34% (p = 0.033) higher in the wood and 20% (p = 0.155) in the vegetable oil based group. Expression on B-lymphocytes was not affected.

Conclusion: Consumption of plant stanol esters induces a higher expression of the LDL receptor on the surface of mononuclear cells. Whether this is due to enhanced receptor synthesis and/or lower degradation remains to be established.

Role of sequestration in hepatic uptake of chylomicron remnants

K.C.-W. Yu[1,2], W. Chen[1], A.D. Cooper[1,2]. [1]*Palo Alto Medical Foundation Research Institute;* [2]*Stanford University Department of Medicine, CA, USA*

Objective: To visualize chylomicron remnant (CR) accumulation in the space of Disse (SD) and determine the role of the LDL receptor, the LDL receptor-related-protein (LRP), hepatic apoE, and HSPG in sequestration in the SD.

Methods: CR were labeled with the fluorescent dye, DiD (DiD-R), and perfused into isolated livers from LDL receptor-knockout (LRKO) mice, apoE-knockout (EKO) mice, apoE/LDLR-double-knockout (DKO) mice and C57BL/6J (wildtype) mice in a single nonrecirculating pass. Livers were processed for immunocytochemistry and confocal laser microscopy. Endothelial cells were labeled with FITC-conjugated anti-von Willebrand factor antibodies. Cellular periphery (F-actin fibers) were labeled with rhodamine-conjugated phalloidin.

Results: In normal livers CR were rapidly internalized with little accumulation in SD. In LRKO livers, the capacity for remnant removal was reduced with substantial accumulation in the SD. To prove CR were not internalized by hepatocytes, endothelial, or Kupfer cells in LRKO, trypan blue was perfused through the liver to quench extracellular fluorescence. The majority of fluoresence in the LRKO animal was between the hepatocyte and the endothelial cells and was quenched. RAP (inhibitor of LRP) virtually eliminated DiD-remnant fluoresence in SD, suggesting the LRP was absolutely required for sequestration. In EKO livers, there was little accumulation of remnants in the SD and internalization into hepatocytes was normal. Accumulation of remnants in SD was increased in DKO livers. Sodium heparin and fibroblast growth factor (ligands of HSPG) are being studied to evaluate the role of HSPG.

Conclusions: 1. There is sequestration of remnants in SD before endocytosis only in the absence of the LDL receptor. 2. Accumulation of remnants in the space of Disse is dependent on the LRP and does not require hepatic apoE. This technique will now allow evaluation of the role of HSPG in this process.

Possible role of SREBP1c in fish oil-mediated regulation of APOC-III gene expression

J. Dallongeville[1], E. Raspé[1,2], E. Baugé[1], J.C. Fruchart[1], B. Staels[1]. [1]*Département d'athérosclérose and INSERM U-325, Lille;* [2]*CRD Lacassagne, Lipha sa, Lyon, France*

Fish oil exert part of its effect by altering the expression of various genes involved in lipid metabolism. The goal of the present study was to assess the effect of fish oil on apoC-III metabolism. To this end, transgenic human apoC-III mice (hTgC-III) and wild-type (WT) controls were fed either coconut oil or fish oil for 2 weeks. Triglyceride and apoC-III levels were lowered in both the fish oil-fed WT and hTgC-III mice. The decrease in TG levels was associated with decrease in TG production rate and an increase in TG catabolic rate. The later effect support the concept that lower levels of apoC-III are associated with improved clearance of TG. Fish oil treatment resulted in lowered levels of liver apoC-III mRNA in both strains suggesting that fish oil decrease apoC-III gene expression. Recently, fish oil has been shown to decrease at least the maturation and hence the transcriptionnal activity of the transcription factor SREBP1c. In order to investigate if such decrease could explain the effects of fish oil on apo C-III and TG levels, cotransfection assays in RK13 cells were conducted. We observed a specific and potent enhancement of the –1415/+24 fragment of the human apo C-III promoter activity by overexpresssing the mature nuclear form of SREBP1c. Specific binding of SREBP on a putative E-Box located in position –87/–82 was confirmed in vitro by gel shift experiments using wild-type or mutated oligonucleotide probes covering this fragment. In conclusion, since SREBP1c activated human apoC-III gene expression, and since fish oil reduces the nuclear SREBP1c level, SREBP1c could be involved in the decrease in plasma apoC-III and liver apoC-III mRNA levels observed with fish oil.

Long-chain N-3 fatty acids improve large artery elasticity in humans; DHA and EPA are equivalent

P. Nestel[1], H. Shige[1], S. Pomeroy[1], M. Cehun[1], D. Raederstorff[2]. [1]*Baker Medical Research Institute, Melbourne, Australia;* [2]*Vitamin Research Human Nutrition, F. Hoffmann-La Roche, Basel, Switzerland*

Objective: To test the relative capacity of the two major fish oil n-3 fatty acids (EPA and DHA) to raise compliance (elasticity) of large arteries, since reduced compliance leads to systolic hypertension and possible coronary insufficiency.

Methods: 38 middle-aged dyslipidemic subjects were randomised into three groups to receive either placebo (Pl) (14), 3 g EPA (12) or 3 g DHA (12) for 7 weeks in a double-blind parallel design trial. The groups were well matched for key variables. Outcome data: systemic arterial compliance (SAC) by noninvasive measurements of arterial pressure pulse waves and aortic flows; plasma lipoproteins; arterial pressures (BP). Comparisons by paired t-test, run-in versus end.

Results: 1. SAC improved with both fatty acids, run-in vs. end: Pl 0.150 and 0.150 units; EPA 0.149 and 0.202 (p < 0.005); DHA 0.147 and 0.186 (p = 0.012). Plasma TG and VLDL TG fell significantly with EPA (28%) and DHA (31%); HDL C rose with DHA (10%, p = 0.002) but not EPA. LDL C and BP were not influenced. Plasma fatty acids: with EPA only EPA rose; with DHA both DHA and EPA rose; oleic fell).

Conclusion: Arterial compliance, a likely new risk factor for cardiovascular disease, was significantly improved when dyslipidemic subjects were given 3 g EPA or DHA.

Lipoprotein profile improved.

Extracellular matrix

Proteoglycans in atherosclerosis and restenosis

T.N. Wight. *University of Washington, Seattle, Washington, USA*

Proteoglycans accumulate within atherosclerotic and restenotic lesions and contribute to increased tissue mass and altered vascular cell phenotypes. Furthermore, these molecules interact with lipoproteins to increase lipid retention throughout vascular lesions. Versican, the major interstitial chondroitin sulfate proteoglycan (CSPG), increases as lesions progress but is rapidly degraded as lesions regress. Versican is synthesized by arterial smooth muscle cells (ASMC) as multiple mRNA spliced variants. Overexpression of versican by cell mediated gene transfer alters ASMC phenotype and influences extracellular matrix (ECM) composition in blood vessels subjected to experimental injury. Versican interacts with hyaluronan to form complexes outside the cell, which are required for these cells to proliferate and migrate. Decorin is a small dermatan sulfate proteoglycan (DSPG) that influences vascular calcification and inhibits TGF-b1 activity when overexpressed by ASMC transduced with decorin cDNA. Transfer of decorin overproducing ASMCs into injured arteries reduces intimal thickening and promotes collagen deposition. Decorin is synthesized also by endothelial cells during sprouting and tube formation in vitro and may, in part, regulate angiogenesis. Biglycan is another DSPG that accumulates in vascular lesions and interacts with lipoproteins. Interference of this interaction in diet induced atherosclerotic animal models blocks lesion formation. Heparan sulfate proteoglycans (HSPGs) are synthesized by ASMCs and endothelial cells and influence vascular cell adhesion, proliferation and migration. Removal of HSPG from injured arteries by heparinase treatment is effective in reducing the mitogenic response induced by bFGF in arterial smooth muscle cells. Collectively, these studies indicate multiple roles for specific proteoglycans in atherosclerosis and restenosis.

Expression of "proteoglycan-binding defective LDL" in transgenic mice

Jan Borén. *Wallenberg Laboratory, University of Göteborg, Sweden*

Subendothelial retention of LDL through their interaction with proteoglycans has been proposed to be a key process in the pathogenesis of atherosclerosis. We have earlier shown that the substitution of the basic amino acids residues in Site B (residues 3359–3369) in apo-B100, the protein moiety of LDL, with neutral amino acids abolished both the LDL receptor-binding activity and the proteoglycan binding activities of the recombinant LDL. To test if the interaction between apo-B100 and proteoglycans is important for atherogenesis, we performed an extensive atherosclerosis study with five groups of transgenic mice expressing different forms of "proteoglycan-binding-defective LDL" or wild-type human LDL. The mice were fed a high-cholesterol diet for 20 weeks. To determine the extent of atherosclerosis, their arteries were stained with Sudan IV and analyzed by an en face procedure. The results showed that arteries of mice expressing "proteoglycan-binding-defective LDL" had less atherosclerotic lesions than mice expressing wild-type human LDL at equal plasma cholesterol concentrations. However, no differences could be seen after the mice were fed a high-cholesterol diet for 30 weeks. We also analyzed the retention of wild-type human LDL and "proteoglycan-binding defective LDL" in mouse and rabbit aortas ex vivo. The results showed that "proteoglycan-binding-defective LDL" are retained to a lesser extent in normal artery wall than normal recombinant LDL. In contrast, both LDL were retained to almost the same extent in artery wall with atherosclerotic lesions. These findings provide direct experimental evidence that interactions between apo-B100 and arterial proteoglycans are key in the initiation of experimental atherosclerotic lesions, and show that other mechanisms come into play as lesions progress.

Secretory sphingomyelinase and atherosclerosis

I. Tabas[1], S. Marathe[1], G. Kuriakose[1], K.J. Williams[2], D. Tribble[3]. [1]Columbia University, New York City, New York; [2]Thomas Jefferson University, Philadelphia, PA; [3]Lawrence Berkeley National Lab, Berkeley, CA, USA

Background: Our laboratory and others have accumulated a large body of evidence from in vitro and cell-culture studies and from human & animal lesional analysis that secretory sphingomyelinase (S-SMase), a product of the acid SMase (ASM) gene secreted by macrophages (Mφs) and endothelial cells, is atherogenic. The proposed mechanisms include S-SMase-induced aggregation and matrix-retention of subendothelial lipoproteins, leading to μφ foam cell formation.

Objective: To determine if S-SMase is atherogenic using induced mutant mice.

Methods: Model #1: ApoE knockout (E0) mice with 0–2 copies of the ASM gene. Model #2: Mφs-targeted SMase transgenic (Tg) mice. Analysis: Proximal aortic cross-sectional lesional area at 25 weeks of age on a chow diet; and aortic LDL retention in vivo using a ^{125}I-LDL/^{125}I-tyramine-cellobiose-LDL assay.

Results: Model #1: ASM1 (heterozyg) mice secreted 30% of wild-type S-SMase and 65% of lysosomal SMase (L-SMase), and ASM0 mice had no S-SMase or L-SMase activity. The plasma cholesterol levels and lipoprotein profiles were very similar among the three different models. Aortic lesional areas (mm^2) were 0.60 for E0/ASM2 (n = 7), 0.27 for E0/ASM1 (46% of E0/ASM2; n = 4; p < 0.002), and 0.22 for E0/ASM0 (37% of E0/ASM2; n = 12; p < 0.000002). This protective effect was observed in both genders and in both early and advanced lesions.

Model #2: Despite identical average plasma LDL concentrations, there was a 1.7–2.3-fold increase in LDL retention & degradation in oxidatively stressed aortae of two lines of Mφ-SMase Tg mice vs. non-Tg mice. Preliminary data with a small number of mice revealed that the Tg mice had ~ 3-fold higher proximal aortic lesion area.

Conclusion: SMase promotes atherogenesis without altering plasma lipid levels, most likely by promoting the arterial retention and degradation of LDL.

Molecular basis for the association of group IIA phospholipase A 2 and decorin in atherosclerotic lesions

Peter Sartipy[1], Berit Johansen[2], Kathrine Gasvik[2], Eva Hurt-Camejo[1]. [1]Wallenberg Laboratory, Göteborg, Sweden; and [2]UNIGEN, Trondheim, Norway

Objective: We recently reported that group IIa secretory nonpancreatic phospholipase A_2 (snpPLA$_2$) is associated to collagen fibers in the extracellular matrix of human atherosclerotic plaques. In the present study we explored if snpPLA$_2$ may be associated to collagen fibers via interaction with decorin.

Methods: The distribution of snpPLA$_2$ and decorin was studied in human atherosclerotic and non-atherosclerotic tissue by immunohistochemistry to compare their relative in vivo localization. In vitro binding experiments were performed to characterize the interaction of snpPLA$_2$ and decorin.

Results: Decorin was detected within the snpPLA$_2$-positive part of the intima close to the media in lesions. Electrophoretic mobility shift assay showed that snpPLA$_2$ binds to decorin isolated from cell cultures of human fibroblasts. In addition, in a solid phase binding assay decorin enhanced the association of snpPLA$_2$ to collagen type I and VI. Digestion of the GAG-moiety with chondroitinase ABC did not change the binding of snpPLA$_2$ to decorin. Furthermore, snpPLA$_2$ bound efficiently to a recombinant decorin core protein fragment B/E (Asp45-Lys359). This binding was competed with soluble decorin and inhibited at NaCl-concentrations above 150 mM. The activity of snpPLA$_2$ increased 2–3-fold in the presence of decorin or GAG-depleted decorin when using phosphatidylcholine containing mixed micelles or low density lipoprotein as substrates.

Conclusions: The results show that snpPLA$_2$ binds to the decorin protein core, and the interaction enhances snpPLA$_2$ activity. As a consequence, this active extracellular enzyme may contribute to the pathogenesis of atherosclerosis by modifying lipoproteins and releasing inflammatory lipid mediators at places of lipoprotein retention in the arterial wall.

Binding of C-reactive protein (CRP) to native and modified low density lipoprotein (LDL) particles

S. Taskinen[1], P.T. Kovanen[1], H. Jarva[2], S. Meri[2], M.O. Pentikäinen[1]. [1] *Wihuri Research Institute, Helsinki;* [2] *Deparment of Bacteriology and Immunology, University of Helsinki, Finland*

C-reactive protein (CRP) is an acute phase reactant, and increased levels of CRP levels are associated with the presence of coronary heart disease is man. Previous studies have shown that CRP protein is present in human coronary arterial intima and suggested that it is colocalized with lipids. Here we studied whether CRP is able to bind native and modified lipoproteins. For this purpose we either immobilized CRP on microtiter wells and studied binding of tritiated lipoproteins to the wells, or immobilized lipoproteins to microtiter wells and studied binding of iodinated CRP to the wells. LDL was modified by vortexing, proteolysis, oxidation, lipolysis by phospholipases A$_2$, C, and sphingomyelinase, and treated by a combination of trypsin and cholesterol esterase. We found that CRP did not bind to native or vortexed LDL, but bound to all the other types of modified LDL. Of the modifications, LDL treated with cholesterol esterase bound most CRP. Binding of CRP to all the modified LDL preparations was found to be calcium-dependent. Interestingly, treatment of the modified LDL particles with cyclodextrin, which removes unesterified cholesterol from the particles, effectively decreased binding of CRP, and phosphoryl choline effectively competed for binding of CRP to modified LDL. Thus, CRP effectively binds to lipoproteins with a modified surface. The presence of CRP on lipoproteins in the arterial intima could be important in modulating the inflammatory resposes elicited by modified lipoproteins in the arterial intima.

PD166793, a matrix metalloproteinase inhibitor, blunts the progression of atherosclerosis in rabbits in the absence of plasma cholesterol lowering

T. Bocan, S. Bak-Mueller, W. Rosebury, H. Hallak, P. O'Brien, C. Dagle, A. Robertson, X. Lu, T. Major. *Parke-Davis Pharm. Res. Div. of Warner-Lambert, Ann Arbor, Michigan, USA*

Objective: Given that matrix metalloproteinases (MMPs) are associated with atherosclerotic lesions and macrophage accumulation, we sought to evaluate the effect of PD166793, an MMP inhibitor, on the progression of atherosclerosis in rabbits.

Methods: Male New Zealand white rabbits were administered 5 mg/kg PD166793 in a 2% cholesterol (C), 3% peanut (PNO), 3% coconut (CNO) oil diet for 8 weeks to assess the compound's effect on lesion progression. Lesions were also preestablished in rabbits by feeding a 0.5%C, 3%PNO, 3%CNO diet for 9 weeks followed by 6 weeks of the chow-fat only diet. Animals were randomized and given 5 mg/kg PD166793 in the chow-fat diet for 8 additional weeks.

Results: Plasma total and lipoprotein cholesterol levels were unaffected by PD166793 in either experimental model. Plasma Cmax levels of PD166793 ranged from 3.2 to 5 µg/ml, i.e., levels consistent with inhibition of rabbit MMP-2 and -9. In rabbits fed the 2% C diet, aortic arch lesion extent and cholesteryl ester (CE) content were reduced 43% and 20%, respectively. Similarly in the model of preestablished disease, thoracic aortic lesion extent and CE content were decreased 38% and 48%, respectively. Cross-sectional lesion and macrophage area were unaffected under either experimental protocol.

Conclusion: We conclude that a bioavailable MMP inhibitor reduced the extent of atherosclerosis irrespective of time of administration; however, lesion size and composition were unaltered.

Oxidized LDL binds to macrophage-secreted extracellular matrix and is taken up by macrophages: an alternative approach to studies on lipoprotein cellular uptake

Marielle Kaplan, Michael Aviram. *The Lipid Research Laboratory, Bruce Rappaport Faculty of Medicine, Technion, The Rappaport Family Institute for Research in the Medical Sciences and Rambam Medical Center, Haifa, Israel*

Objective: To analyze 1) whether macrophages can secrete an extracellular matrix (ECM) layer, 2) if oxidized LDL (Ox-LDL) can bind to this macrophage-derived ECM layer, and 3) whether binding of Ox-LDL to the macrophage-derived ECM leads to its uptake by macrophages.

Results: Macrophages were shown to produce an ECM layer as illustrated by electron-microscopic, as well as optic-microscopic studies. Macrophage derived ECM could bind native LDL, as well as oxidized LDL (by 3-fold more than native LDL), in the presence of lipoprotein lipase. The uptake of ECM-retained Ox-LDL by PMA-activated macrophages was found to be specific, dose- and time-dependent, and it was higher by 1.5 fold than the uptake of ECM-retained native LDL. Following labeling of the ECM glycosaminoglycans (GAGs) with ^{35}S, the cellular uptake of ECM-retained Ox-LDL, as well as that of ECM-GAGs were obtained in parallel, illustrating that ECM-retained Ox-LDL is taken up by the macrophages together with the ECM-GAG which is bound to the lipoprotein. These results were confirmed in vivo by using ECM layer from mouse peritoneal macrophages (MPM) that were harvested from the atherosclerotic apolipoprotein E deficient mice (E^0). During mice aging (10–24 weeks) and development of atherosclerosis, the GAG content of their MPM-derived ECM increased by up to 52%, the ability of their MPM-derived ECM to bind Ox-LDL increased by up to 57%, and the uptake by J-774 A.1 macrophages of Ox-LDL that was retained in MPM-derived ECM increased by up to 86%.

Conclusions: Thus, the present study demonstrated for the first time: (A) that macrophages can secrete an ECM layer; (B) that Ox-LDL can bind to this macrophage-derived ECM and (C) that binding of Ox-LDL to ECM can lead to its uptake by activated macrophages. This may represent a physio/pathological phenomenon, leading to cholesterol and oxysterols accumulation in arterial wall macrophages, the hallmark of early atherosclerosis.

Plaque instability and acute coronary syndromes

Pathology of vulnerable plaques

E. Falk. *Aarhus University Hospital (Skejby), Aarhus, Denmark*

Coronary atherosclerosis is by far the most frequent cause of ischemic heart disease, and plaque disruption with superimposed thrombosis is the main cause of the acute coronary syndromes of unstable angina, myocardial infarction, and sudden coronary death.

The risk of plaque rupture depends more on plaque vulnerability (plaque type) than on degree of stenosis (plaque size); lipid-rich and soft plaques are more vulnerable and prone to rupture than collagen-rich and hard plaques. Furthermore, they are highly thrombogenic after disruption.

There seem to be three major determinants of a plaque's vulnerability to rupture: 1) size and consistency of the lipid-rich atheromatous core (the "gruel"); 2) thickness of the fibrous cap covering the core; and 3) ongoing inflammation and repair processes within the fibrous cap. Lipid accumulation, cap thinning, loss of smooth muscle cells (smc), and macrophage-related inflammation destabilize plaques, making them vulnerable to rupture. In contrast, smc-related healing and repair processes stabilize plaques, protecting them against disruption. Plaque size or stenosis severity tell nothing about a plaque's vulnerability. Many vulnerable plaques are invisible angiographically due to their small size and compensatory vascular remodeling.

The most feared consequence of plaque disruption is thrombotic occlusion of the artery. There are three major determinants of the thrombotic response to plaque rupture: 1) local thrombogenic substrate; 2) local flow disturbances; and 3) systemic thrombotic propensity.

To study the devastating consequences of atherosclerosis we have tried to develop an animal model of plaque rupture with superimposed thrombosis. Until now, we have failed to induce rupture of "vulnerable-looking" aortic root plaques in more than 200 middle-aged (> 1 year old) apoE−/− mice exposed to extremely stressful stimuli.

Is there a mouse model of plaque rupture?

C.L. Jackson. *Bristol Heart Institute, University of Bristol, Bristol, UK*

Objective: To determine the incidence of atherosclerotic plaque rupture at arterial branch points in apolipoprotein E knockout (apoε−/−) mice.

Methods: Six male and five female apoε−/− mice were fed a diet supplemented with 21% lard and 0.15% cholesterol for up to 14 months. In animals that died, the principal branch points in the carotid arteries and aorta were removed and analysed. Sections were examined histologically, using haematoxylin and eosin. Miller's elastin stain, or Martius Scarlet Blue, and by immunocytochemistry, using an antibody directed against a-smooth muscle action to identify smooth muscle cells.

Results: Four of the male mice and four of the female mice died, after 46 ± 3 weeks of feeding (range 37−59 weeks). Lumenal thrombus associated with atherosclerotic plaque rupture was observed in three male and all four female mice. In six of these seven mice, an atherosclerotic plaque rupture was found where the brachiocephalic artery branches into the right common carotid and right subclavian arteries. The ruptures were characterised by fragmentation and loss of elastin in the fibrous caps of relatively small and lipid-rich plaques overlying large complex lesions, with intraplaque haemorrhage. Immunocytochemical analysis revealed loss of smooth muscle cells from ruptured caps.

Conclusions: These data suggest that long-term fat-feeding of apolipoprotein E knockout mice is a useful and reproducible model of atherosclerotic plaque rupture, and that these ruptures occur predominantly in the brachiocephalic artery.

Visualization of the vulnerable plaque

G. Pasterkamp. *Department of Cardiology, University Medical Center Utrecht, Utrecht, The Netherlands*

The composition of the atherosclerotic lesion rather than the degree of stenosis is currently considered to be the most important determinant for acute clinical events. Modalities capable of characterizing the atherosclerotic lesion may help to understand its natural history and detect lesions with high risk for acute events. Grossly, three histological features of the vulnerable plaque have been reported: size of the atheroma, thickness of the fibrous cap and inflammation. Imaging techniques are currently being deployed and under development to visualize these characteristics of the vulnerable coronary plaque. Most of these diagnostic modalities have the potential to locally detect one or more of the three histologically defined features of the vulnerable plaque. The highest resolutions are achieved by catheter based techniques like IVUS and Raman spectroscopy. Except for optical coherence tomography, however, the resolution of current techniques is still too limited to discriminate the thin fibrous cap. The non invasive imaging modalities like MRI suffer from inadequate resolutions but their unlimited penetration depth and its noninvasive nature are advantages. Imaging techniques that visualize the plaque locally may provide new insight into the etiology of sudden progression of atherosclerotic disease or acute events. However, due to their local applicability, it is not expected that they will have prognostic properties for the development of acute clinical syndromes that often originate from non haemodynamically significant lesions. Therefore, systemic markers for inflammation may have more prognostic value for the identification of patients suffering from clinical events as a result of plaque rupture.

Increased serum MMP-9 concentrations in patients with angiographically assessed coronary artery disease

A. Kalela[1], T.A. Koivu[1], J. Kanervisto[1], P. Sillanaukee[1,2], T. Lehtimäki[2], S.T. Nikkari[1,2]. *[1]University of Tampere, Medical School; and [2]Centre for Laboratory Medicine, University Hospital of Tampere, Finland*

Objectives: Matrix metalloproteinases (MMPs) are upregulated in unstable atherosclerotic plaques. We examined whether MMP serum levels reflect the progression of coronary artery disease (CAD).

Methods: Serum matrix metalloproteinase-9 (MMP-9) concentrations were determined by ELISA in 61 patients (39 males, 22 females, mean age 56.5 years), who had narrowing in one or more coronary arteries assessed by coronary angiography. The control group consisted of 19 patients (9 males, 10 females, mean age 50.9 years), who had no pathological findings in coronary angiography.

Results: Serum MMP-9 concentrations tended to increase in the order; controls (32.2 ± 16.1 mg/l), 1 or 2 vessel CAD (40.4 ± 25.1 mg/l) and 3 vessel CAD (57.3 ± 39.1 mg/l) (p = 0.011, ANOVA). In a logistic regression model adjusting for known CAD risk factors, serum MMP-9 was the strongest predictor of CAD (p = 0.013). In a 10 year follow-up, the serum MMP-9 concentration, taken before coronary bypass surgery, did not predict subsequent mortality from coronary events.

Conclusions: These results suggest that serum MMP-9 concentration is associated with severity of coronary narrowing and may have diagnostic value in evaluating the extent of CAD.

Lipoprotein-associated phospholipase A2 (Lp PLA₂), an inflammatory marker and novel independent risk factor in the West of Scotland Coronary Prevention Study (WOSCOPS)

C.J. Packard[1], D. O'Reilly[1], M.J. Caslake[1], G. McIntosh[1], C.H. Macphee[2], K.E. Suckling[2], M. Krishna[3], A. Rumley[1], G. Lowe[1]. *On behalf of WOSCOPS Group;*
[1] *Depts of Biochemistry and Medicine, Robertson Centre, Glasgow University;*
[2] *SmithKline Beecham Labs, Harlow, UK; and* [3] *DiaDexus, Santaclara, USA*

Objective: To determine the usefulness of chronic inflammation markers as predictors of risk in WOSCOPS.

Methods: A nested case-control study was designed from within the WOSCOPS cohort. 580 cases with CHD were age and smoking matched with 1160 controls. C Reactive Protein (CRP), Lp PLA₂ mass, fibrinogen (Fib) and white cell count (WCC) were measured at baseline or on frozen, stored samples. Relationship to risk was tested in Cox proportional hazards models. Risk ratios were estimated for quintiles (Q) of each variable.

Results: All four markers were strong predictors of risk in univariate analysis with about a 2-fold increase in risk comparing subjects in the highest vs. lowest quintile. CRP correlated with Fib, WCC, body mass index, HDL and plasma triglyceride and in multivariate analysis its predictive capacity (like that of Fib and WCC) was much reduced. Lp PLA₂ was not correlated with other inflammatory markers and remained a strong independent risk factor in multivariate analysis. For Lp PLA₂, risks in Q 2-4 relative to Q1 were 1.26 (CI 0.83−1.92), 1.58 (1.04−2.4), 1.73 (1.16−2.60) and 1.66 (1.10−2.50) adjusting all other risk factors.

Conclusions: Chronic inflammation is a strong determinant of risk in asymptomatic, moderately hypercholesterolemic men. Lp PLA₂, an entity distinct from Group II secretory PLA₂, is identified as a new, independent marker of CHD risk.

Genetics of risk factors for CVD

Genomic searches for genes that influence risk factors for CVD

J.E. Hixson. *Dept. of Genetics, S.W. Found. for Biomed. Res., San Antonio, Texas, USA*

Objective: To identify quantitative trait loci (QTLs) that influence CVD risk factors using genomic screens in families.

Methods: Our general approach is to perform genome-wide searches in large extended families that are not selected according to any particular disease. The genetic markers that are used for genomic searches are random microsatellite markers distributed throughout the human chromosomes at approximately 10 cM intervals. These markers are used for linkage analysis with variance component methods to identify chromosomal regions containing QTLs for CVD risk factors.

Results: We have conducted a genomic search in 480 family members from 10 large extended pedigrees of Mexican Americans in San Antonio. Our first published finding was the identification of a major QTL on chromosome 2 that influences serum levels of leptin hormone, an important risk factor for obesity. We have also identified QTLs on chromosomes 3 and 4 that influence LDL size class, an important CVD risk factor. In addition to lipid risk factors, we are measuring levels of gene products involved in atherogenesis in the arterial wall. For example, we have found strong evidence for genetic control of serum levels of soluble P-selectin ($h^2 = 0.70$), and have detected major QTLs on chromosome 15 (LOD = 3.8) and chromosome 12 (LOD = 2.6).

Conclusions: Genomic searches in families are a powerful strategy to identify new QTLs that influence CVD risk factors.

Genetic factors and the response of CVD risk factors to regular exercise

C. Bouchard. *Pennington Biomedical Research Center; Baton Rouge, Louisiana, USA*

Objective: To review the evidence for familial aggregation and the contribution of specific genes in the response of CVD risk factors to regular physical activity.

The 1996 USA Surgeon General's Report on physical activity and health reviews several prospective studies concerning the relationship between levels of physical activity, CVD outcomes and CVD mortality rates. Collectively, these studies indicate that physically active adults are, on the average, less prone to CVD and have lower death rates from CVD than sedentary people. There are considerable individual differences in the changes observed in lipids and lipoproteins, blood pressure and other CVD risk factors as a result of exposure to exercise programs. A handful of twin studies and more recently the HERITAGE Family Study have shown that there is strong familial aggregation for the response pattern to regular exercise. The heritability for the changes in maximal oxygen uptake to a standardized exercise training program attained about 50 percent in HERITAGE. A genomic scan performed has revealed that several QTLs are linked to the responsiveness to regular exercise for cadiorespiratory endurance. However, thus far, candidate gene studies have evidenced only weak associations with the changes in CVD risk factors with regular exercise. The genetic dissection of the familial component of the response to regular exercise will be a complex undertaking requiring a variety of genomic and expression technologies.

Gene environment interaction in determining risk of ischaemic heart disease

S.E. Humphries[1], P.J. Talmud[1], J. Cooper[2], D.M. Waterworth[1], I.N.M. Day[1], G.J. Miller[2]. [1]British Heart Foundation Centre for Cardiovascular Genetics, Royal Free and University College London Medical School, London; and [2]MRC Epidemiology and Medical Care Unit, London, UK

In understanding the impact of risk of thrombosis and Ischaemic Heart Disease (IHD), the modifying effects of different environmental factors experienced by individuals on the predisposition that they have inherited is particularly important. IHD risk has been determined in the second Northwick Park Heart Study, at ten candidate gene loci; apolipoprotein (apo) CIII (C3238G [SstI]) and C-482T [insulin responsive element, IRE]), apoAIV (Thr347Ser), apoE (E2, E3, E4), apoB (C7672T [XbaI]), Lipoprotein Lipase (Ser447Stop), beta-fibrinogen (G-455A), factor VII (Arg353Gln), ACE (I/D), eNOS (intron 4) and stromelysin-1 (5A/6A). DNA was available on 2743 middle-aged men, free of IHD at baseline, recruited for prospective cardiovascular surveillance. Carriers of the apoAIV gene Ser347 allele had a Relative Risk (RR) of 1.57 (95% CI: 1.07—2.31, p = 0.04) compared to Thr347 homozygous men, while stromelysin 6A6A homozygous men had a RR of 1.91 (1.11—3.28, p = 0.02) compared with those with genotype 5A5A. Overall, men who were current smokers had a 2.20 (1.52—3.17, p < 0.0001) fold higher risk of IHD, and there was evidence for interaction between smoking and genotype in modulating risk at the stromelysin (p = 0.09), apoE (p = 0.02) and apoCIII (p = 0.002) loci. In particular, smoking was not associated with increased risk in the apoE3E3 group, but markedly augmented risk in apoE4 carriers (RR = 2.22 (1.33—3.72) in smokers compared with 0.58 (0.32—1.05) in nonsmokers). Estimates of all of the genotype-associated IHD risk effects remained essentially unchanged after adjustment for the classical risk factors, suggesting that risk is not mediated through effects on plasma levels of measured lipids or clotting factors. Since men with the stromelysin genotype 5A5A and those who carry the apoE4 allele each represent 25% of the general population, this provides a strong argument for smoking avoidance in these individuals.

Linkage of blood pressure to a locus on chromosome 4 in dutch dyslipidemic families

H. Allayee[1], T.W.A. de Bruin[2], R.M. Cantor[1], B.E. Aouizerat[1], A.J. Lusis[1], J.I. Rotter[3]. [1]Department of Human Genetics, UCLA; [3]Division of Medical Genetics, Steven Spielberg Research Center, Cedars-Sinai Medical Center, Los Angeles, USA; and [2]Department of Medicine, Academic Hospital, Maastricht, The Netherlands

Genes contributing to the common forms of essential hypertension and blood pressure (BP) variation are largely unknown. This may result from the underlying genetic heterogeneity of this disorder. One approach to reduce such heterogeneity is to conduct gene finding efforts in families ascertained for common metabolic syndromes with associated hypertension. Familial combined hyperlipidemia (FCHL), a metabolic syndrome associated with insulin resistance, central obesity, and an increased frequency of hypertension, is such a disorder. Insulin resistance, defined by fasting insulin levels and more direct measures, is both associated with hypertension in cross-sectional studies and predictive in prospective studies. Furthermore, insulin resistance and FCHL are also accompanied by increased free fatty acid (FFA) levels. In the present study, we analyzed a 10 cM genome-wide scan in 18 Dutch FCHL pedigrees (n = 240) to search for genes contributing to BP in this metabolic syndrome. A multipoint genome scan of systolic (S) BP and diastolic (D) BP identified a region on chromosome 4 exhibiting a LOD score of 3.9 with SBP (peak marker D4S2639). Interestingly, FFA levels mapped to this region, with a LOD score of 2.4. Two-point linkage with markers under the peak also yielded evidence for linkage of SBP (p < 0.0008) and FFA (p < 0.009) to this locus, supporting the multipoint results. Alpha adducin, a gene involved in renal sodium handling, resides within this locus and has been associated with elevated blood pressure in both human populations and in animal models of hypertension. However, there is no evidence for an association between two intragenic polymorphisms within a-adducin and SBP in our Dutch population. In conclusion, this genome scan for BP has identified a chromosomal region harboring a potentially novel gene that contributes to hypertension associated with insulin resistant dyslipidemia.

A quantitative trait locus for vascular cellular adhesion molecule-1 levels on chromosome 19

M.C. Mahaney[1], L. Almasy[1], A.G. Comuzzie[1], S.A. Cole[1], J.E. Hixson[1], J.W. MacCluer[1], M.P. Stern[2], J. Blangero[1]. [1]Southwest Foundation for Biomedical Research; and [2]University of Texas Health Science Center, San Antonio, Texas, USA

Objective: To detect, characterize and localize quantitative trait loci (QTLs) influencing serum vascular cellular adhesion molecule-1 (VCAM-1) levels in Mexican Americans from San Antonio, Texas.

Methods: We assayed serum levels of VCAM-1 in 471 Mexican Americans from 10 extended pedigrees using a commercially available ELISA kit. Initial statistical genetic analyses and a two-point, 20 cM whole genome linkage screen was accomplished using a maximum-likelihood based, variance-decomposition approach. We followed these analyses with a multipoint, 15 cM, whole genome linkage screen.

Results: Our initial analyses showed that variation in VCAM-1 levels was influenced by additive genes ($h^2 = 0.26$), sex, diabetes, smoking, and menopause and provided suggestive evidence for QTLs on chromosomes 19 (LOD = 2.36) and 14 (LOD = 2.02). The 15 cM multipoint linkage screen yielded a maximum multipoint LOD score of 3.25 (p = 0.000122) on chromosome 19p. The 95% confidence interval localizes this QTL to 19p13.3 and subsumes a region containing excellent candidate loci for vascular biology; including loci for the mucosal addressin cell adhesion molecule-1 (MAdCAM-1), the thromboxane A2 receptor (TBXA2R), and intercellular adhesion molecules-1 and-3 (ICAM-1 and ICAM-3).

Conclusions: A small-but-significant proportion of the phenotypic variance in normal serum levels of VCAM-1 is due the additive effects of genes. A QTL responsible for most of the additive genetic effect on VCAM-1 levels in this population is located on chromosome 19p13.3.

Acute coronary event risk-increasing polymorphisms of α_{2B} adrenergic receptor and serum paraoxonase genes. Demonstration of a gene-gene instruction

T.-P. Tuomainen[1], T.A. Lakka[1], A. Snapir[2], R. Malin[3], T. Lehtimäki[3], M. Koulu[2], M. Scheinin[2], J.T. Salonen[1]. *[1]University of Kuopio, Kuopio; [2]University of Turku, Turku; [3]University of Tampere, Tampere, Finland*

Objective: We hypothesised that multiple gene polymorphisms which predispose to the same disease may have a synergistic rather than an additive effect.

Methods: We studied the associations between an α_{2B}-adrenergic receptor polymorphism, a serum paraoxonase polymorphism and the risk of developing an acute coronary event (ACE) in the 2682 men prospective KIHD study. All men for whom both genotypic data were available and who were CHD-free at the baseline were included in the present analyses.

Results: Of the 1118 men, 48 (4.3%) developed an ACE during the follow-up. 16/240 (6.7%) subjects that were α_{2B}-AR del/del homozygotes, 11/119 (9.2%) PON 54 Met/Met homozygotes and 4/25 (16%) that were homozygous for both developed an ACE. In multivariate Cox models adjusting for age, smoking, hypertension, blood lipids, obesity, diabetes, alcohol consumption, socioeconomic status and physical fitness, α_{2B}-AR deletion homozygotes had 1.8-fold (95% CI 1.0−3.4, p = 0.045), PON 54 methionine homozygotes 2.4-fold (95% CI 1.2−4.9, p = 0.011) and homozygotes for both 5.0-fold (95% CI 1.8−14.2, p = 0.002) risk of developing an acute coronary event during the maximum 7.6 years of follow-up.

Conclusions: These data demonstrate the importance of simultaneous studying of multiple genes when assessing the effect of gene polymorphisms on cardiovascular diseases.

A poymorphism of the Cholesteryl Ester Transfer Protein (CETP) gene predicts Cardiovascular (CV) events in the West of Scotland Coronary Prevention Study (WOSCOPS)

D.J. Freeman[1], V. Wilson[1], A.D. McMahon[2], C.J. Packard[3], D. Gaffney[3]. *[1]Durham University, Durham; [2]Glasgow University, Glasgow; [3]Glasgow Royal Infirmary University NHS Trust, Glasgow, UK*

Objective: To assess the importance of polymorphisms in the CETP and hepatic lipase (HL) genes in predicting CV events.

Methods: Subjects were participants in WOSCOPS. Lifestyle and lipid data were collected at baseline. DNA from 580 cases (experiencing a CV event) and 1160 controls (age and smoking matched) were typed for the *Taq*IB CETP and C-480T HL gene polymorphisms.

Results: Homozygotes for the rare CETP *Taq*IB allele (B2B2), had a higher HDL cholesterol and a 30% reduced risk of suffering a CV event (odds ratio [OR] 0.70, p = 0.03) compared to B1B1 homozygotes. When confounding factors, including HDL cholesterol, were accounted for in a multivariate analysis this association was lost. When HDL cholesterol was excluded from the multivariate model, the significant association between B2B2 genotype and CV events was retained. Benefit of pravastatin treatment was not significantly different in B1B1 (OR 0.71), B1B2 (OR 0.65) and B2B2 (OR 0.61) individuals. There was no association between the HL polymorphism and CV risk.

Conclusions: There was a significant association between *Taq*IB genotype and risk of a CV event. The relationship was not independent of HDL cholesterol and we suggest that the HDL raising effect of the B2B2 genotype, at least in part, accounts for the mechanism of the association. There was no evidence for an interaction between the *Taq*IB genotype and pravastatin treatment.

New aspects of pharmacological treatment

Cholesterol absorption: mechansims and inhibitors

S.D. Wright, M. Hernandez, S. Patel, M. Steinger, D. Kim, J. Montenegro, J. Lisnock, C. Sparrow, P.A. Detmers, Y.S. Chao. *Merck Research Laboratories, POB 2000, Rahway, New Jersey, 07065, USA*

Absorption of intestinal cholesterol involves a linear sequence of steps: emulsification, passage of cholesterol from bile salt micelles into the brush border membrane of enterocytes, transit to the endoplasmic reticulum, esterification, packaging into chylomicrons, and secretion from the basolateral surface. We have gained a high resolution view of the process by following both radioactive cholesterol and a fluorescent cholesterol analog in hamsters and have used these methods to map the site of action of cholesterol absorption inhibitors (CAI). Chemical modifications have led to very potent sterol glycosides CAI, and we find that these agents act by blocking the movement of cholesterol from bile acid micelles into the apical membrane of enterocytes. Moreover, radioactive CAI bind saturably and specifically to the brush border of enterocytes, and affinity varies with CAI potency. We conclude that sterol glycoside CAI bind to an intestinal transporter that moves cholesterol from bile acid micelles into the membranes of enterocytes.

HDL modifying agents: from small molecules to recombinant proteins for intervention in vascular disease

Roger S. Newton. *Esperion Therapeutics, Ann Arbor, Michigan, USA*

Over the past three decades, the discovery and development of HDL modulating agents has been limited mostly to the "fraudulent fatty acid" class of drugs known as fibrates. More recently, with the discovery of specific nuclear receptors (e.g., PPARs), HDL receptors (e.g., SRB1) and the ABC-1 gene cassette in the regulation of HDL metabolism, new opportunities have been presented to the worldwide pharmaceutical industry for discovering new, more effective drugs for elevating HDL, promoting reverse lipid transport and benefitting vascular disease. In addition to the focus on small molecule research, an unexploited area of research is the use of recombinant apo A-I proteins in phospholipid vesicles as synthetic HDL particles for the acute and chronic treatment of vascular disease complications (restenosis, unstable angina, ischemia, etc.) In addition to transgenic animal experiments involving knockout and overexpression of specific HDL-related genes, studies involving infusion of wild-type apo A-I, recombinant pro-apo A-I or variant forms (e.g., recombinant apo A-I Milano) in animal models of restenosis and atherosclerosis have confirmed the beneficial effects of this therapy for mobilizing cholesterol from arteries and/or reducing complications of vascular disease. Lastly, preliminary studies involving human subjects support the testing of different forms of apo A-I complexed to phospholipid as a new therapeutic for mobilizing and redistributing cholesterol, promoting its elimination through increased bile acid production and secretion, and potentially for treatment of atherosclerosis. A thorough review of the studies and their supporting data will be presented for this exciting new area of drug discovery research.

HDL mutants and mimetics for the direct treatment of vascular disease

Cesare R. Sirtori. *Center E. Grossi Paoletti, Institute of Pharmacological Sciences, University of Milan, Italy*

Objective: The use of HDL or analogues for the treatment of vascular disease has come of age. ApoA-I liposomes have been shown to mobilize tissue cholesterol in patients with familial hypercholesterolemia (Eriksson et al. Circulation 1999;100:594), by way of recruitment of cell cholesterol and formation of nascent small HDL (Nanjee et al. ATVB 1999;19:979). Availability of the mutant apoA-IMilano in large amounts allows the direct evaluation of the potential therapeutic benefit of enhancing the reverse cholesterol transport system.

Methods: The recombinant apoA-IMilano (r apoA-IM) dimer, formulated with phospholipids, resembles the structure of native HDL. The product is a disk shaped complex of dipalmitoyl PC or oleoyl PC with r apoA-IM dimer; it is stable and well tolerated after iv injection.

Results: Preclinical data have been obtained in rabbit models of arterial restenosis and of neo-intimal proliferation induced by perivascular manipulation, and are supported by a direct antagonism toward aortic atherosclerosis in apoE KO mice (Sirtori et al. Atherosclerosis 1999;142:29). The r apoA-IM/PL complex also improves endothelial dysfunction in apoE KO mice and exerts an antithrombotic effect in the ferric chloride lesioned abdominal aorta in rats. More recently, data have been obtained indicating that the r apoA-IM/PL, given intrapericardially to minipigs prior to PTCA, significantly inhibits intimal proliferation, giving a benefit in diameter stenosis of 52% compared to placebo. Finally, a single 1—2 h infusion of the r apo A-IM/PL complex has proved effective in a rabbit model of soft carotid plaque. Initial clinical evaluation of the product in volunteers is forthcoming.

Bay 13-9952 (implitapide), an inhibitor of the Microsomal Triglyceride Transfer Protein (MTP), blocks secretion of Apo-B-lipoproteins

R. Gruetzmann, M. Beuck, U. Mueller, U. Nielsch. *Cardiovascular Research, Bayer AG, Aprather Weg 18 a, D-42096 Wuppertal, Germany*

Objective: The aim was to identify inhibitors of lipoprotein secretion that are suitable as cholesterol and triglyceride lowering drugs.

Methods: In order to find such inhibitors we used the human hepatoma cell line HepG2, which shows differentiation-associated functions of parenchymal liver cells such as secretion of ApoB-containing VLDL-like lipoproteins and of α-2-macroglobulin.

Results: BAY 13-9952 is an αa-carboline derivative and was found to inhibit the secretion of apoB-associated particles from HepG2 cells with an IC 50 value of 1.1 nM. Cell viability of HepG2 cells and general inhibition of secretory processes are not affected as indicated by the unchanged levels of α-2-macroglobulin secretion. MTP is a heterodimer composed of an unique 97-kDa subunit and the multifunctional protein disulfide isomerase (PDI). MTP is involved in the cotranslational translocation of lipids to nascent triglyceride-rich lipoproteins, a process required for VLDL and chylomicron synthesis in hepatocytes and enterocytes, respectively. BAY 13-9952 potently inhibits the MTP-catalysed transport of lipids between synthetic small unilamellar vesicles. In this in vitro system, triglyceride transport is inhibited with an $IC_{50} = 27$ nM for partially purified MTP from porcine liver and with an $IC_{50} = 10$ nM for recombinant human MTP/PDI complex.

Conclusion: These studies demonstrate that BAY 13-9952 is a potent inhibitor of MTP with a potential use for the treatment of hyperlipidimias. Targeting this new mechanism may offer a new therapeutic principle for the treatment and prevention of CAD.

Probucol increases hepatic expression of High Density Lipoprotein (HDL) receptor, scavenger receptor class B type I (SR-BI), in vitro and in vivo — enhancement of reverse cholesterol transport (RCT)

K. Tsujii, K. Hirano, F. Matsuura, Y. Nakagawa-Toyama, T. Sugimoto, A. Matsuyama, K. Matsumoto, S. Yamashita, Y. Matsuzawa. *Osaka University, Osaka, Japan*

Objective: SR-BI is an established HDL receptor to mediate the selective uptake of HDL-lipids. The overexpression of SR-BI in the liver decreased plasma HDL-cholesterol levels and reduced atherosclerosis in murine models. Therefore, it is obvious that the enhancement of SR-BI-mediated pathway is one of the important therapeutic targets for atherosclerosis. Probucol is a potent hypolipidemic drug to reduce xanthoma formation in both human and rabbit low density lipoprotein receptor-deficient mutants and is unique in that this compound causes the reduction of plasma HDL-cholesterol levels. In the present study, we have examined the effect of probucol on the hepatic expression of SR-BI.

Methods: For in vivo and in vitro experiments, rabbit and human hepatoma cell lines, HepG2, were selected as experimental models, respectively.

Results: Prubucol treatment decreased plasma HDL-cholesterol levels and induced smaller-sized HDL in rabbits. Hepatic expression of rabbit SR-BI mRNA expression was up-regulated by probucol-treatment. Next, we have examined the regulation of human SR-BI in HepG2 cells. By the addition of probucol into the media, both mRNA and protein levels of human SR-BI were increased in a dose-dependent manner with significantly increased uptake of Dil-labeled HDL-lipids.

Conclusion: These observations demonstrate that probucol up-regulated the hepatic expression of HDL receptor, SR-BI, in vitro and in vivo, suggesting that this compound increases the hepatic uptake of HDL-lipid, as well as activates cholesteryl ester transfer as previously reported. In conclusion, probucol has a unique property to enhance the major protective system against atherosclerosis, RCT.

Rapid normalization of pre-established hypercholesterolemia in rhesus monkeys by the potent cholesterol absorption inhibitor ezetimibe (SCH58235)

D.S. Compton, H.R. Davis, M. van Heek. *Schering-Plough Research Institute, Kenilworth, New Jersey, USA*

Objective: To determine if the cholesterol absorption inhibitor ezetimibe (SCH58235) reduces pre-established hypercholesterolemia (HC) and prevents diet induced HC in rhesus monkeys fed a "Western" diet.

Methods: The effect of ezetimibe (0.3, 1, 3, 10, 30 and 100 µg/kg/day, admixed in diet) on plasma lipids and lipoprotein composition was evaluated in rhesus monkeys fed a high fat/cholesterol Western diet containing 0.25% cholesterol and 22% fat for 3 weeks (n = 5/group). In one study, a crossover of the control and 100 µg/kg ezetimibe treatment groups was employed to study the duration of action of the drug and the time course of the reversal of pre-established HC.

Results: Rhesus monkeys fed a Western diet for 3 weeks results in an increase in plasma cholesterol (147–294 mg/dl) and LDL cholesterol (54–161 mg/dl). Ezetimibe at 3 µg/kg/day completely prevented these increases without significant changes in HDL or triglycerides (ED50 = 0.5 µg/kg). In a related study, a single dose of an analog of ezetimibe was shown to decrease postprandial chylomicra cholesteryl-esters by 69% without changes in other lipid components. In the crossover experiment, treating pre-established HC monkeys with 100 µg/kg ezetimibe reduced plasma cholesterol levels by 57% within 3 days of treatment and normalized plasma cholesterol within 10 days (294–148 mg/dl) and LDL (161–53 mg/dl). Despite a daily intake of 375 mg of dietary cholesterol, plasma cholesterol remained unchanged for 3 days after discontinuing ezetimibe treatment.

Conclusion: Ezetimibe rapidly reverses pre-established HC in rhesus monkeys predominantly through the normalization of LDL cholesterol. Removal of ezetimibe treatment results in a 3 day lag in plasma cholesterol rise due to its long duration of action. Ezetimibe will likely be effective in the treatment of hypercholesterolemia in humans.

The effect of metoprolol CR/XL on atherosclerosis

G. Bondjers[1], O. Wiklund[1], J. Hulthe[1], C. Schmidt[1], S.O. Olofsson[2], J. Wikstrand[1,3].
[1] Wallenberg Laboratory; [2] Department of Med. chemistry; and [3] Göteborg University, Astra Zeneca, Gothenburg, Sweden

Objective: To investigate whether metoprolol CR/XL treatment might affect subclinical atherosclerosis in subjects with hypercholesterolemia.

Methods: Subjects with primary hypercholesterolemia (total cholesterol ⩾ 6.5 and LDL cholesterol ⩾ 5.5 mmol/l) and also fulfilling the following ultrasound criteria: a maximum intima-media thickness (IMT) > 1.0 mm and/or a measurable plaque in the far wall of the carotid artery were recruited to the present three-year prospective, randomised, placebo controlled, double-blind study. A total of 103 subjects started double blind treatment; 47 in the metoprolol CR/XL (100 mg) group and 56 in the placebo group. Twelve patients in each group withdrew from treatment. Results are reported for the remaining 79 subjects. Subclinical atherosclerosis was measured by B-mode ultrasound in the carotid artery each year during follow-up.

Results: Thirty-nine subjects in the placebo group and 33 subjects in the metoprolol CR/XL group were treated with statins with similar dose levels and total cholesterol was reduced from 9.4 to 6.0 mmol/l in the metoprolol CR/XL group and from 8.7 to 6.2 mmol/l in the placebo group. Furthermore, IMT of the common carotid artery in the metoprolol CR/XL group decreased from 0.905 ± 0.232 mm to 0.869 ± 0.169 mm and increased from 0.892 ± 0.177 mm to 0.922 ± 0.188 mm in the placebo group ($p < 0.05$ for difference in change between groups). The decrease in IMT in the metoprolol CR/XL group was obvious already after the first year of follow-up.

Conclusion: In subjects with hypercholesterolemia treated with lipid lowering drugs, the addition of 100 mg of metoprolol CR/XL seems to beneficially affect atherosclerosis development, as measured by IMT. This may reflect direct effects of metoprolol on arterial tissue.

Genetic animal models of lipoprotein metabolism

Multifunctionality of apolipoprotein E in lipoprotein metabolism as studied in transgenic mice

Louis M. Havekes, Bart J.M. van Vlijmen, Miek C. Jong, Marten H. Hofker, Ko Willems van Dijk. *TNO-PG, Gaubius Laboratory, Leiden; Leiden University Medical Center, Leiden, The Netherlands*

Studies with apolipoprotein E (APOE) deficient and APOE transgenic mice has revealed that apoE has various major functions in lipoprotein metabolism:

Ligand for lipoprotein receptors: ApoE is a ligand for receptor-mediated uptake of apoB-containing lipoproteins by the liver. ApoE2 and ApoE3 Leiden proteins are both defective in binding to the LDL receptor. However, in APOE*2 and APOE*3 Leiden transgenic mice, the LDL receptor still constitutes the predominant route for clearance of VLDL remnants. These apoE variants can also still bind to the LRP and VLDL receptor. However, as compared to binding to the LDL receptor, for binding to the LRP a relatively high amount of apoE per particle is needed.

Inhibitor of LPL-mediated VLDL-triglyceride lipolysis: Above a certain amount per particle apoE leads to a dose-dependent inhibition of LPL-mediated lipolysis, whereas an apoE variant-specific inhibition of VLDL lipolysis has also been found. If lipolysis of VLDL is inhibited, binding of VLDL to the LRP is severely hampered.

Stimulator of hepatic VLDL assembly and secretion: In apoE-deficient mice the newly secreted VLDL particles are smaller in size due to less triglyceride in the core. The hampered VLDL-triglyceride secretion in these mice could be enhanced upon introducing physiologically relevant APOE gene expression in the liver by APOE-adenovirus transduction, indicating a regulating role for apoE in hepatic VLDL secretion.

The muliple roles of macrophage scavenger receptors in vivo

Hiroshi Suzuki, Youichiro Wada, Takao Hamakubo, Tatsuhiko Kodama. *Molecular Biology and Medicine, RCAST#35, The University of Tokyo, Japan*

Macrophage scavenger receptors (MSR) are implicated in the pathologic deposition of cjolesterol during atherogenesis. More than 10 types of MSRs are reported and their roles in vivo have been studied using several knockout mice strains and human genetic disorders. The targeted disruption of the type I and II class A MSR gene (SRA-KO) results in a reduction in the size of atherosclerotic lesions in apo E deficient mice (60%) and in LDL receptor deficient mice wth high fat diet (about 20%). De Winther reported that in ApoE3 Leiden mice, SRA deficiency caused development of more severe lesions. We found that SR-A KO in C57B6 with high cholesterol diet developed smaller atherosclerotic lesion, supporting the hypothesis that SR-A mediates the development of atherosclerosis in vivo. Davignon reported a Canadian Family with increased SRA expression indicated xanthomatosis. SRA KO macrophages exhibit a marked decrease in modified LDL uptake in vitro, whereas modified LDL clearance from plasma occurs at a normal rate, suggesting that there are alternative mechanisms for the uptake of mLDL from the circulation. SRA-KO macrophages had reduced phagocytic activity and impaired adhesion function. Oxidized LDL can induce macrophage growth stimulation, but the activity is weak in SRA-KO. In addition, MSR-A knockout mice show increased susceptibility to

Listeria monocytogenes infection and herpes simplex virus type-1 (HSV-1) infection, indicating a role for MSR-A in host defense against various pathogens. Krieger et al. reported that the targeted disruption of SR-B1 resulted in impaired HDL metabolism and enhanced atherosclerosis. Matsuzawa et al. reported that human CD36 deficiency caused higher rate of atherosclerotic events. These results suggest that the protective role of class B scavenger receptors against atherosclerosis.

VLDL or LDL cholesterol: which is more atherogenic?

Stephen G. Young. *Gladstone Inst. of Cardiov. Disease, San Francisco, California, USA*

Apo-E deficient "apo-B100-only" mice (Apoe$^{-/-}$ Apob$^{100/100}$) and LDL receptor deficient apo-B100-only mice (Ldlr$^{-/-}$ Apob$^{100/100}$) have similar total plasma cholesterol levels on a chow diet (~ 300 mg/dl) and virtually identical HDL cholesterol levels. However, nearly all of the cholesterol in the Apoe$^{-/-}$ Apob$^{100/100}$ plasma is contained in VLDL particles, while nearly all of the cholesterol in the Ldlr$^{-/-}$ Apob$^{100/100}$ plasma is contained in smaller LDL particles. In this study, we sought to compare the sizes and numbers of apo-B100-containing lipoproteins in these mice, and then determine whether the differences were associated with different susceptibilities to atherosclerosis. The mean size of the apo-B100-containing lipoprotein particles in Apoe$^{-/-}$ Apob$^{100/100}$ plasma was 53.4 nm. while it was 22.1 nm in Ldlr$^{-/-}$ Apob$^{100/100}$ plasma; the smallest 10% of particles in the Apoe$^{-/-}$ Apob$^{100/100}$ plasma was larger than the largest 10% of particles in Ldlr$^{-/-}$ Apob$^{100/100}$ mice. The plasma levels of apo-B100 were $\sim 450\%$ higher in the Ldlr$^{-/-}$ Apob$^{100/100}$ mice, compared with the Apoe$^{-/-}$ Apob$^{100/100}$ mice. After 40 weeks on a chow diet, $14.0 \pm 2.9\%$ of the aortic surface in Ldlr$^{-/-}$ Apob$^{100/100}$ mice was covered with atherosclerotic lesions, versus only $4.8 \pm 2.5\%$ in the Apoe$^{-/-}$ Apob$^{100/100}$ mice ($p < 0.0001$; $n > 40$ mice in each group). We conclude that large numbers of small apo-B100-containing lipoproteins (the Ldlr$^{-/-}$ Apob$^{100/100}$ phenotype) are much more atherogenic than smaller numbers of large lipoproteins (the Apoe$^{-/-}$ Apob$^{100/100}$ phenotype).

Creation and initial characterization of apo B48 receptor knockout mouse

J. Smith[1], M. Brown[2],W. Bradley[2], S. Gianturco[2]. *[1]Rockefeller Univ., New York; [2]Univ. of Alabama, Birmingham, USA*

Objective: To determine the in vivo and ex vivo effects of knocking out the monocyte, macrophage, and endothelial cell specific apoB48 receptor (B48r) gene.

  Methods and Results: The human B48r cDNA was cloned from a THP-1 cell library using a probe derived from peptide sequence of the purified protein. The mRNA codes for a polar protein of 1088 amino acid residues with 2 hydrophobic domains. The cDNA and protein sequence are not closely related to previously identified genes. Transfection of full-length cDNA into CHO cells results in uptake of remnant lipoproteins. A mouse genomic clone was isolated from a phage library, and a targeting vector was constructed which deleted the promoter, first exon, first intron, and a portion of the second exon. Transfection into ES cells resulted in three cell lines with gene disruption via homologous recombination, two of which yielded germline transmitting chimeric mice after blastocyst microinjection Heterozygous mice were bred and yielded the expected ratio of wildtype, heterozygous, and knockout mice. The knockouts appear healthy and are being bred back to C57BL6 stock and with apoE-deficient mice. Bone marrow derived macrophages derived from the wildtype, heterozygous, and knockout mice were treated with DiI labeled apoE-deficient βVLDL alone and in the presence of excess human LDL as competitor. βVLDL uptake was observed by all cells, with the notable exception that in the presence of excess LDL, the B48r knockout macrophages failed to take up any βVLDL.

Conclusion: The B48r may play an important role in macrophage uptake of triglyceride rich and remnant lipoproteins, and may play a role in macrophage foam cell formation during atherogenesis, especially when apoE is compromised.

Disturbances of fatty acid and cholesterol metabolism in peroxisome proliferator-activated receptor-alpha (PPARa) deficient mice

D. Patel[1], B. Knight[1], S. Humphreys[2], G. Gibbons[3]. *[1]Lipoprotein Group, MRC Clinical Sciences Centre, London; [2]Oxford Lipid Metabolism Group; [3]Metabolic Research Laboratory, Oxford, UK*

Objectives: To establish whether PPARa deficiency affects the co-ordinate regulation by food intake and the normal diurnal cycles of hepatic fatty acid oxidation, fatty acid synthesis (FAS) and cholesterogenesis (CS).

Methods: PPARa null mice and their respective controls were maintained on a 12 h dark/12 h light cycle with free access to food. Plasma lipids were determined at 4 h intervals and livers removed for measurement of mRNA. In vitro rates of hepatic FAS and CS were determined by incorporation of tritiated water.

Results: Plasma levels of free fatty acids (NEFA), cholesterol, ketone bodies and triacylglycerol were increased in the $-/-$ mice and did not follow the circadian variation seen in $(+/+)$ animals. In the $(+/+)$ mice, the rates of FAS and CS were significantly higher during the dark phase (D6) than during the light phase (L6). These differences were abolished in the $-/-$ mice. The lower rate of FAS at D6 in the $-/-$ mice was associated with a decreased expression of acetyl CoA carboxylase (ACC) mRNA and could be related to the increased level of plasma NEFA. Surprisingly, the increased rate of hepatic CS in the $-/-$ mice was associated with a marked decline in the expression of hydroxymethylglutaryl CoA reductase (HMGR) mRNA. PPARa deletion did not appear to have any effect on the expression of LDL-receptor or cholesterol 7-alpha hydroxylase mRNAs.

Conclusions: Deletion of PPARa attenuates or abolishes the circadian rhythm of hepatic and plasma lipid metabolism. The rate of hepatic CS is increased whilst that of FAS is diminished. The FAS change may be explained by a decreased expression of ACC mRNA. The effects on CS do not appear to result from changes in HMGR mRNA but may be related to changes in the demand for a common substrate, acetyl-CoA.

Generation of adult LPL-deficient mice

Juliane G. Strauss[1], Sasa Frank[2], Gabriele Knipping[2], Rudolf Zechner[1]. *Institutes of [1]Biochemistry; and [2]Medical Biochemistry, Karl-Franzens University, A-8010 Graz, Austria*

Objective: The transient adenovirus-mediated expression of LPL during the suckling period to rescue LPL knock-out mice (L0) from neonatal death and generate adult LPL deficient mice.

Methods: A total of 5×10^9 plaque forming units (pfu) of LPL-expressing adenovirus was injected intraperitoneally into mouse litters from matings of heterozygous LPL knock-out mice immediatley after birth.

Results: Over 90% of treated L0-mice survived the first days of life. In 3% of all cases L0-mice survived the suckling period and stayed alive for at least one year. Rescued L0-mice were smaller than their control littermates until 3 months of age and had strongly elevated triglyceride levels in the fed (5000 mg/dl) and in the fasted state (2000 mg/dl). Total cholesterol levels were also increased in both conditions due to increased VLDL-cholesterol. L0-mice lacked HDL-cholesterol indicating that LPL is essential for the HDL biogenesis. Glucose levels of L0-mice were normal, whereas ketone bodies and FFA were elevated.

Conclusion: Adult L0-mice will provide a valuable model to study the role of LPL deficiency in rodents.

Apolipoprotein (apo) E modulates hepatic very low density lipoprotein (VLDL) assembly and secretion

Y. Huang[1,2], W.J. Brecht[1], X.Q. Liu[1], Y. Wang[1,2], J.M. Taylor[1,2], S.C. Rall Jr.[1], R.W. Mahley[1,2]. [1]*Gladstone Institute of Cardiovascular Disease;* [2]*University of California, San Francisco, California, USA*

Objective: To investigate apoE's regulatory effect on hepatic VLDL assembly/secretion in transgenic animals and transfected hepatoma cells.

Methods and Results: In transgenic mice (apoE-null background) and rabbits expressing medium (10–20 mg/dl) or high (> 20 mg/dl) levels of human apoE3 in the liver, hepatic VLDL triglyceride (TG) and VLDL-apoB production rates were determined with the Triton-WR1339 method. Compared with wild-type mice, apoE3 medium- and high-expressing mice had increases of 29% and 56% in VLDL-TG production and 20% and 42% in VLDL-apoB production, respectively; apoE-null mice had decreases of 47% in VLDL-TG and 53% in VLDL-apoB production. Compared with nontransgenic rabbits, apoE3 medium- and high-expressing rabbits had increases of 2- and 4-fold in VLDL-TG production and 1.5- and 3-fold in VLDL-apoB production, respectively. The increased hepatic VLDL production contributed largely to hypertriglyceridemia in high-expressing mice and combined hyperlipidemia in high-expressing rabbits. After 2 h of incubation with ^{3}H-glycerol, ^{35}S-methionine, and 0.4 mM oleic acid, stably transfected McA-RH7777 cells overexpressing apoE3 (1.2 µg/mg cell protein/h) secreted 2.5-fold more VLDL-^{3}H-TG and twofold more VLDL-35 S-apoB into the medium than nontransfected cells; transfected cells also had 75% higher 3 H-TG content, most of which accumulated in the lumen of the endoplasmic reticulum, where VLDL assembly occurs. Microsomal TG transfer protein activity was about twofold higher in transfected than nontransfected cells and may have helped to mobilize TG to the endoplasmic reticulum.

Conclusion: ApoE overexpression stimulates the synthesis and mobilization of TG to the endoplasmic reticulum and increases hepatic assembly/secretion of TG-rich VLDL. Thus, apoE appears to be a powerful modulator of hepatic VLDL assembly and secretion.

Proteolysis and plaque rupture

Divergent roles of extracellular proteases in plaque stabilization and rupture; what are the molecular switches?

A. Newby, T. Izzard, M. Bond, S. Hussein, A. Chase. *Bristol Heart Institute, Bristol Royal Infirmary, Bristol, UK*

Basement membrane degrading metalloproteinases (MMPs-2 and -9) may be essential to allow vascular smooth muscle cells (VSMC) to migrate and proliferate in response to injury and inflammation. The molecular events which need to take place before quiescent VSMC in the artery wall can migrate and proliferate are however ill-defined. The presentation will identify the important events taking place during the G1 phase of the cell cycle, which have been compared in isolated rat VSMC and segments of rat aorta. The studies identify molecular switches that may be controlled by injury and extracellular proteolysis, which permit proliferation.

MMPs with activity against interstitial matrix, MMPs-1, -3, -7, -12 and -13, for example, have been associated with plaque rupture rather than stabilisation. We have sought to identify common and divergent features of the regulation of the MMP genes in VSMC. These studies may identify whether plaques prone to rupture produce an unfavourable complement of MMPs, and, if so, by what mechanisms. We also hope to identify potential inhibitors so as to stabilise plaques.

Why is it that some plaques rupture and others don't?

A.E. Becker, A.C. van der Wal, O.J. de Boer, C.M. van der Loos. *Academic Medical Center, University of Amsterdam, Amsterdam, The Netherlands*

Plaque rupture is defined as the condition in which the fibrous cap of an atherosclerotic (AS) plaque is torn apart producing a fissure into the lipid core, associated with intra-plaque hemorrhage and adherent mural thrombosis. This is the most common pathology underlying acute myocardial infarction (AMI).

Over the past decade it has been shown that plaques prone to rupture are characterized by a large lipid core, an attenuated fibrous cap and a dense inflammatory infiltrate composed of macrophages and T lymphocytes and, to a lesser extent, mast cells.

It is presently acknowledged that the immune system is involved; AS plaques contain an inflammatory cell-mediated (Th1)-like response, responsible for the release of a variety of cytokines, growth factors and enzymes. It appears as if the balance between these products may be responsible for the eventual effects on the tissues. The release of a cascade of matrix metalloproteinases, for instance, may lead to excessive collagen breakdown and this process, in the presence of high tissue tensile forces and rheological factors, may produce plaque rupture.

Why then is it that some AS plaques with characteristics alluded to above remain intact and others rupture?

Atherectomy specimens from patients with AMI show recent onset activation of T lymphocytes. This fits with clinical observations of increased inflammatory markers in peripheral blood. We have isolated T cells from AS plaques, which were tested against particular antigens, such as C. pneumoniae. Our preliminary results have shown that in some patients T cells cloned from plaques respond to C. pneumoniae. This boosts our belief that an additional stimulus serves as "the last straw that breaks the camel's back".

A novel adipocyte-derived plasma protein, adiponectin, suppresses lipid accumulation and class a scavenger receptor expression in human macrophages

N. Ouchi, S. Kihara, Y. Arita, A. Matsuyama, M. Nishida, Y. Okamoto, T. Nakamura, S. Yamashita, T. Funahashi, Y. Matsuzawa. *Department of Internal Medicine and Molecular Science, Graduate School of Medicine, Osaka University, Suita, Osaka, Japan*

Objectives: Obesity is the most common nutritional disorder and one of the major risk factors of atherosclerosis. However the molecular basis for the link between obesity and atherosclerosis has not been fully elucidated. We found an adipocyte-specific secretory protein, adiponectin, and developed an ELISA system to determine adiponectin concentrations. Plasma adiponectin level negatively correlated with body mass index (BMI) (Arita et. al. BBRC 1999) and was significantly low in patients with coronary artery disease compared with BMI-adjusted control subjects (Ouchi et. al. Circulation 1999). Here we showed the effects of adiponectin on lipid accumulation and macrophage scavenger receptor (MSR) expression in human macrophages.

Methods: Human monocytes were differentiated in human type AB serum for 7 days and then studied with adiponectin. The intracellular cholesteryl ester content was determined by the enzymatic, fluorometric method. Lipid droplets were stained with oil red O. The expression of class A MSR was analyzed by immunoblotting and northern blotting. The expression of CD36 was quantified by flow cytometry. The class A MSR ligand binding and uptake activities were examined by flow cytometry using Dil-AcLDL.

Results: Treatment with physiological concentration of adiponectin reduced intracellular cholesteryl ester content. Adiponectin-treated macrophages contained smaller lipid droplets. Adiponectin suppressed the expression of class A MSR at both mRNA and protein level without affecting the expression of CD36. Adiponectin treatment dose-dependently decreased both binding and uptake of Dil-AcLDL.

Conclusions: Adiponectin suppresses lipid accumulation in macrophages through inhibition of class A MSR expression.

Macrophage P53-deficiency leads to enhanced atherosclerosis in APOE*3-Leiden mice

B. van Vlijmen[1], G. Gerritsen[1], A. Franken[2], B. van de Water[3], M. Kock[4], J. von der Thüsen[1], M. Gijbels[5], M. van Eck[1], L. Havekes[1], T. Van Berkel[2]. *[1]TNO-PG/Gaubius Laboratory, Leiden; [2]Dept. of Biopharmaceutics; [3]Toxicology, LACDR, Leiden; [5]Dept. of Human Genetics, LUMC, Leiden, The Netherlands; and [4]Dept. of Pathology, Middelheim Hospital, Antwerp, Belgium*

Cell proliferation and cell death (either necrosis or apoptosis) are key processes in the progression of atherosclerotic plaques. The tumor suppressor gene p53 is an essential gene in cell proliferation and death, and is upregulated in human plaques. We investigated the importance of macrophage p53 in the progression of atherosclerotic lesions using bone marrow (BM) transplantation in APOE*3-Leiden transgenic mice, an animal model for human-like atherosclerosis. Reconstitution of APOE*3-Leiden mice with p53 deficient (p53–/–) BM did not cause any blood or splenic abnormalities within the period studied (i.e., a total of 16 weeks). Mice reconstituted with p53–/– BM showed a strong exacerbation of the progression of atherosclerotic lesions as compared to mice reconstituted with control (p53+/+) BM. Plaques in APOE*3-Leiden mice reconstituted with p53–/– BM had significantly larger total lesion area as compared to mice reconstituted with p53+/+ BM (186 ± 127 versus 82 ± 72 μm 2, p = 0.006); in addition, these plaques contained more necrosis (necrotic index: 1.1 ± 1.3 versus 0.2 ± 0.7; p = 0.04) and more lipid-loaded macrophages (macrophage area: 113 ± 56 vs. 54 ± 68 μm 2 ; p = 0.05). Importantly, these observations coincided with a decrease in apoptosis (TUNEL-positive nuclei going from 0.42 ± 0.39 to 0.14 ± 0.15%, p = 0.06), while the number of proliferating cells (BrdU-positive nuclei) was not affected. These studies indicate that p53 is important in the progression of atherosclerotic plaques due to its effect of macrophage cell death.

Functional 5A/6A polymorphism in human stromelysin-1 gene is in age-dependent relation to autopsy-verified calcified coronary lesions

Perttu Pöllänen[1], Pekka J. Karhunen[4], Jussi Mikkelsson[4], Kari M. Mattila[1], Kirsi Syrjäkoski[2], Seppo T. Nikkari[1,3], Timo Koivula[1], Terho Lehtimäki[1,3]. *[1]Laboratory of Aterosclerosis Genetics; [2]Cancer Genetics, Department of Clinical Chemistry, Centre for Laboratory Medicine Tampere University Hospital, Tampere; [3]The Medical School, University of Tampere; [4]Tampere University Hospital, Tampere, Finland*

Objective: We studied the association between human stromelysin-1 promoter 5A/6A genotype and autopsy-verified coronary atherosclerotic lesions in a cohort of 300 men, average age 53 years, range 33 to 70 years.

Methods: The allelic variation was detected from purified DNA by PCR and by automated minisequensing method. The right and left anterior descending coronary arteries (RCA and LAD) were stained for fat, and areas covered with fatty streaks, fibrotic plaques and complicated lesions were measured.

Results: A significant stromelysin promoter genotype-by-age association was observed with areas of calcified lesions of the coronary arteries (p = 0.0395). In the RCA and LCX arteries of men > 53 years, carriers of the 5A/5A, 5A/6A had on average a 101% and a 79% increase, respectively, in the area of calcified lesions, when compared with the carriers of 6A/6A genotype.

Conclusions: In men, the stromelysin 5A-allele is a significant genetic risk factor for calcified atherosclerotic lesion rupture at late middle age.

Genetic regulation of the MMP-7 and MMP-12 gene expression

Sofia Jormsjö[1], Shu Ye[2], Joseffa Moritz[1], Barbro Burt[1], Adriano Henney[2], Anders Hamsten[1], Per Eriksson[1]. *[1]Atherosclerosis Research Unit, King Gustaf V Research Institute, Karolinska Institute, Stockholm, Sweden; and [2]The Wellcome Trust Center for Human Genetics, Oxford, UK*

Degradation of extracellular matrix within the aortic wall by matrix metalloproteinases has been implicated in several pathological conditions such as development of atherosclerosis, plaque rupture, high blood pressure and aneurysm formation. To elucidate the role that elastolytic enzymes may play in these conditions, we scanned the metalloelastase (MMP-12) and the matrilysin (MMP-7) gene for polymorphisms by single strand conformational polymorphism (SSCP) analysis. Two common polymorphic consisting of an A to G substitution were found in the metalloelastase gene, one located in exon 6 and one in the promoter region. The exon 6 mutaion was a silent mutation. The promoter A/G polymorphism was located 82 bp upstream from the transcription start site adjacent to an activator protein-1 (AP-1) consensus sequence. The allele frequnecy of the G allele was 0.19 and in linkage disequilibrium with the exon 6 polymorphism. By EMSA studies we established that the promoter polymorphism influences the binding of transcrition factor AP-1 with a higher affinity for the A allele. Furthermore, transfection studies showed that the polymorphism influences the transcriptional activity of the MMP-12 promoter and that there is an allele-specific effect on arterial luminal dimensions in a cohort of patients undergoing PTCA with stent implantation.

At present, we have found two promoter polymorphsims in the MMP-7 gene and studies are ongoing in order to analyse the functional significance of these mutations.

Cerebrovascular disease

Strategies to prevent stroke: lessons for developing countries

Ruth Bonita. *Noncommunicable Disease Surveillance, WHO, Geneva, Switzerland*

Cerebrovascular disease (stroke) is the second leading cause of death worldwide, responsible for approximately 9.5% of all deaths. Although we have access to almost 50 years of epidemiological research and knowledge about appropriate interventions, the global burden of stroke is still increasing, with most of the stroke deaths now occurring in the poorer regions of the world. Although many lessons have been learnt, the strategies adopted to date have been only partially effective in preventing and controlling the stroke epidemic.

Given the increasingly global nature of the stroke epidemics, a global response is required. This presentation describes the dimensions of the global burden of stroke, the evolution of the global stroke epidemic and its several patterns, summarizes current understanding of the determinants of the stroke epidemics at both the individual and population levels, and identifies appropriate policies for the primary prevention and control of stroke with a specific focus on developing countries.

Neuroprotection in acute brain infarction — where do we stand?

Kennedy R. Lees. *Acute Stroke Unit, University Department of Medicine & Therapeutics, Western Infirmary, Glasgow, UK*

Severe cerebral ischaemia rapidly leads to cell death but moderate ischaemia can be withstood for several hours. Reperfusion with alteplase or ancrod improves clinical outcome and specialist care is of proven value. Experimental data suggest that infarct size can be limited by early administration of NMDA antagonists, ion channel blockers or anti-inflammatory measures. Unfortunately, neuroprotective strategies have so far failed to live up to their initial promise. Selfotel, aptiganel, gavestinel and eliprodil represent antagonists at various sites of the NMDA receptor, and each has been unsuccessful in clinical trials. Free radical scavenging with tirilazad, an anti-inflammatory approach with enlimomab and ion channel blockade with lubeluzole fared no better. Closer analysis of the preclinical data and the trial results reveals many potential explanations for the disappointing results so far. These include a lack of robust animal data to support neuroprotective efficacy, a low therapeutic index that precluded adequate dosing in man, and failures of trial design. A major factor may be the discrepancy between the effective time window in animals and the delay to treatment in man. More rigorous guidelines for development have recently been established, and the lessons learned are now being applied. These include strategies to enhance dose selection, to "enrich" the trial population with potential responders, to control for confounding factors, to optimise trial endpoints or to use surrogate imaging measures. Drugs presently in development include the GABA agonist, clomethiazole, a potassium channel opener (BMS 204352), magnesium, a neutrophil inhibitory factor (NIF), and a nitrone, NXY-059. Inhibitors of the proteasome, such as PS-519, and of PARP will shortly be available. Finally, experimental approaches are being revised to consider if generic brain protection rather than specific neuroprotection may improve outcome.

Carotid atherosclerosis and lipoprotein(a) levels in CHD patients

M. Ezhov, A. Lyakishev, O. Afanasieva, G. Benevolenskaya, T. Balakhonova, S. Pokrovsky. *Cardiology Research Center, Moscow, Russia*

Objective: Of our study was to assess whether lipoprotein (a) [Lp(a)] levels are associated with carotid atherosclerotic lesions in CHD patients.

Methods: We have included 230 male patients (aged 24 to 68 years) with proven coronary atherosclerosis (accordant to angiographic findings one or more major coronary arteries had stenosis $> 50\%$). Duplex scan with a linear array transducer at a frequency of 7.5 MHz was used for imaging of carotid arteries. The severity of carotid atherosclerosis was scored according to the following criteria: 0 — no atherosclerotic lesions (n = 33); 1 — intima-media thickening from 1 to 2 mm (n = 33); 2 — stenoses $< 50\%$ (n = 140); 3 — stenoses $> 50\%$ in one or more branches (n = 24). We have examined plasma lipid values [total cholesterol (TC), triglycerides (TG), HDL cholesterol (HDL-C), LDL cholesterol (LDL-C)]. Lp(a) concentration was measured by ELISA.

	0	1	2	3
Lp(a), mg/dl	22 ± 22	29 ± 31	33 ± 40	48 ± 63*
TC, mmol/l	6.4 ± 1.2	6.5 ± 1.4	6.6 ± 1.1	7.1 ± 1.3*
LDL-C, mmol/l	4.2 ± 0.9	4.6 ± 1.3	4.6 ± 1.2	5.0 ± 1.3 *

*$p < 0.05$ vs. group 0. Values are M ± SD.

Concentrations of TC, LDL-C and Lp(a) steadily increased, reaching statistical significance in the group 3. There were not differences in the prevalence of classic factors and concentrations of HDL-C, TG, fibrinogen among the groups. Patients with plaques (groups 2 + 3) were older [54 ± 7 vs. 50 ± 8 in groups 0 + 1, $p < 0.001$] and had a trend toward higher Lp(a) level (36 ± 43 vs. 26 ± 27 mg/dl, p = 0.07). This difference in Lp(a) is concerned only patients younger than 55 years but not the older ones.

Conclusion: Elevated Lp(a) levels are associated with severe carotid atherosclerosis and the presence of plaques in carotid arteries in CHD patients younger 55 years.

Lp(a), homocysteine and hemostatic risk factors in children with a family history of early ischaemic cerebral stroke

B. Torbus-Lisiecka, H. Bukowska, M. Jastrzebska, K. Honczarenko, M. Naruszewicz. *Pomeranian Medical University, Szczecin, Poland*

Objective: The aim of this study was 1) to evaluate the concentration of homocysteine depending on severity of ischaemic cerebral stroke and 2) to search for a correlation between children and parents as to Lp(a) and homocysteine levels.

Material and Methods: The study was performed in 35 patients with early ischaemic cerebral stroke (ICS) and their children (FH-ICS). Patients were grouped according to the form of ICS: transient (TIA), progressive (PRIND) or complete (CS). Concentrations of Lp(a), homocysteine (HCY), fibrinogen (Fb), factor VII (FVII) and uric acid (UA) were measured in parents and children.

216

Results:

	TIA	PRIND	CS	FH-TIA	FH-PRIND	FH-CS
Lp(a)	19 ± 20.4	16 ± 9.4	50 ± 53	16 ± 9.7	12 ± 5.9	25 ± 34
HCY	9.9 ± 2.6	11 ± 3.4	15 ± 4.0	8.0 ± 0.7	10.0 ± 2.6	10 ± 3.1
Fb	3.8 ± 0.7	3.8 ± 0.9	4.1 ± 0.7	3.2 ± 0.7	3.2 ± 0.6	3.8 ± 0.5

The following correlations between parents and children were noted: Lp(a) (r = 0.77, p < 0.0001), UA (r = 0.71, p < 0.001), HCY (r = 0.45, p < 0.05) FVII (r = 0.45, p < 0.05), Fb (r = 0.42, p = 0.06). A correlation between Lp(a) and HCY (r = 0.47, p < 0.05) and between Fb and FVII (r = 0.60, p < 0.01) was found in children.

Conclusions: 1. HCY levels correlate with severity of ICS; 2. In families with a history of ICS the levels of risk factors in children are determined by levels in parents.

Functional significance of G-33A mutation in the promoter region of thrombomodulin gene and its association with carotid atherosclerosis

Y.H. Li[1], P.S. Yeh[2], H.J. Lin[2], C.H. Chen[1], B.I. Chang[1], J.C. Lin[1], H.L. Wu[1], G.Y. Shi[1], M.L. Lai[1], J.H. Chen[1]. [1]National Cheng Kung University Medical Center; [2]Chi-Mei Foundation Hospital, Tainan, Taiwan, China

Objective: We have previously reported that G-33A promoter mutation of thrombomodulin (TM) gene is associated with coronary atherosclerosis. This study was conducted to determine whether the TM G-33A mutation is a genetic risk factor for ischemic stroke or carotid atherosclerosis. The functional significance of this mutation was also examined.

Methods: We investigated 333 patients (mean age 65 years, 59% male) with ischemic stroke and 257 age- and sex-matched control subjects. In all study participants, carotid atherosclerosis was assessed by Duplex scanning and TM G-33A promoter mutation was detected by single-strand conformation polymorphism. To assess the influence of this mutation on TM promoter activity, TM promoter/luciferase reporter gene plasmids containing normal sequence or G-33A mutation were constructed and transfected into endothelial cell culture.

Results: There was no significant difference (18.3% vs. 24.1%, p = 0.105) in the TM G-33A mutation frequency (GA + AA genotypes) between stroke and control group, even only in younger (age ≤ 60 years) subjects (20.9% vs. 22.0%, p = 0.991). All study participants were reclassified into 2 groups according to the presence or absence of significant carotid atherosclerosis. The TM G-33A mutation frequency was similar between the subjects with and without carotid atherosclerosis (22.2% vs. 19.8%, p = 0.550). But when only younger subjects were included, the mutation occurred more frequently in carotid atherosclerosis group (33.3% vs. 17.3%, odds ratio [OR] = 2.38, p = 0.027). Logistic regression analysis demonstrated that only diabetes mellitus (OR = 3.11, 95% confidence interval [CI] = 1.33–7.30, p = 0.009) and G-33A mutation (OR = 2.46, 95% CI = 1.14–5.29, p = 0.021) were independently associated with carotid atherosclerosis in younger subjects. As assessed by luciferase reporter gene assays, the activity of the constructs bearing the G-33A mutation showed a significant decrease –36 ± 12%) in transcriptional activity compared with the wild type constructs.

Conclusions: These findings suggest that the TM G-33A promoter mutation reduces the endothelial TM synthesis and is related to carotid atherosclerosis in younger subjects.

A possible role of thermolabile methylenetetrahydrofolate reductase in the occurrence of vascular dementia

Jun-Hyun Yoo[1], Gyu-Dong Choi[2], Soo-Sang Kang[3]. *[1]Family Medicine, Samsung Medical Center, Sungkyunkwan University School of Medicine, Seoul; [2]Geriatric Medicine, Inchon Eun-Hye Hospital, Neuropsychiatric Hospital, Inchon, Korea; and [3]Genetics, Pediatrics, Rush Medical College and Rush-Presbyterian-St. Luke's Medical Center, Chicago, Illinois, USA*

Objective: To investigate the relationship of the TT genotype of MTHFR and hyper-homocyst(e)inemia in the development of cerebral infarction with and without cognitive impairment.

Methods: We assessed the status of hyperhomocyst(e)inemia and the C677T genotypes of MTHFR in 143 patients with vascular dementia, 122 nondemented patients with cerebral infarction and 306 healthy subjects matched for age and gender, in a hospital-based setting.

Results: Proportion of moderate hyperhomocyst(e)inemia (plasma homocyst(e)ine $\geqslant 15$ μmol/l) as higher in patients with vascular dementia or cerebral infarction than in normal controls (42.6%, 20%, 10.1%, p = 0.001). In contrast, a higher frequency of the TT genotype of MTHFR was found only in demented patients compared to non-demented patients or controls (25.3%, 9.8%, 12.1%, p = 0.01), with odds ratio of 2.70 (95% CI; 2.05–3.53, p = 0.0002) adjusted for hypertension, smoking, diabetes mellitus, age, and gender. Demented patients with multiple infarct had a higher frequency of TT genotype (OR 3.1, 95% CI; 2.2–4.4, p = 0.0007), whereas those with single infarct did not (OR 2.0, p = 0.15). When subjects were stratified according to homocyst(e)ine levels, MTHFR TT genotype was significantly associated with risk of vascular dementia in hyperhomocyst(e)inemia groups (OR 3.03, 95% CI, 1.80–5.10, p = 0.03), compared to with CT/CC genotype, but not in normohomocysteinemic groups.

Conclusions: Findings provide evidence that thermolabile variant of MTHFR enzyme is associated with the severity of cerebral infarction and the occurrence of vascular dementia, furthermore homocyst(e)inemia may not be the only pathogenic factor in MTHFR deficiency. Analysis of both plasma homocyst(e)ine and C677T genotype of MTHFR is probably necessary for the risk evaluation of cerebrovascular disease.

Triglycerides and CVD

Hypertriglyceridemia and the metabolic syndrome

S. Grundy. *University of Texas Southwestern Medical Center, Dallas, Texas, USA*

Most patients with hypertriglyceridemia have other cardiovascular risk factors that are typical of the metabolic syndrome. These include elevations of apolipoprotein B, remnant lipoproteins and small LDL particles; reduced HDL cholesterol; elevated blood pressure; insulin resistance and glucose intolerance; and coagulation abnormalities. Thus, elevated serum triglycerides are a marker for the metabolic syndrome. This is especially the case when patients have abdominal obesity. Rarely patients will have hypertriglyceridemia in the absence of abdominal obesity and insulin resistance, but such cases are an exception, and not the rule. Hypertriglyceridemia in patients with insulin resistance is usually secondary to fatty liver, which in turn is the result of elevated plasma nonesterified fatty acids (NEFA). Elevations of NEFA can be due either to obesity or to insulin resistance in adipose tissue. In addition to being a marker for the metabolic syndrome, elevated triglycerides may be directly or indirectly atherogenic. Some triglyceride rich lipoproteins, particularly VLDL remnants, appear to be directly atherogenic; also elevated triglycerides give rise to small LDL particles and low HDL levels, both of which may be atherogenic. The primary treatment of hypertriglyceridemia is weight control plus physical activity; both reduce insulin resistance and mitigate the metabolic syndrome. A question of great importance is whether triglyceride-lowering drugs will also reduce risk for coronary heart disease. Several clinical trials give strongly suggestive evidence of risk reduction from these triglyceride-lowering drugs.

Twenty-year cardiovascular disease mortality in the familial forms of hypertriglyceridemia

M.A. Austin, B. McKnight, K.L. Edwards, C.M. Bradley, M.J. McNeely, B.M. Psaty, J.D. Brunzell, A.G. Motulsky. *University of Washington, Seattle, Washington, USA*

Background: Familial combined hyperlipidemia (FCHL) and familial hypertriglyceridemia (FHTG) are two of the most common familial forms of hyperlipidemia. The purposes of this study were to estimate 20-year cardiovascular disease (CVD) mortality among relatives in these families, and to evaluate plasma triglyceride as a predictor of CVD mortality.

Methods: The study was based on lipid and medical history data from 101 families ascertained in two studies conducted in the early 1970s. Vital status and cause-of-death was determined during 1993–1997 for 685 family members, including first degree relatives of the probands and spouse controls.

Results: Compared to spouse controls, CVD mortality was increased among sibs and offspring in FCHL (relative risk = 1.7, p = 0.02) after adjustment for baseline covariates. Baseline triglyceride was associated with increased CVD mortality independent of total cholesterol among relatives in FHTG families, (relative risk = 2.7, p = 0.02), but not in FCHL families (relatives risk = 1.5, p = 0.16), after adjustment for baseline covariates.

Conclusions: This prospective study establishes that relatives in FCHL families are at increased risk for CVD mortality and that triglyceride predicts CVD mortality among relatives in FHTG families. The findings add to the growing evidence for the importance of hypertriglyceridemia as a risk factor for CVD.

Diurnal triglyceridemia: a surrogate of postprandial lipemia?

M. Castro Cabezas, C.J.M. Halkes, S. Meijssen, D.W. Erkelens. *Univ. Hosp. Utrecht, Dpt. of Intern. Med., The Netherlands*

Background: Postprandial hypertriglyceridemia is regarded as an independent risk factor for atherosclerosis. Large prospective studies have not been performed due to the workload and the costs involved in performing oral fat loading tests. We evaluated the feasibility of determining ambulatory diurnal capillary TG (TGc) profiles compared to standardized oral fat loading tests (OFLT) in 18 subjects and we determined the variability of diurnal triglyceridemia in a larger cohort of 106 subjects.

Methods: In 18 subjects with a wide range of fasting plasma TG, results of OFLT (50 g/m^2 ; 10 hrs) were compared to diurnal TGc profiles measured in an out-patient clinic setting. In an observational study, 106 healthy volunteers (54 females and 52 males) measured TGc. Food intake was recorded in a diary and fasting blood was drawn once at inclusion. Diurnal TGc profiles were estimated as the mean area under the TGc curve of 6 time-point measurements on 3 different days.

Results: Plasma TG clearance after the acute OFLT correlated well with the diurnal TGc-AUC (r = 0.77; $p < 0.01$; n = 18). In addition, hyperTG subjects (plasma TG > 2.0 mM) had a higher diurnal triglyceridemia (49.8 ± 15.4 h.mM) as well as a higher response of plasma TG to the OFLT (42.1 ± 15.4 h.mM), than the subjects with normal fasting plasma TG (29.8 ± 11.8 h.mM ($p < 0.05$) and 20.8 ± 5.9 h.mM ($p < 0.01$), respectively). In the cohort of 106 subjects, repeated measurements of diurnal triglyceridemia tended to be less variable than fasting capillary TG (mean coefficients of variation 15% (range: 0.60%—46%) and 25% (range: 1.4%—73%), respectively; p = 0.09) for the whole group and in males (19% (0.60%—46%) and 24% (1.4%—58%), respectively; p = 0.07). Stepwise multiple regression analysis with TGc-AUC as dependent variable showed that the best predictors were fasting TGc, gender, systolic blood pressure and mean daily energy intake, explaining 72% of the variation of diurnal triglyceridemia.

Conclusion: Diurnal capillary TG profiles may be used to estimate the total daily load of potential atherogenic triglyceride rich particles to which individuals are subjected during the day without the need for metabolic ward studies.

Application of a sandwich ELISA for apo B48

Y. Saika[1], S. Yamashita[1], N. Sakai[1], K. Hirano[1], Y. Utida[2], S. Itou[2], Y. Matsuzawa[1].
[1]*Department of Internal Medicine and Molecular Science, Graduate School of Medicine, Osaka University; and* [2]*Fujirebio, Inc., Japan*

Object: Chylomicron (CM) remnants are assumed to play important roles in atherogenesis. However, there have been no appropriate methods to sensitively evaluate the fasting levels of CM remnants. The object of the current study was to raise monoclonal antibodies (mAbs) against human apo B-48 and to establish a sensitive ELISA for measuring serum apo B-48 levels in normolipidemic and hyperlipidemic subjects.

Methods and Results: mAbs were raised against human apo B-48 by immunizing synthetic peptides. These mAbs specifically reacted with the C-terminal of apo B-48, but not B-100. Using these mAbs, a sandwich ELISA was established to measure serum apo B-48 levels, using recombinant apo B-48 as a standard (kindly provided by Dr. Yao). The CV of the assay was approximately 10%. After oral fat loading in normolipidemic subjects, serum apo B-48 increased with a peak at 3-4 h. In the normolipidemic subjects (n = 369), fasting serum apo B-48 levels were 41 ± 28 (Mean ± SD) arbitrary units (AU)/ ml (100 AU/ml ~ 1 mg/dl). Serum apo B-48 concentration positively correlated with serum triglyceride levels (r = 0.72, p < 0.05), while there was no significant correlation between serum apo B-48 and cholesterol levels. Apo B-48 was detected in ultracentrifugally separated lipoproteins including CM, VLDL, IDL and even LDL. In dyslipidemic subjects with apo E2/2, apo B-48 was extremely increased even if they were normolipidemic. In patients with diabetes mellitus, apo B-48 was also increased, suggesting the impairment of CM metabolism. Furthermore, we used the mAbs to examine the presence or absence of apo B-48 in human aortic tissues. Immunohistochemical analysis demonstrated a strong positive staining of apo B-48 mainly in the extracellular matrices of aterosclerotic aorta.

Conclusion: These data suggest that this apo B-48 ELISA provides a useful tool to estimate the impairment of CM metabolism and that the deposition of CM remnants could contribute partly to the pathogenesis of atherosclerosis.

Metabolic risk factors for CHD in the elderly

L.A. Simons, J. Simons, Y. Friedlander, J. McCallum. *The Dubbo Study, St Vincent's Hospital, Sydney, NSW, Australia*

Objective: To identify metabolic risk factors for coronary heart disease (CHD) in the elderly.

Methods: A 10 year follow-up in a prospective study of cardiovascular disease in the Australian elderly. The cohort, first examined in 1988–1989, was composed of 2,805 men and women 60 years and older. The prediction of CHD was examined in a Cox proportional hazards model.

Results: CHD outcomes (ICD-9 410–414) occurred in 448 men (36%) and 435 women (28%). The hazard ratios (95% CI) for men and women respectively were: total cholesterol 1.09 (1.01–1.18) and 1.09 (1.02–1.17); HDL cholesterol 0.64 (0.46–0.90) and 0.62 (0.46–0.83); total/HDL cholesterol 1.05 (1.01–1.09) and 1.04 (1.01–1.09); log triglycerides 1.07 (0.89–1.29) and 1.42 (1.14–1.76); LDL cholesterol 1.14 (1.04–1.25) and 1.08 (0.99–1.17); serum apo-B 1.64 (1.15–2.34) and 1.60 (1.16–2.21); apo-AI 0.74 (0.53–1.03) and 0.81 (0.59–1.10) (per 1 unit change in each continuous variable); Lp(a) 1.52 (1.13–2.02) and 1.25 (0.91–1.71) (Quintile V vs. Quintile I); diabetes 1.18 (0.87–1.59) and 1.95 (1.44–2.63). Hazard ratios by age for total cholesterol (sexes combined) were: 60–69 years, 1.17 (1.08–1.27); 70–79 years, 1.02 (0.94–1.11); 80+ years, 1.05 (0.88–1.25).

Conclusions: Lipids and lipoproteins still predict CHD in the elderly, but with some attenuation as the population ages.

Paraoxonase activity in primary hypertriglyceridemia

F. Brites[1], J. Verona[1], J.C. Fruchart[2], G. Castro[2], R. Wikinski[1]. *[1]School of Pharmacy and Biochemistry, Univ. of Buenos Aires, Argentina; and [2]Institut Pasteur de Lille, France*

Objective: The aim of the present study was to evaluate paraoxonase (PON) activity in primary hypertriglyceridemia (HTG), whose independent relationship with atherosclerosis still remains controversial.

Methods: We studied a group of well-characterised men with primary hypertriglyceridemia (Triglycerides, TG ⩾ 200 mg/dl) and low HDL-cholesterol levels (HDL-C ⩽ 35 mg/dl) (n = 12) in comparison to normotriglycridemic (NTG) subjects with (n = 12) or without low HDL-C concentration (n = 12). The lipid, lipoprotein and apolipoprotein profiles were evaluated by standardised methods and previously reported (Brites et al. Atherosclerosis, in press). PON was evaluated following the original method of Furlong et al. and employing two different substrates: paraoxon (PON activity) and phenylacetate (arylesterase, ARE activity), the latter being a better indicator of the enzyme mass. PON activity was also measured in the presence and in the absence of 1 M NaCl (PON 1 M).

Results: PON, PON 1 M and ARE activities were significantly reduced only in patients who combined HTG and low HDL-C levels in comparison to NTG subjects with normal HDL-C (PON = 166 ± 63 vs. 247 ± 69 hmol/ml.min, $p < 0.01$; PON 1 M = 201 ± 115 vs. 376 ± 180 μmol/ml.min, $p < 0.05$; ARE = 760 ± 199 vs. 950 ± 216 μmol/ml.min, $p < 0.01$; respectively). All the three activities showed positive and significant correlations with total HDL-C, HDL 2 -C, HDL 3 -C, apo A-I and LpA-I:A-II level s.

Conclusions: HDL antiatherogenic capacity is not only limited to its role in reverse cholesterol transport, but also to its antioxidant potential, mainly attributed to PON. In patients with primary HTG and low HDL-C, the low PON activity, evaluated by different ways, could reflect a reduced antioxidant capacity, thus contributing to the association between hypertriglyceridemia and atherosclerosis.

Cellular stress and gene regulation

Hemodynamic forces, endothelial gene regulation and atherogenesis: an overview

M.A. Gimbrone Jr. *Vascular Research Div, Dept. of Pathology, Brigham & Women's Hospital, Harvard Medical School, Boston, Massachusetts, USA*

The localization of atherosclerotic lesions to arterial geometries associated with disturbed flow patterns suggests an important role for hemodynamic forces in atherogenesis. There is increasing evidence that the endothelium can discriminate among different bio-mechanical forces and transduce these stimuli into genetic regulatory events. At the level of individual genes, this regulation is accomplished via the interaction of transcription factors such as NF-kB with promoter elements such as the shear-stress-response element (SSRE), in the PDGF-B gene. Several such biomechanical force-sensitive transcriptional mechanisms appear to exist. At the level of multiple genes, distinct patterns of up- and down-regulation appear to be elicited by exposure to physiological levels of steady laminar shear stress (LSS), compared with similar magnitudes of turbulent shear stress (TSS), versus cytokine (IL-1) stimulation. LSS appears to elicit a distinct pattern of endothelial gene expression, not observed with TSS or IL-1. Certain of the genes upregulated by steady LSS, such as ecNOS, MnSOD, COX-2, support vaso-protective (anti-inflammatory, anti-thrombotic, anti-oxidant, anti-apoptotic) functions in endothelium. The selective and sustained upregulation of these "atheroprotective genes" in the endothelial lining of lesion-protected areas may be a mechanism by which hemodynamic forces can influence lesion formation and progression. The application of genome-wide, high-throughput technologies for the analysis of endothelial phenotypic modulation by biomechanical stimuli promises to afford new insights into the signaling networks that orchestrate endothelial gene regulation in atherogenesis. These new insights may enable novel strategies for early diagnosis, treatment and prevention of atherosclerotic vascular disease.

Focal atherogenesis, hemodynamics, and heterogeneous endothelial gene expression

P.F. Davies, C. Shi, R. Riley, D. Polacek. *Institute for Medicine and Engineering, University of Pennsylvania, Philadelphia, USA*

Atherosclerosis originates at predictable focal loci that have long been known to be associated with regions of disturbed blood flow. Improved precision in experimental models of spatially defined flow has recently been combined with regional and single-cell gene-expression ("transcriptional profiling") to investigate the relationships linking haemodynamics to vessel wall pathobiology. We have proposed that a limited number of proatherosclerotic genes expressed in only a few endothelial cells may play a dominant role in focal pathogenesis and vascular regulation. However, their identity may be masked because of message dilution in mRNAs isolated from a larger pool of cells. To begin to address the hypothesis, we have applied an amplified antisense mRNA technique to the cardiovascular system. Quantitative profiles of gene expression, including the use of high-throughput hybridization to screen many genes simultaneously, now allow endothelial heterogeneity to be addressed in a detailed (single cell) yet comprehensive (multiple genes, high-throughput) approach that increases the probability of finding new therapeutic targets.

Supported by NIH grants HL62250, HL36049, and a grant from AstraZeneca Pharmaceuticals.

Gene regulation by hypoxia

C. Pugh, G.-W. Chang, S. Clifford, M. Cockman, A. Epstein, P. Jaakkolla, N. Masson, P. Maxwell, D. Mole, P. Ratcliffe, Y.-M. Tian, E. Vaux. *The Wellcome Trust Centre for Human Genetics, University of Oxford, UK*

Tissue hypoxia underlies the pathophysiology of much human disease. Erythropoietin gene expression has provided a paradigm for transcriptional regulation in response to hypoxia. The erythropoietin $3'$ enhancer is activated in hypoxia in specialised cells by the binding of an inducible DNA binding complex, hypoxia inducible factor-1 (HIF).

HIF is widely expressed and has a key role in other cellular responses to hypoxia, binding the DNA consensus sequence BRCGTGV of genes involved in a variety of processes including energy metabolism, angiogenesis, vasomotor tone and apoptosis and regulating their expression. Furthermore, tumour transplantation experiments indicate that HIF is activated by hypoxia within solid tumours and that this activation has a critical bearing on tumour angiogenesis and growth.

HIF is a heterodimer of basic-helix-loop-helix PAS domain containing alpha and beta chains, each of which exist as gene families. We have mapped functional domains within the HIF-1 alpha and HIF-2 alpha chains. Two mechanisms of regulated transactivation are revealed, one involving the carboxyl terminus, which interacts with the co-activator P300, and the other involving an internal domain responsible for rapid degradation of the molecule by the proteasome in normoxia. Degradation is prevented by hypoxia, cobaltous ions or iron chelators.

Experiments with mutant cell lines and model organisms have allowed molecular dissection of the HIF alpha degradative pathway. We have demonstrated a critical role for the von Hippel-Lindau tumour suppressor protein, pVHL, in the degradation process. The interaction between these molecules requires part of the internal oxygen dependent degradation domain of HIF alpha chains and is disrupted by tumour associated mutations in the beta domain of pVHL. Loss of this interaction is associated with a failure to ubiquitylate HIF alpha chains and consequently, a failure to regulate HIF and HIF-dependent genes.

Mechanical stress-induced HSP70 expression in SMC via RAS/RAC G-proteins, but not MAPK

Y. Hu[1], C. Li[2], G. Sturm[2], G. Wick[2], Q. Xu[2]. *[1]Inst. for Exp. Pathology, University of Innsbruck; and [2]Inst. for Biomed. Aging Research, Austrian Academy of Sciences, Innsbruck, Austria*

Objective: Previous reports documented that acute elevation in blood pressure results in heat shock protein 70 (hsp70) mRNA expression followed by hsp70 protein production in rat aortas. The present study was designed to study whether mechanical stress per se induces HSP70 expression in smooth muscle cells (SMCs).

Methods and Results: Western blot analysis demonstrated that hsp70 protein induction peaked between 6 and 12 h after treatment with cyclic stain stress (60 cycles/min, 5–

30% elongation). Elevated protein levels were preceded by hsp70 mRNA transcription, which was associated with HSF1 phosphorylation and activation stimulated by mechanical forces, suggesting that the response was regulated at the transcriptional level. Conditioned medium from cyclic strain-stressed SMCs did not result in HSF-DNA binding activation. Furthermore, mitogen-activated protein kinases (MAPKs), including extracellular signal-regulated kinases, c-Jun NH2-terminal protein kinases or stress-activated protein kinases and p38 MAPKs, were also highly activated in response to cyclic strain stress. Inhibition of ERK and p38 MAPK activation by their specific inhibitors (PD98059 and SB 202190) did not influence HSF1 activation.

Interestingly, SMC lines stably expressing dominant negative rac (rac N17) abolished hsp production and HSF1 activation induced by cyclic strain stress, while a significant reduction of hsp70 expression was seen in ras N17 transfected-SMC lines.

Conclusions: Our findings demonstrate that cyclic strain stress induced-hsp70 expression is mediated by HSF1 and regulated by rac/ras GTP-binding proteins. Induction of hsp70 could be important in maintaining SMC homeostasis during vascular remodeling stimulated by hemodynamic stress.

Genotype dependent and environmental specific effects on endothelial nitric oxide synthase (eNOS) gene expression and enzyme activity

X.L. Wang[1,2], A.S. Sim[2], M.X. Wang[3], G.A.C. Murrell[3], B. Trudinger[4], J. Wang[1,4].
[1] Southwest Foundation for Biomedical Research, San Antonio, Texas, USA;
[2] Cardiovascular Genetics Laboratory; [3] Orthopaedic Research Institute, University of New South Wales; and [4] Department of Obstetrics and Gynaecology, Westmead Hospital, Australia

Objective: We have shown that the rare 4 27bp repeat allele at intron 4 of the eNOS is associated with an elevated risk for coronary artery disease (CAD) in smokers but higher basal NO levels in healthy nonsmokers. In the present study, we explored the interactive effects of eNOS genotypes and cigarette smoking on the eNOS gene expression and enzyme activity.

Methods: We measured levels of the eNOS mRNA (quantitative RT-PCR) and protein (Western blotting), and eNOS enzyme activity (L-arginine conversion) in 33 postpartum placentas.

Results: We found that the eNOS protein levels were significantly lower among those with the rare 4 repeat allele (0.48 ± 0.11, n = 9) compared to the common allele (1.05 ± 0.10, n = 24, $p < 0.01$). In contrast, the eNOS enzyme activity was about 7-fold higher in the rare allele (4556.2 ± 255.4 cpm/mg/min) than that in the common allele (621.8 ± 180.5 cpm/mg/min). Whilst cigarette smoking decreased the eNOS protein levels in both the common allele (nonsmokers vs. smokers: 1.09 ± 0.12 vs. 0.90 ± 0.27) and the rare allele (0.42 ± 27 vs. 0.27 ± 0.28), it had an interactive effect on eNOS activities. Cigarette smoking reduced the eNOS activities for more than half of the value in the rare allele placentas (nonsmokers: 6143.8 ± 251.2, n = 5, smokers: 2968.5 ± 259.4, n = 4). But the enzyme activities for the common allele placentas were even modestly elevated (nonsmokers: 521.3 ± 110.8, n = 19, smokers: 722.2 ± 251.1, n = 5).

Conclusion: Although the rare allele may generate more NO when not exposed to cigarette smoking, the capacity of NO production by eNOS is seriously compromised when the rare allele carriers smoke, which does not occur for the common allele. We established a genotype dependent and environmental specific model in eNOS regulation.

25-hydroxycholesterol modulates an inflammatory response in human macrophages

M.C.O. Englund, P.I. Morelli, L. Mattsson Hultén, O. Wiklund, B.G. Ohlsson. *The Wallenberg Laboratory for Cardiovascular Research, Göteborg University, Göteborg, Sweden*

Objective: Several different oxysterols and Tumor Necrosis Factor-α (TNFα) have been found in atherosclerotic plaques. Oxysterols have in earlier studies been shown to have regulatory effects on expression of different genes. The aim of this study was to examine the impact of these oxysterols on the TNFα secretion in human monocyte-derived macrophages (hMDM) and to investigate the regulatory pathway.

Methods: Binding of transcription factors to DNA was studied by Electrophoretic Mobility Shift Assay (EMSA) and TNFα protein secretion was assayed by Enzyme-Linked Immuno-Sorbent Assay (ELISA). Intracellular levels of H_2O_2 were determined and Western Blot was used to analyze activity of Stress Activated Protein Kinase/Jun N-terminal Kinase (SAPK/JNK).

Results: An increased TNFα secretion was found when hMDM were treated with 25-OH (5 µg/ml) in combination with IFNγ (500 U) for 24 h. Other oxysterols assayed did not increase the TNFα secretion in combination with IFNγ. The DNA-binding of the transcription factor complex Activating Protein-1 (AP-1) was increased when treating cells with 25-OH. However, no NFκB was induced to bind to the TNFα promoter. The AP-1 complex is activated by JNK/SAPK. We found that 25-OH caused an increase in SAPK/JNK activity, in contrast to 7-ketocholesterol (7-keto), which did not activate SAPK/JNK. 25-OH, but not 7-keto, increased the intracellular levels of H_2O_2. Transfection studies showed that the primary action of IFNγ is on the 3′ UTR of the TNFα gene.

Conclusion: 25-OH might influence the expression of TNFα through activation of the SAPK/JNK pathway.

Gene expression in atherosclerotic lesions analyzed by DNA array

Mikko O. Hiltunen[1], Tiina Tuomisto[1], Mari Niemi[1], Jan Bräsen[1], Tuomas T. Rissanen[1], Seppo Ylä-Herttuala[1,2,3]. *[1] A.I. Virtanen Institute; [2] Department of Medicine; and [3] Gene Therapy Unit, University of Kuopio, Kuopio, Finland*

Objective: DNA arrays are revolutionizing the analysis of gene expression. Currently, the expression of 10−15% of human genes can be analyzed simultaneously in a single experiment. With the aid of DNA array it is possible to identify multiple, simultaneous, transcriptional events that ameliorate or contribute to atherogenesis.

Methods and Results: We analyzed the gene expression patterns of vessel wall during atherogenesis using DNA array techniques. GenomeSystem's DNA filter arrays of 18,000 cDNA clones were used. Arterial samples were collected from vascular surgery operations (n = 3) or immediately after death (n = 2). Normalization of the data was carried out using the expression intensity of all genes. A large number of activation and inactivation in gene expression patterns was identified in atherosclerotic lesions which were previously unknown or not connected to the pathogenesis of atherosclerosis. Changes in gene expression of selected identified genes were confirmed using in situ hybridization.

Conclusions: Many of the novel genes, which were activated in atherosclerotic lesions, have a role in monocyte differentiation.

Reverse cholesterol transport

Synthesis of HDL by apolipoprotein-cell interaction: its molecular mechanism and physiological importance

S. Yokoyama. *Biochemistry 1, Nagoya City University Medical School, Nagoya, Japan*

Helical apolipoproteins interact with various types of cells to generate new HDL particles with cellular lipids. This is an important reaction as one of the two major pathways for the release of cellular cholesterol to maintain cholesterol homeostasis both in a cell and for a whole body and also as a major source of plasma HDL.

Two major molecular machanisms are involved in this reaction. 1) An apolipoprotein-interaction site of the cell surface. This site involves a protein component(s) and is inducible by cAMP and other compounds in certain types of cells. Probucol inhibits its function and ABC1 is not absolutely required to compose this site. 2) Intracellular cholesterol mobilization specific for its incorporation into the HDL. This is triggered by the apolipoprotein-cell interaction, perhaps mediated by a signal transduction system. Newly synthesized cholesterol is preferably mobilized, and caveolin-1 is responsible for its trafficking. Cholesterol-poor HDL is generated when this part is lacking or insufficient in the cells. A sphingomyelin-rich domain of plasma membrane seems a site for cholesterol incorporation into the HDL.

This reaction seems a major source of plasma HDL. Impairment of the apolipoprotein-cell interaction causes the decrease of plasma HDL. This is suggested not only by Tangier disease, but also the effect of probucol in reduction of HDL. In vitro, it completely inhibits apolipoprotein-cell interaction. In mice, it rapidly reduce the HDL level without changing the major HDL-regulatory parameters such as the messages of apoA-I, E, LCAT, SRB1 and PLTP or CETP activity and plasma HDL-CE clearance rate, except for the reduction of cellular interaction with apolipoprotein and the increase of HDL apoprotein clearance rate, both being consistent with the findings with Tangier disease.

Lipid transfer proteins and receptors in HDL in metabolism

Alan R. Tall, David Silver, Xian-cheng Jiang, Phillipe Costet, Yi Luo. *Division of Molecular Medicine, Department of Medicine, New York City, New York, USA*

The reverse cholesterol transport pathway is initiated in the arterial wall, by the interaction of HDL or apoA-I with cholesterol-loaded macrophages. The latter is facilitated by ABC1. Cholesterol may be directly transported in HDL to the liver and removed from the circulation by interaction with scavenger receptor BI (SRBI), or transferred to other lipoproteins by cholesteryl ester transfer protein (CETP). Recent studies on the mechanism of sterol-mediated up-regulation of CETP gene transcription indicate that this involves the hydroxysterol-activated transcription factors, the LXRs. LXRs may coordinately induce several different molecules involved in reverse cholesterol transport, including ABC1, CETP and cyp7a. In the circulation HDL is also modified by transfer of phospholipids derived from triglyceride-rich lipoproteins. This process is mediated by the phospholipid transfer protein (PLTP); knock-out of PLTP results in reduced HDL levels, but also has unexpected effects on the metabolism of apoB-lipoproteins and atherosclerosis. The final step of RCT involves the excretion of HDL cholesterol into bile. Although SRBI has been thought to primarily mediate selective uptake of HDL CE at the cell surface, recent studies indicate that SRBI also functions as an endocytic receptor. In hepatocytes, SRBI mediates internalization and recycling or transcytosis of HDL particles across the liver cell to the bile canaliculus. Thus, SRBI mediates selective transcytosis of HDL cholesterol across the hepatocyte.

Mechanisms of cholesterol movement between high density lipoproteins (HDL) and cells

Michael C. Phillips. *Children's Hospital of Philadelphia, Philadelphia, USA*

HDL plays a central role in reverse cholesterol transport because it is capable of mediating both the delivery to and removal from cells of cholesterol. Scavenger receptor class B, type I (SR-BI) plays a central role in the mechanisms of these processes. The presence of SR-BI in the plasma membrane (PM) is essential for the phenomenon of cholesteryl ester (CE) selective uptake. The binding of CE-containing HDL particles to SR-BI allows diffusion of CE molecules down a concentration gradient along a non-aqueous channel, created by the extracellular domains of SR-BI, between the bound HDL and the PM. The apolipoprotein (apo) A-I in HDL is a ligand for the SR-BI and the structural motif recognized by receptor is the amphipathic α-helix. Binding of HDL to SR-BI can also facilitate the bidirectional flux of unesterified cholesterol (C) molecules between HDL and the cell PM. The direction of net flux is determined by the C concentration gradient. Independent of HDL binding, SR-BI also enhances efflux of C from cells by causing a reorganization of the PM so that C can desorb more readily into the extracellular aqueous phase and be absorbed by HDL particles.

The dual role of HDL in macrophage lipid processing and immune regulation

G. Schmitz. *Institute for Clinical Chemistry, University of Regensburg, Germany*

Activation of CD14 has been shown to be modulated by a complex interaction of endotoxin and plasma components including HDL, LBP and CETP while ceramide (Cer) which structurally resembles LPS has been postulated as a naturally occurring ligand. As CD14 is a GPI-anchored protein, signal transduction is assumed to occur within cholesterol and sphingolipid rich microdomains (rafts) via clustering with proteins such as the β2-integrin CD11b/CD18. Using fluorescence resonance energy transfer (FRET) we were able to demonstrate no significant co-association between CD14 and CD11b in resting monocytes. Both LPS and Cer, in contrast, induced a significant co-association between CD14 and CD11b suggesting an activation-dependent conformational change of the receptor complex due ligand binding. Integrin Associated Proteins (IAP, CD47 and CD81) and the FcγRIII (CD16) were identified as further components of the multimeric functional receptor complex. LPS and Cer have been shown to be associated to HDL lipoproteins in a process mediated via lipid transfer proteins including LBP and PLTP. Recently, an apo-AI/LBP containing particle has been demonstrated, facilitating cellular responses to LPS. Based on our data we propose CD14 to be a raft receptor for LPS/Cer enriched apo-AI/LBP-containing HDL-particles in the acute phase response. The increase in LBP and PLTP activities in inflammation may further enhance the transfer of LPS to HDL. Together with the recent report of an increased expression of CD14 on monocytes in myocardial infarction, this suggests the targeting of proinflammatory HDL particles to rafts and an signaling through an innate immunity receptor complex as important cellular activation processes in the acute phase response.

Age-related decline of the expression of a Rho GTPases family, CDC42Hs, in human skin fibroblasts in association with reduction of HDL-mediated cholesterol efflux

K. Tsukamoto, K. Hirano, F. Matsuura, N. Sakai, A. Matsuyama, S. Yamashita, Y. Matsuzawa. *Osaka University, Osaka, Japan*

Objective: Reverse cholesterol transport (RCT) is one of the major protective system against atherosclerosis. The initial step of RCT is named "cholesterol efflux", where HDL particles take up cholesterol from the lipid-laden cells. Recently, we have found that the expression of a member of RhoGTPases, Cdc42Hs, is decreased in association with the abnormal actin cytoskeleton, slow cell proliferation, and cholesterol efflux, in cells from patients with Tangier disease, a model for the impairment of RCT (Hirano K et al.). Although it is obvious that senescence is the unescapable risk factor for atherosclerosis, the effect of aging on the RCT has not been fully clarified yet. The aim of the present study is to know whether or not aging affects the initial step of RCT, cholesterol efflux.

Methods: We have analyzed HDL-mediated cholesterol efflux as well as the expression levels of RhoGTPases in passaged human skin fibroblasts obtained from seven subjects whose age are ranging from 24 to 86 years old.

Results: The expression levels of Cdc42Hs were decreased in proportion to aging, which was associated with altered actin cytoskeletons and slow cell proliferation. HDL-mediated cholesterol was reduced in proportion to aging. There was a close correlation between the expression levels of Cdc42Hs and cholesterol efflux.

Conclusion: The present study demonstrates that aging may decrease HDL-mediated cholesterol efflux in conjunction with the decreased expression of the small G protein, suggesting that aging affects the reverse cholesterol transport system. The present data support our recent finding that the small G protein may play an important role as one of the physiological key components for cholesterol efflux.

cAMP regulates apolipoprotein-mediated cholesterol efflux by induction of expression of the tangier protein ABC1

D. Wade[1], M. Garvin[1], K. Schwartz[1], X. Wang[1], A. Vaughan[2], J. Oram[2], R. Lawn[1].
[1]CV Therapeutics Inc, Palo Alto; [2]University of Washington, Seattle, USA

The ATP-binding cassette transporter ABC1 was identified as the defective gene in Tangier Disease and a key component of the regulation of cellular cholesterol efflux. This was accomplished by a comparison of gene expression in Tangier and normal fibroblasts by hybridisation to microarray chips, and biochemical studies that demonstrated that over-expression of the gene increased, and ABC1 antisense oligonucleotide treatment decreased specific cellular efflux of cholesterol to apolipoprotein A-I. In previous studies apoA-I mediated cholesterol efflux from RAW 264.7 macrophages was shown to be absolutely dependent on treatment of the cells with permeable cAMP analogs. Here we show by quantitative RT-PCR of ABC1 mRNA that transcription of the gene in RAW cells is rapidly induced from very low levels by cAMP treatment, in parallel with the cells' capacity to efflux cholesterol to apoA-I. Immunoprecipitation of ABC1 protein from pulse-chase labelled cells also showed that cAMP confers a marked increase in protein half-life compared to untreated cells. The acquisition of the cells ability to efflux cholesterol is therefore dependent on the induction of ABC1 expression, and stabilisation of the protein. Assays of reporter gene activity in RAW cells transfected with wild-type and mutated ABC1-promoter-luciferase fusion constructs have enabled us to identify important regulatory elements in the promoter including those responsible for the transcriptional response to cAMP.

Oxidation of specific Met residues does not decrease anti-atherogenic activities of apolipoprotein A-I

U. Panzenböck[1], M. Raftery[2], L. Kritharides[1], K.-A. Rye[3], R. Perry[4], G. Francis[4], R. Stocker[1]. *[1]Heart Research Institute; [2]University of NSW, Sydney; [3]Royal Adelaide Hospital, Adelaide, Australia; and [4]Lipid and Lipoprotein Research Group, University of Alberta, Edmonton, Canada*

In human lesions, lipids in high- (HDL) and low-density lipoproteins (LDL) are oxidized to comparable extents (ATVB 1999;19:1708). HDL may become oxidized directly or accept preformed lipid hydroperoxides (LOOH) from oxidized LDL via cholesteryl ester transfer protein (JLR 1995;36:2017). Once present in HDL, LOOH are detoxified to the corresponding alcohols (FRBM 1995;18:421), a process associated with the oxidation of two Met residues of apolipoprotein A-I (apoA-I) to Met sulfoxides (Met(O); JBC 1998;273:6080; ibid 273:6088). Formation of such specifically oxidized apoA-I (apoA-I +32) may affect reverse cholesterol transport as Met residues are implicated in cholesterol efflux and activation of lecithin: cholesterol acyltransferase (LCAT). Mass spectrometry of intact and proteolytic fragments revealed that Met[86] and Met[112] are present as Met(O) in apoA-I$_{+32}$. Circular dichroismshowed that the alpha-helical content of lipid-free and lipid-associated apoA-I and apoA-I$_{+32}$ were comparable, as was the affinity for LCAT for reconstituted HDL containing apoA-I$_{+32}$ or apoA-I. By contrast, lipid-free apoA-I$_{+32}$ displayed a greater affinity for liposomal phospholipid, and cholesterol, phospholipids, and vitamin E present in human macrophages loaded with acetylated LDL. HPLC-analysis indicated the presence of apoA-I$_{+32}$ in HDL isolated from human atherosclerotic lesions. Such lesion HDL remained capable of promoting cellular cholesterol efflux, independent of the severity of atherosclerosis. Together, the results suggest that mild oxidation does not diminish known anti-atherogenic activities of apoA-I, consistent with our hypothesis that detoxification of pro-atherogenic LOOH by HDL may be anti-atherogenic.

Immune and inflammatory mechanisms in atherosclerosis

Biological significance of autoantibodies to oxidative neoepitopes

W. Palinski, S. Hörkkö, P. Shaw, S. Tsimikas, G. Silverman, J.L. Witztum. *Dept. of Medicine, University of California San Diego, La Jolla, USA*

Adducts of reactive aldehydes or oxidized phospholipids formed during lipid peroxidation with (apolipo) proteins or other phospholipids trigger extensive humoral and cellular immune responses in vivo. Titers of autoantibodies against "oxidation-specific epitopes" generally correlate with the extent and rate of progression of atherosclerosis in humans and murine models. However, antigen formation is not limited to atherosclerotic lesions, but also occurs in other chronic inflammatory diseases or aging cells. Immunization of rabbits and mice with oxidized LDL reduces the progression of atherosclerosis, suggesting that modulation of specific humoral or cellular immune responses may be beneficial. Naturally occurring antibodies cloned from nonimmunized atherosclerotic apoE$^{-/-}$ mice ("EO"-antibodies) provide insights into the nature of antigens formed in vivo and on biological effects of selected antibody populations. For example, EO antibodies binding to oxidized phospholipid adducts inhibit macrophage uptake of oxidized LDL by blocking scavenger receptors. Similar antibodies in human subjects with "antiphospholipid-antibody syndrome" may also affect thrombosis. Cloning of the V_H and V_L genes of four EO antibodies to oxidized phospholipids that had been independently selected for binding to copper-oxidized LDL showed that these antibodies were identical to classical T-15 antibodies, evolutionarily selected, B1-lymphocyte dependent antibodies that protect against pneumococcal infection. Antibodies against oxidation-specific epitopes can also be used to quantify atheroscleorsis. Murine studies indicated that the in vivo uptake of ^{125}I-labeled antibodies correlated with several conventional measures of atherosclerosis but was more sensitive to regression of lesions rich in oxidation-specific epitopes. An oxidation-specific human Fab antibody cloned from a phage display library, IK17, may be particularly useful for diagnostic purpos, because it mainly recognizes epitopes in lipid-rich core regions of human and animal atheromas.

Autoimmunity to heat shock protein 60/65 as an initiating mechanism in the atherosclerosis development

G. Wick. *Institute for Biomedical Aging Research of the Austrian Academy of Sciences, Innsbruck, Austria*

In the last decade, we have developed a new "autoimmune" concept for the pathogenesis of atherosclerosis that is supported by solid experimental and clinical data. In essence, we have shown that heat shock protein 60 (HSP60) expressed by stressed arterial endothelial cells at known predilection sites for the development of atherosclerotic lesions (i.e., branching points of arteries) form the target for cellular and humoral immunity against highly conserved HSP60 epitopes in various forms of microbes (viruses, bacteria, parasites). We are thus "paying" for protective immunity in younger age by the development of atherosclerosis in older age in case vascular endothelial cells are subjected to classical risk factors for atherosclerosis, notably hypertension, oxidized low-density lipo-proteins (oxLDL), toxins, etc. We now show that the life-long exposure of arterial endothelial cells to the high arterial blood pressure makes these cells more vulnerable to the effect of other stressors that lead to a simultaneous expression of HSP60 and certain adhesion molecules (ICAM-1, VCAM-1, ELAM-1). In this context, the question will be addressed which are the cellular sensors for mechanical stress that may be responsive for inflammatory arterial changes and even advanced severe vascular lesions in older age. Furthermore, results of a prospective clinical study will be presented to show that immunity to HSP60 is not only a parameter for morbidity but also for mortality.

Supported by the Austrian Science Fund, Grant No 12213-MED

Pro- and anti-inflammatory balance and atherosclerosis

A. Tedgui, Z. Mallat. *INSERM U541, Hopital Lariboisière, Paris, France*

Atherosclerosis has been recognized as an inflammatory disease. Proinflammatory cytokines, including TNFα, IL-1, IL-8, IL-12, oncostatin M and IFNγ are all present within the human atherosclerotic plaque, and participate in the activation of macrophages, lymphocytes and vascular cells. However, the inflammatory response is known to be balanced by anti-inflammatory cytokines, including IL-4, IL-10 and IL-13. Among the anti-inflammatory cytokines produced by Th2 cells, IL-10 is also produced by macrophages and has potent deactivating properties. Whereas IL-4 and IL-13 can be barely found in human atherosclerotic plaques, IL-10 mRNA and protein are highly expressed, mainly by macrophages. IL-10 expression is associated with a marked decrease in NOS II expression and low levels of apoptosis, suggesting that locally produced IL-10 has an anti-inflammatory role and protects from excessive cell damage and death in the plaque. Indeed, endothelial NF-κB activation and expression of VCAM-1 and ICAM-1 that are markedly increased in C57BL/6J mice after a short period of time (10 days) on an atherogenic diet, can be totally prevented by in vivo transfer of murine IL-10 cDNA. On the other hand, IL-10-deficient C57BL/6J mice fed an atherogenic diet and raised under specific-pathogen-free conditions exhibit a significant 3-fold increase in atherosclerotic lesions compared with wild type mice. Interestingly, the susceptibility of IL-10-deficient mice to atherosclerosis is exceedingly high (30-fold increase) when the mice are housed under conventional conditions. Moreover, atherosclerotic lesions of IL-10-deficient mice show increased T-cell infiltration, abundant IFNγ expression, and decreased collagen content. Therefore, IL-10 appears to have critical roles in both atherosclerotic lesion formation and stability, and might be crucial as a protective factor against the effect of environmental pathogens on atherosclerosis.

Human vascular smooth muscle cells express an endogenous inhibitor of Caspase-1

U. Schönbeck, J.L. Young, G.K. Sukhova, P. Libby. *Brigham and Women's Hospital, Harvard Medical School, Boston, MA, USA*

Objective: Caspase-1 regulates key steps in inflammation and immunity, by either activating the pro-inflammatory cytokines IL-1beta and IL-18 or mediating apoptosis, processes associated with the chronic inflammatory disease, atherosclerosis. We recently provided evidence for the regulation of Caspase-1 activity via an endogenous inhibitor expressed by human vascular smooth muscle cells (SMC). However, the molecular identity of this endogenous inhibitor remained undefined, rendering Caspase-1 inhibitors restricted to either synthetic peptides or viral proteins.

Methods and Results: We report here, that the serine proteinase inhibitor (Serpin) PI-9 accounts for the endogenous Caspase-1 inhibitory activity in human SMC and prevents processing of the natural substrates, IL-1beta and IL-18 precursor, as determined by Western blot analysis. Treatment of SMC lysates with anti-PI-9 antibody abrogated the Caspase-1 inhibitory activity and co-precipitated the enzyme, demonstrating protein-protein interaction. Furthermore, PI-9 antisense oligonucleotides coordinately reduced PI-9 expression and promoted IL-1beta release. Since SMC comprise the majority of cells in the vascular wall, and Caspase-1 and IL-1 are firmly implicated in atherogenesis, we tested the biological validity of our findings within human atheroma in situ. The unaffected arterial wall contains abundant, homogeneously distributed, PI-9. In human atherosclerotic lesions, however, PI-9 expression correlated inversely with immunoreactive IL-1beta, supporting a potential role of the endogenous Caspase-1 inhibitor in this chronic inflammatory disease.

Conclusions: Our results provide new insights into the regulation of Caspase-1, an enzyme involved in immune and inflammatory processes of chronic inflammatory diseases, and point to an endogenous anti-inflammatory action of PI-9, dysregulated in the human prevalent disease, atherosclerosis.

Contrasting effects of AT1 and AT2 antagonism on angiotensin II induced atherosclerosis and abdominal aortic aneurysms

Alan Daugherty, Lisa Cassis. *University of Kentucky, Lexington, KY, USA*

Objective: Previously, we have demonstrated that infusion of angiotensin II (AngII) into apolipoprotein E−/− mice leads to the rapid formation of atherosclerotic lesions and development of abdominal aortic aneurysms (AAA). The aim of the present study was to define the effects of specific AngII receptor antagonism on the development of vascular pathology.

Methods: Mature apoE−/− mice were infused via osmotic pumps for 28 days with either an AT1 (losartan, 30 mg/kg/day) or AT2 (PD 123319, 3 mg/kg/day) antagonist, either alone, or with combined administration of AngII (1 μg/kg/min).

Results: AngII infusion increased the extent of atherosclerosis and generated AAA in 70% on mice. Losartan totally ablated the AngII induced atherosclerosis and AAA. PD123319 failed to influence the AngII induced development of atherosclerosis. However, it increased the incidence of aneurysms to 100%. Furthermore, the aneurysms formed were larger and had a more complex appearance. Administration of losartan or PD123319, in the absence of AngII infusion, had no effect on the development of atherosclerotic lesions or AAA.

Conclusion: AT1 receptor antagonism profoundly decreased AngII induced vascular pathology, while blockade of AT2 receptors unexpectedly promoted effects on AAA.

Anti-atherosclerotic effect of SB-244323, a lipoprotein associated phospholipase A2 inhibitor, in WHHL rabbits

G.M. Benson[1], D. Grimsditch[1], K. Milliner[1], K. Moores[1], H. Boyd[2], D. Tew[2], D. Hickey[3], R. Ife[3], K. Suckling[1], C. Macphee[1]. *Departments of [1] Vascular Biology; [2] Molecular Recognition; [3] Medicinal Chemistry, SmithKline Beecham Pharmaceuticals, NFSP(N), Harlow, Essex, UK*

Lipoprotein-associated phospholipase A_2 (Lp-PLA$_2$), PAF-acetylhydrolase, is expressed by macrophages in atherosclerotic lesions and is responsible for generating significant quantities of the pro-inflammatory mediator lyso-PC during the oxidation of LDL. We therefore investigated the potential anti-atherogenic properties of the potent Lp-PLA$_2$ inhibitor SB-244323 (ethyl ester pro-drug of SB-245713, IC$_{50}$ = 8 nM) in WHHL rabbits. A dose of compound was selected that reduced aortic Lp-PLA$_2$ activity to that observed in aortas of normal NZW rabbits. Male WHHL rabbits (n = 21/grp) were treated with 20 umol/kg/d of SB-244323 in the diet or diet alone for 12 weeks. The rabbits were then killed, their aortas were removed and the atherosclerotic lesions were measured and characterised. SB-244323 reduced Lp-PLA$_2$ activity in rabbit plasma and aortas by 99% and 54%, respectively, and there were no adverse reactions to treatment. Whereas plasma lipids were unaffected by treatment, concentrations of plasma PAI-1 were significantly reduced by 41% by SB-244323 after 6 weeks of treatment. The total cross-sectional area, thickness and macrophage content of aortic atherosclerotic lesions were measured in histological sections. Treatment reduced all parameters measured with larger lesions; SB 244323 reduced median lesion cross-sectional area and thickness significantly by 38% and 24% respectively in sections taken from just below the coeliac artery.

Conclusion: These results support the view that Lp-PLA$_2$ plays a significant role in the development of atherosclerotic plaque.

Adoptive transfer of b2-glycoprotein I (b2GPI)-reactive lymphocyte enhances atherosclerosis in LDL receptor deficient mice

D. Harats, J. George, B. Gilburd, A. Afek, A. Shaish, Y. Shoenfeld. *Institute of Lipid and Atherosclerosis Research, Sheba Medical Center, Tel Hashomer, Sackler Faculty of Medicine, Tel Aviv University, Israel*

Background: It has been proposed that autoimmune factors can influence the progression of atherosclerosis. We have previously shown that immunization of LDL-receptor-deficient (LDL-RD mice) with b2 glycopotein I (b2GPI; a principal target of "autoimmune" anti-phospholipid antibodies) enhances early atherosclerosis. In the current study we tested the hypothesis that adoptive transfer of b2GPI reactive T-cells can accelerate atherogenesis in LDL-RD mice.

Methods and Results: LDL-RD mice were immunized with human b2GPI. An additional group of mice were immunized with b2GPI and boosted with the same antigen 3 weeks later. Control mice with immunized with human serum albumin (HSA). Lymphocytes obtained from the draining lymph-node cells or from splenocytes of b2GPI or HSA immunized mice were stimulated in-vitro with b2GPI or with the mitogen Concavaline A, respectively. The cultured lymphocytes were transferred intraperiteneally to syngenic LDL-RD mice and fed for 5 weeks a high-fat "Western" diet until sacrifice. Mice injected with lymphocytes from draining lymph nodes or spleens of b2GPI-immunized animals displayed larger atherosclerotic lesions as compared to those induced by control treated animals. T-cell depleted splenocytes from b2GPI were unable to promote lesion formation in the mice. Lymphocytes that mediated lesion enhancement displayed a predominant T helper 1 phenotype evident by increased secretion of g interferon in-vitro priming with b2GPI.

Conclusion: This is the first direct evidence for a role of antigen (b2GPI)-reactive T cells in promoting atherosclerotic lesions in mice.

Hormones and cardiovascular disease

A clinical overview with focus on growth hormone

K.J. Osterziel. *Franz-Volhard-Klinik/Charité, Humboldt University of Berlin, Germany*

Ischemic and dilated cardiomyopathies are characterized by ventricular dilatation, thin ventricular walls and impaired systolic function. Recently, it could be shown that the activity of the somatotrophic system is decreased in heart failure. Cardiac cachexia is characterized by low IGF-I. The decrease of insulin-like growth factor I (IGF-I), one of the mediators of growth hormone (GH) effects, correlates to left ventricular ejection fraction and inversely to left ventricular size. Subtle, yet unknown alterations of the somatotrophic system may lead to the decrease of serum IGF-I levels. Several pilot studies have shown hemodynamic and clinical improvement after treatment with human recombinant growth hormone (GH) for 3 months. Larger randomized, double-blind and placebo-controlled trials could not confirm the expected clinical improvement. A subgroup of patients showed hemodynamic improvement, most likely due to an increased NO-formation. The significant increase of myocardial mass by GH was related to the increase of IGF-I. When IGF-I increased by more than 80 pg/ml a significant increse of ejection fraction could be shown.

Summary: The somatotrophic axis is altered in patients with heart failure. Short-term treatment with GH leads in a subgroup of patients to an improvement of left ventricular function.

Cellular and molecular mechanisms of the atheroprotective effects of estrogens

F. Bayard. *INSERM U397, Institut L. Bugnard, CHU Rangueil, 31403 Toulouse Cedex, France*

Objective: The mechanism(s) whereby the atheroprotective effect of estrogens is mediated has been thought to be due to potentially favorable changes in blood lipids and lipoproteins but a number of animal studies strongly suggest a direct effect on the vascular wall.

Methods: Estradiol-1β (E_2) prevents fatty streak formation in apolipoprotein E-deficient (apoEKO) mice. We used this animal model under variable experimental conditions of diet, pharmacological and genetic manipulations, to characterize the mechanisms which mediate E2 effects in this process.

Results: Studies of the lesion-serum cholesterol relationships confirm that the main action of E_2 is on cells of the vascular wall. Endothelial cell turn over and production of EDRF are under estrogen control but do not constitute a main target. Using apoEKO mice also deficient in other cell populations of the inflammatory/immune system, we show that T lymphocytes are involved, possibly by conditioning the behavior of monocytes/macrophages. However, contrary to our expectation, E_2 increases the macrophage production of pro-inflammatory cytokines such as IL-12 and INF-γ and decreases the production of IL-10. The relationships between development of this pro-inflammatory profile and the atheroprotective effect, together with the respective roles of estrogen receptor α (ERα) and ERβ as mediators of these effects, are under current investigation.

Conclusion: The apoEKO mice model enabled us to determine the target cell populations which mediate the atheroprotective effect of E_2.

The role of the estrogen receptor-β for the vascular effects of estrogen

J.-Å. Gustafsson. *Dept. of Med. Nutrition, Karolinska Institute NOVUM, Huddinge Univ. Hospital, Huddinge, Sweden*

The recent discovery of a second estrogen receptor, ERβ, has radically changed our view on how estrogens act. It appears that ERβ in many contexts counteracts ERα so that the two receptors can be said to have a yin/yang relationship. Interestingly, this ERα controlling activity of ERβ seems to be exerted not only by wtERβ but also by at least one variant form of ERβ, namely ERβcx. This ERβ isoform has a different last exon than wtERβ making it incapable of binding steroid but still able to heterodimerize with ERα thereby somehow inactivating this receptor. These fundamental properties of ERβ and its isoform ERβcx are of vital physiological importance as judged from some phenotypical characteristics of ERβ (–/–) mice, namely hyperproliferative tendencies in prostate as well as uterus. Indeed, ERβ seems to exert antiproliferative actions in these tissues. In other contexts ERβ may mediate other estrogenic effects than ERα, such as in the immune system and bone, where we also use ERβ –/–) as well as ERα –/–) mice to dissect ERβ and ERα controlled signal transduction pathways. Also, it turns out that the issue of estrogen receptors in breast needs to be thoroughly revisited in view of these new concepts. Finally, ERα/ERβ mediated signal transduction may be involved in some of the estrogenic effects on vessels.

Estrogen receptor-b expression in male coronary arteries

E. O'Brien[1], B. Han[1], C. Hoffert[1], R. Jankowski[1], H. Miller[1], M. Labinaz[1], P. Saunders[2]. [1]*Ottawa Heart Institute, Canada; and* [2]*Centre for Reproductive Biology, Edinburgh, UK*

Objective: The purpose of this study was to examine the expression of the novel estrogen receptor beta (ERb) in normal and diseased human and porcine coronary arteries of both sexes.

Methods: ERb mRNA and protein expression was assessed using reverse transcription PCR and immunocytochemistry, respectively. Pairs of normal (internal mammary artery) and diseased (coronary endarterectomy specimens) human vascular tissues from patients undergoing coronary artery bypass surgery (five males, one female), as well as porcine coronary arteries (n = 24 pigs) subjected to balloon injury were studied.

Results: There was no difference in the abundance of ERb mRNA expression amongst the pairs of normal and diseased human arteries. ERb protein was immunodetected in endothelial cells, smooth muscle cells and adventitial cells of normal human and porcine coronary arteries. For 14 days post-balloon injury, there was transient over-expression of ERb in porcine coronary arteries, despite very low levels of circulating estradiol (<100 pmol/l). Human coronary arteries with complex atherosclerotic lesions, also expressed ERb protein, however, at low abundance. Overall, there was no apparent gender difference in ERb expression. To extend these findings we tested the ability of smooth muscle cells from male and female pigs to respond to estradiol in vitro. Both populations of cells responded to estradiol administration by showing decreased levels of proliferation, as assessed by tritiated thymidine incorporation.

Conclusion: ERb mRNA and protein are expressed in normal and disease arteries. The abundance of ERb expression does not appear to be sex-related, and smooth muscle cells of both males and females are responsive to estradiol. Taken together, these data suggest that strategies to develop estrogen therapies should be considered for, not only female but also male populations that are at risk for coronary artery disease.

Free plasma testosterone and estradiol and the extent of coronary artery disease in males

P. Lercher[1], A. Fahrleitner[2], K. Stoschitzky[1], H. Dobnig[2], J.C. Piswanger-Sölkner[2], O. Luha[1], G. Leb[2], W. Klein[1]. [2]*Department of Medicine/Divisions of Cardiology and Endocrinology,* [1]*Karl Franzens University Graz, Austria*

Objective: Male sex may be an important risk factor of coronary artery disease. It has been suggested that sexual hormones may influence the development and progression of coronary artery disease (CAD). The objective of the present study was to investigate the relationship of free plasma testosterone, estradiol and coronary atherosclerosis.

Methods: 237 consecutive male patients who underwent elective coronary angiography were included. Exclusion criteria were previous angioplasty, coronary artery bypass grafting or diabetes mellitus in the history. Blood samples were taken in a fasting state prior to the procedure. The extent of coronary atherosclerosis was determined by the number of affected vessels (vessel score) (stenosis > 50% in a vessel area) and the number of stenoses > 50% (stenosis score) (0 = 0; 1 = 1—2; 2 = 3—4; 3 > 4).

Results: 49 (21%) patients had one vessel disease, 37 (16%) two vessel disease, 50 (21%) three vessel disease and 101 (42%) showed normal coronary angiograms. Free plasma testosterone significantly differed between the groups with lowest values in patients with severe CAD (vessel score $p < 0.03$; stenosis score $p < 0.04$; ANOVA). No significant differences were observed regarding estradiol ($p = 0.69$; $p = 0.73$).

	0	1	2	3	
Vessel score	15.1	16.0	14.3	12.5	$p < 0.03$
Stenosis score	15.3	15.4	14.2	12.3	$p < 0.04$

mean values of free testosterone (pg/ml) depending on the different atherosclerosis scores

Conclusions: Our results indicate that the extent of angiographically documented atheriosclerotic lesions defined by two different scores is significantly associated with free plasma testosterone levels. Estradiol, however, had no influence on the atherosclerotic process in this cohort. In conclusion, low plasma testosterone levels might be an additional risk factor in the development and extent of CAD.

Sexual steroids upregulate thrombin receptor expression in cultured vascular smooth muscle cells: Role of the glucocorticoid receptor

O. Herkert[1], H. Kuhl[2], R. Busse[1], V.B. Schini-Kerth[1]. [1]*Institut für Kardiovaskuläre Physiologie;* [2]*Abteil. für Gynäkologische Endokrinologie, Klinikum der JWG-Universität, Frankfurt/Main, Germany*

Objectives: Both the estrogen and the progestogen component of oral contraceptives are thought to be involved in the development of thromboembolic diseases in women. This study examines whether sexual steroids affect the expression of thrombin receptors which mediate numerous proinflammatory responses in vascular smooth muscle cells (SMC).

Methods: Experiments were performed with confluent cultures of serum-deprived rat aortic SMCs. Thrombin receptor expression in SMC was assessed by Northern blot analysis and thrombin receptor function by the thrombin-induced release of 6-keto-prostaglandin F1alpha.

Results: 3-keto-desogestrel time-dependently increased the steady state level of thrombin receptor mRNA after a delay of 4 h and thrombin receptor mRNA levels remained elevated for at least 48 h. Increased thrombin receptor mRNA levels were also obtained with medroxyprogesterone acetate (MPA), gestodene and progesterone and with the glucocorticoid dexamethasone, whereas levonorgestrel, norethisterone, norgestimate and 17 alpha-ethinylestradiol had no effect. Increased thrombin receptor mRNA levels were associated with a significant greater thrombin-induced release of 6-keto-prostaglandin F1alpha. The stimulatory effect of MPA and dexamethasone was reduced by the glucocorticoid and progesterone receptor antagonist RU 38486.

Conclusions: These findings indicate that several progestogens increase the expression of thrombin receptors in cultured vascular SMCs through activation of the glucocorticoid and/or progesterone receptor whereas estrogens were inactive. The upregulation of thrombin receptors in the vascular wall may represent a mechanism which contributes to the increased risk of vascular diseases in users of oral contraceptives.

Hypertensive pregnancy and LDL-subfractions: Remnant disease like dyslipoproteinemia in preeclampsia

K. Winkler[1], B. Wetzka[2], M.M. Hoffmann[1], I. Friedrich[1], M. Kinner[2], M.W. Baumstark[3], H. Wieland[1], H.P. Zahradnik[2], W. März[1]. *Departments of [1]Clinical Chemistry; [2]Obstetrics and Gynecology; [3]Sports Medicine, University of Freiburg, Germany*

Introduction: Disturbances of lipoprotein metabolism are an important risk factor for the development of atherosclerosis and may cause endothelial cell dysfunction. Endothelial damage is also an essential part in the pathophysiology of preeclampsia (PE).

Methods: In a longitudinal study, fasting serum was obtained from 23 women during normal pregnancies in the 1st, 2nd and 3rd trimester. From 10 women with severe PE, serum was collected immediately before delivery. Lipid and apolipoprotein (apo) B-100 concentrations were measured in plasma, in the very low density (VLDL), intermediate density (IDL) and low density (LDL) fractions as well as in each of 6 LDL subfractions separated by equilibrium density ultracentrifugation.

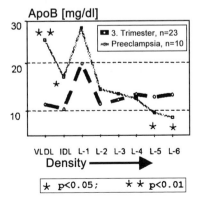

238

Results: During normal pregnancy, LDL-1 ("buoyant LDL") dominates the LDL-profile in the 3rd trimester (see Figure). The serum from patients with PE showed a significantly different lipoprotein profile compared to normal pregnancy of the same gestational age (34 weeks) with a higher proportion of VLDL, IDL, and LDL-1. The most striking finding, however, was the significant decrease of dense LDL particles, most probably due to the decreasing lipolytic activity during late gestation.

Conclusion: The lipoprotein pattern in preeclampsia is similar to that well-known for remnant disease like dyslipoproteinemia, in which triglyceride-rich lipoproteins accumulate and denser apoB containing particles, namely LDL are depleted. This study is the first to describe the remnant-disease like nature of the lipoprotein metabolism of pre-eclampsia and may thus provide new insights in the pathophysiology of this life-threatening condition.

Psychosocial mechanisms in CVD

Social stress, sympathetic nervous system regulation and atherosclerosis

N. Schneiderman. *University of Miami, Coral Gables, Florida, USA*

Negative affect, including hostility, distress and depression are associated with tonic eleva-tions in catecholamines and cortisol as well as decreases in vagal tone and platelet aggre-gation. Clinical studies indicate that persons who are easily provoked to anger show increased atherosclerosis measured by diagnostic angiography. In order to document causal associations between psychosocial factors and atherosclerosis, research has been conducted upon animal models. Thus, mice raised in socially deprived environments reveal thickening of the coronary arteries when interacting with mice reared under nor-mal social conditions. Also, we have found that Watanabe rabbits either raised alone (rela-tive social isolation) or exposed to a new cage mate each week, develop pronounced ath-erosclerosis as compared to a rabbit continually reared with a sibling. Similarly, others have found that dominant male cynomolgus monkeys reared on a cholesterol-containing diet develop atherosclerosis when periodically subjected to redistribution of the living group. Regular administration of a sympathetic antagonist (beta blocker) attenuates the atherosclerosis. A clinical trial is now underway in post-myocardial infarction patients to determine whether a group based psychosocial intervention that decreases distress improves diet and increases exercise in post myocardial infarction patients, has a positive impact on stress hormones, sympathetically mediated brachial artery vasodilation and traditional coronary risk factors.

Stress and coronary disease in Swedish women

K. Orth-Gomér. *Department of Public Health Sciences, Karolinska Institutet, Stockholm, Sweden*

Coronary heart disease (CHD) is almost as common in women as in men. Our knowl-edge about risk factors in women is surprisingly scarce. This is particularly true for psychosocial factors.

The Stockholm Female Coronary Risk Factor Study (Fem Cor Risk) was designed to study both standard and psychosocial risk factors, with an emphasis on mechanisms which mediate psychosocial influences on the heart. It was designed as a population based case control study including all female cases of acute events of CHD (acute myo-cardial infarction and unstable angina pectoris) who were 65 years or under, and who were hospitalised in the greater Stockholm area during a three year period. For each case an age matched control woman was obtained from the City Census Register. Around 600 women were examined for standard and psychosocial risk factors by means of ques-tionnaires, interviews, laboratory mental stress testing, blood samples, cardiological examination, exercise stress testing, and (in a subsample) quantitative coronary angiogra-phy. All but two women were employed, and only two house wives were found. All women were followed for five years. Among clinical factors, a history of diabetes and dyslipid-emia were the strongest predictors of poor outcome. Of psychosocial factors, perceived mental stress from family life, but not stress from working life, was a strong predictor of risk. In addition, depressive symptoms, social isolation, and low socio-economic status

(SES) further increased the risk in Stockholm women. Furthermore, low SES and social isolation were strongly associated with the Metabolic Syndrome, suggesting a major pathway of psychosocial influences on CHD in women.

Social stress, behavioral mechanisms, and atherosclerosis

P. Kaufmann. *National Institutes of Health, Bethesda, Maryland, USA*

Objective: To review mechanisms through which social stress influences progression of atherosclerosis.

Methods: Research review of mechanisms through which acute psychological stress promotes atherosclerosis. Acute vasospasm begins to be evident in the early, subclinical stages of atherosclerotic disease. Chronic stress accelerates the rate of atherosclerosis in animal models, while stress reduction enhances regression of atherosclerosis and facilitates rehabilitation. A positive mental stress test is prognostic of future cardiac events. In the presence of atherosclerosis, vasodilation of epicardial vessels and the coronary microcirculation is reduced or absent in response to mental stress. Endothelial function begins to be compromised early in the atherosclerotic process, and its assessment provides a powerful non-invasive approach to identifying individuals at risk as well as their response to interventions. All major lifestyle risk factors — mental stress, diet, smoking, and exercise — influence endothelial function, in part through the action of numerous neurohumoral substances, some of which also mediate responses to stress.

Conclusions: The beneficial effects of lifestyle changes including stress management for patients with atherosclerosis may be mediated by reduced neurohumoral influences on the endothelium and improved vascular function.

Triggering of acute coronary syndrome at work in people free of coronary heart disease. Final results of a case-crossover Israeli experience

N. Lipovetzky, H. Hod, A. Rot, Y. Kishon, Sh. Sclarovsky, M.S. Green. *Department of Epidemiology and Preventive Medicine, Sackler Faculty of Medicine, Tel-Aviv University, Israel*

Objective: To study extreme episodes at work as triggers for the onset of an acute coronary syndrome (ACS).

Methods: A case-crossover study design was used where each patient serves as his/her own control. We interviewed 209 patients (194 men and 15 women) an average of two days after an acute ischaemic event that occurred at work. Emotional events were assessed by the positive and negative affect scale questionnaire (PANAS), comprising two nine-item, three-level, mood scales. Physical exertion was measured by an eight-item metabolic equivalents (MET) scale. Anger was measured by the Onset Anger Scale. Intellectual activity, overeating and lack of sleep were assessed by a standard 5 level scale. Patients were asked about the occurrence of these activities in the hours preceding the onset of ACS (hazard period) and for two types of control data: (1) the same period during the previous day, (2) the estimated usual frequency during the previous year.

Results: 24% of the study population report one trigger at least in the hour who preceded the symptoms of ACS. The odds ratio for an ACS in the first hour after the exposure to a potential trigger compared to the same period in the day before the ACS, was 3.5 (95% CI 0.7—16.8) for positive emotions, 14 (95% CI 1.8—106.5) for negative emotions, 14 (95% CI 1.6—30.8) for physical exertion, 9 (95% CI 1.1—71) for anger, 2.5 (95% CI 0.5—12.9) for intellectual activity, 7 (95% CI 0.75—65.8) for overeating and 1.85 (95% CI 0.97—3.56) for lack of sleep. By conditional logistic regression negative emotions and physical exertion were the only two significant triggers for ACS.

Conclusions: Episodes of extreme negative emotions and heavy physical exertion at work can trigger the onset of an ACS. Possible preventive strategies in the workplace should be explored.

Quality of life in genetic disease: The example of familial hypercholesterolemia

G. Hollman[1], A.-C. Ek[1], M. Eriksson[2], A.G. Olsson[1]. [1]Dept of Medicine and Care Linköping; and [2]Centre for Metabolism and Endocrinology Huddinge University Hospital Stockholm, Sweden

Objective: The influence of information of having genetic disease on quality of life is increasingly relevant. We have studied familial hypercholesterolemia (FH) with regard to quality of life, anxiety, depression, coping and perceived health in comparison with normocholesterolemic controls.

Methods: Patients with FH older than 18 years of age were included in the study. All had received lifestyle advice and medical treatment for their FH. One hundred and ninety patients (97 female) attending lipid clinics in two Swedish university hospitals participated by filling out questionnaires. Quality of life, anxiety and coping were estimated by established instruments and perceived health by a questionnaire constructed for FH patients. The study was performed in close connection with the MED-PED FH (Make Early Diagnosis- Prevent Early Death in Familial Hypercholesterolemia) program. A randomly selected control group of 278 individuals 18—80 years of age were drawn from the Swedish population register for comparison. They were asked by mail to complete the same questionnaires regarding to quality of life, anxiety, depression and coping as the patients.

Results: FH patients stated that their mothers and fathers had had heart attack in 12% and 35% and had died in heart attack 11% and 33% respectively. Among the FH patients, mean age 51 years, mean of quality of life was slightly but significantly higher than controls (21.8 ± 3.8 [SD] vs. 20.9 ± 4.1, t test p < 0.01). There were no differences in anxiety, depression or coping. Perceived health was similar in both groups. Fear for having a heart attack was expressed in 50% among FH patients.

Conclusions: Quality of life was higher among FH patients than controls. Half of the FH patients expressed fear for a heart attack. The higher quality of life among FH patients may be due to the treatment and care of the patients.

Socioeconomic status and superoxide dismutase levels in a Spanish female population

M.I. Covas, R. Elosua, M. Fitó, J. Benach, J. Vila, J. Marrugat. Unitat de Lípids i Epidemiologia Cardiovascular. Institut Municipal d'Investigació Mèdica. Barcelona, Spain

Objective: To explore whether levels of the antioxidant scavenger enzyme superoxide dismutase were associated with socioeconomic and educational status in a female Spanish population.

Methods: Cross-sectional study in 434 Spanish women aged 18 to 60 years. Superoxide dismutase in erythrocytes (E-SOD) activity levels were measured as described previously (Covas M.I. et al. Clin Chem 1997;43:562—568). Socioeconomic status was assessed on the basis of occupation. Occupation was recorded into five categories based on the British Classification of occupations. Educational level was classified into four categories from "primary school" to "tertiary education". In a subsample of 150 women lipid peroxidation was assessed by the thiobarbituric acid reactive substances (TBARS) method (Vasankari T. et al. Clin Chim Acta 1995;234:63—69).

Results: In bivariate analysis a negative association was found between TBARS and E-SOD ($r = -0.317$, $p = 0.001$). TBARS were directely associated with socioeconomic status ($r = 0.288$, $p = 0.002$) and educational status ($r = 0.295$, $p = 0.001$). Multiple regression analysis showed that higher socioeconomic ($p = 0.005$) and educational status ($p = 0.003$) were associated with low E-SOD activity levels after adjustment for age, body mass index, tobacco consumption, and physical activity.

Conclusions: Socioeconomic status appear as a determinant of E-SOD activity levels. From our results a high-ranking position in work is a factor which could promote oxidative stress in our female population.

Regulation of endothelial function

Phosphorylation of NO synthase. Impact on endothelial function

R. Busse, I. Fleming. *Klinikum der J.W.G-Universität, Frankfurt am Main, Germany*

The endothelial NO synthase (eNOS) was, until recently, thought to be regulated solely by changes in the intracellular Ca^{2+} concentration ($[Ca^{2+}]_i$). It is now clear that eNOS can be phosphorylated on serine, threonine and tyrosine residues and that a battery of protein kinases is involved in the regulation of eNOS activity in both, the presence and the absence of an increase in $[Ca^{2+}]_i$.

Tyrosine kinases modulate endothelial NO production, especially in response to mechanical stimuli and growth factors. However, the tyrosine kinases responsible and the residues targeted remain to be identified.

Of the potential phosphorylation sites within the eNOS sequence, most is known about the CaM-binding domain (CBD) and the carboxy terminal region of the reductase domain. Phosphorylation of serine by PKC, or threonine by the AMP-activated protein kinase (AMPK) within the CBD decreases eNOS activity, presumably by interfering with the binding of Ca^{2+}/CaM.

Phosphorylation of the second eNOS regulatory site (Ser^{1177}) by AMPK, CaM kinase II, or Akt/PKB enhances NO production. AMPK and CaM kinase II phosphorylate eNOS only following an increase in $[Ca^{2+}]_i$, but Akt can phosphorylate eNOS in the absence of Ca^{2+}. Indeed, the physiologically most important endothelial stimulus, fluid shear stress, known to elicit the activation of eNOS in an apparently Ca^{2+}-independent manner, achieves this effect by activating phosphatidylinositol 3-kinase which subsequently activates Akt. The phosphorylation of Ser^{1177} by Akt is sufficient to enhance enzyme activity at sub-physiological levels of $[Ca^{2+}]_i$. This Akt-induced activation of eNOS, which results in the maintained production of NO, is implicated not only in the adjustment of local vascular tone, but also in the regulation of gene expression, angiogenesis and endothelial cell migration.

Regulation of endothelial function by cardiovascular risk factors and race

D.S. Celermajer. *Department of Cardiology, Royal Prince Alfred Hospital, Sydney, Australia*

Endothelial dysfunction is an important early event in atherosclerosis, preceding discrete plaque formation and also determining vascular reactivity at the sites of established stenosis.

The influence of various risk factors on endothelial function, particularly release of nitric oxide by the vessel wall, is now being explored, with potential diagnostic and therapeutic implications. We have recently described the effects of cholesterol, active and passive cigarette smoking, diabetes mellitus and hyperhomocysteinaemia amongst others on endothelial function, and also elucidated some racial differences in the susceptibility of the vessel wall to these various risk factors, in different populations. For example, Chinese subjects appear less prone to the deleterious effects of aging and smoking on endothelial function, compared to white populations.

In vivo endothelial function testing is useful for the assessment of preventive strategies, when applied to serial studies. Strategies such as L-arginine therapy, antioxidants, ACE inhibition and folate therapy (for high homcysteine levels) have been assessed in clinical trials, and these results will be reviewed.

Differential regulation of ET-1 and ecNOS expression in human vessels exposed to complex mechanical forces

L. Gan, U. Hägg, A. Johansson, R. Doroudi, L. Sjögren, S. Jern. *Clinical Experimental Research Laboratory, Sahlgren's University Hospital/Östra, Göteborg, Sweden*

Objectives: To investigate how combined shear and pressure modulate the opposing vascular factors, NO and ET-1 in intact conduit vessels.

Methods: In a novel computerized perfusion system, human umbilical veins were perfused with high vs. low shear stress (25 vs. < 4 dyn/cm^2) at identical intraluminal pressure (20 mmHg) or high vs. low pressure (40 vs. 20 mmHg) at identical shear stress (10 dyn/cm^2) for 1.5, 3 or 6 h. Endothelial ecNOS and ET-1 gene expressions were quantified by real-time RT-PCR with b-actin as endogenous control. Semi-quantification of the protein expression by immunohistochemistry. The vascular NO producing capacity was measured with an amperometric NO probe. The vasoactivity was measured continuously as vascular resistance (pressure drop/flow) during the perfusion experiments.

Results: After a transient slight 28% down-regulation, ET-1 gene expression returned to base-line level after 6 h high shear perfusion, while high pressure up-regulated ET-1 expression by 111 $\pm$ 54% after 6 h (p = 0.02). The temporal regulation patterns of ecNOS gene by shear and pressure was significantly different (p $<$ 0.05). High shear up-regulated ecNOS gene expression gradually by 114 $\pm$ 56% (p = 0.035) after 6 h, while high pressure induced only a transient up-regulation of ecNOS by 205 $\pm$ 90% (p $<$ 0.05) after 3 h perfusion. These transcriptional events were accompanied by increased protein expressions, enhanced enzymatic activity and synchronal changes in vascular tone.

Conclusions: Vascular production of NO and ET-1 is differentially regulated by shear and pressure and the balance between these two pathways appears to be important for the regulation of the vascular tone.

Lysophosphatidylcholine induces early growth response factor-1 and activates the core promoter of PDGF-A chain in cultured vascular endothelial cells

M. Morimoto[2], N. Kume[1], S. Miyamoto[2], Y. Ueno[2], H. Kataoka[2], M. Minami[1], N. Hashimoto[2], T. Kita[1]. *[1]Department of Geriatric Medicine; [2]Neurosurgery, Kyoto University, Kyoto, Japan*

Objectives: Lysophosphatidylcholine (Lyso-PC), a bioactive phospholipid component increased in atherogenic oxidized low density lipoprotein, has been shown to induce various genes relevant to atherogenesis including PDGF-A chain. We therefore sought to define whether lyso-PC can induce expression of Egr-1, an inducible transcription factor which regulates gene expression including PDGF-A chain in cultured vascular endothelial cells.

Methods and Results: Northern blot analyses showed that lyso-PC (10—20 μmol/l) transiently (30 min—1 h) induced expression of Egr-1 mRNA. Induced expression of

Egr-1 mRNA by lyso-PC was associated with increased amounts of Egr-1 protein in nuclei as shown by western blot analyses. Transient transfection of the oligonucleotide corresponding to the proximal core promoter of the PDGF-A chain (oligo A) linked to the luciferase reporter gene revealed that lyso-PC activates the core promoter of the PDGF-A chain by 5-fold. Mutation in the nucleotide sequence of oligo A abolished the lyso-PC-induced increases in luciferase activities. Electrophoretic mobility shift assay using radiolabeled oligo A showed a lyso-PC-inducible shift band, which was suppressed by excess amounts of unlabeled oligo A and an anti-Egr-1 antibody. Induced expression of Egr-1 by lyso-PC appeared to precede the lyso-PC-induced expression of the PDGF-A chain mRNA by Northern blot analysis.

Conclusion: Induced expression of Egr-1 by lyso-PC may be a key regulator in the transcription of various endothelial genes relevant to atherogenesis.

Inhibition of mitochondrial complex I reduces TNF-alpha-stimulated superoxide anion generation and VCAM-1 expression in endothelial cells (EC) to mimic the effect of adenovirus-mediated overexpression of manganese sod

J. Oliver-Krasinski, Richard A. Cohen, A.J. Cayatte. *Boston University Medical Center, Vasclar Biology Unit, Evans Biomedical Research Center, Boston, Massachusetts, USA*

Objective: To investigate the role of mitochondrial superoxide anion generating system, as a regulatory signal in the expression of cell surface adhesion molecules in response to TNF-alpha stimulation.

Methods: We determined the effect of complex I inhibitor rotenone on endogenous superoxide anion measured by cytochrome C reduction and VCAM-1 expression by immunofluorescence.

Results: Rotenone (10 uM) inhibited TNF-alpha-stimulated ECI release of superoxide anion (0.139 ± 0.037 vs. 0.025 ± 0.01, nmoles/min/ug $p < 0.05$), and VCAM-1 expression (1131 ± 94 vs. 387 ± 50, AFU, $p < 0.05$). Unlike oxypurinol (300 µM) or superoxide dismutase (2500 units/ml), rotenone (50 µM) did not inhibit the reduction of cytochrome C by xanthine oxidase generated superoxide anion in a cell-free system indicating that is not a direct superoxide scavenger nor an inhibitor of xanthine oxidase. This effect was mimicked by DPI, a flavoprotein inhibitor, or by 48 h transfection of EC with an adenoviral expression vector that increased Mn^{2+} superoxide dismutase activity (from 4 to 38 units/mg), reduced superoxide anion (0.098 ± 0.019 vs. 0.071 ± 0.022, $p < 0.05$) and VCAM-1 expression (508 ± 48 vs. 282 ± 80 units, $p < 0.05$). However, antimycin A, which blocks mitochondrial electron transport chain downstream from the ubiquinone-cytochrome c reductase cycle, failed to affect superoxide anion or VCAM-1 expression.

Conclusions: These results suggest that the effect of rotenone on TNF-alpha-induction of VCAM-1 expression is explained by its ability to inhibit the superoxide anion generation by NADH dependent enzymes, including NAD(P)H oxidases and/or mitochondrial NADH oxido-reductases.

In vivo gene transfer of endothelial nitric oxide synthase to carotid arteries from hypercholesterolemic rabbits enhances endothelium-dependent relaxations

J. Sato, T. Mohácsi, A. Noel, C. Jost, P. Gloviczki, G. Mozes, Z. Katusic, T. O'Brien.
Mayo Foundation, Rochester, Minnesota, USA

Objective: Hypercholesterolemia is associated with abnormal endothelium dependent vasorelaxation due to decreased nitric oxide bioavailability. Our aim was to examine the effect of adenoviral-mediated gene transfer of eNOS to the hypercholesterolemic rabbit carotid artery in vivo. In addition, we examined whether adenoviral-mediated gene transfer was associated with vascular dysfunction.

Methods: Rabbits were fed a 1% cholesterol diet for 4 weeks followed by a 0.5% cholesterol diet for 6 weeks. Vascular reactivity was assessed in non-transduced carotid arteries from chow-and cholesterol-fed animals. In addition, carotid arteries were surgically isolated and two separate doses of adenoviral vectors encoding eNOS (AdeNOS) or β-galactosidase (AdβGal) on the contralateral side were delivered to the lumen (1×10^{10} pfu/ml and 5×10^{10} pfu/ml).

Results: Abnormal acetylcholine-mediated endothelium dependent-vasorelaxation was detected in the carotid artery from cholesterol fed animals, while responses to calcium ionophore and DEA NONOate were normal. Vascular reactivity was similar in non-transduced and Adβ-gal transduced hypercholesterolemic vessels. In vessels transduced with eNOS, transgene expression was demonstrated by immunostaining in both the endothelium and adventitia and also by Western Analysis. High dose but not low dose eNOS gene transfer enhanced endothelium dependent relaxation in vessels from cholesterol-fed rabbits.

Conclusions: Thus, adenoviral mediated gene transfer of eNOS to carotid arteries of cholesterol-fed animals improves endothelium dependent relaxation when an optimal viral titer is administered.

Lipoprotein(a)

Assembly of lipoprotein(a)

S.P.A. McCormick. *Department of Biochemistry, University of Otago, Dunedin, New Zealand*

The assembly of lipoprotein(a) [Lp(a)] is a two-step process. The first step is thought to be a noncovalent interaction between apolipoprotein (apo) B and apolipoprotein(a), while the second step comprises a disulphide link between apoBCys4326 and apo(a)Cys4057. Evidence for the initial noncovalent interaction comes from studies of two forms of apoB that lack apoBCys4326 (mouse apoB and human apoBCys4326) which can associate with apo(a) in the plasma. The protein interactions involved in the initial binding between apoB and apo(a) are not fully understood. The aim of our current research is to identify the apoB sequences that are important for its initial binding to apo(a).

Recent work targeting the Cys4326 residue into the mouse apoB sequence in a human/mouse hybrid apoB has shown that variation in the carboxyl-terminal sequences of apoB affects the efficiency of Lp(a) formation. In addition, studies of Lp(a) assembly with carboxyl-terminally truncated human apoB proteins have indicted that apoB amino acids 4330–4397 are important for the initial interaction with apo(a). Within the 4330–4397 region, we have identified a stretch of amino acids (residues 4372–4392) that are highly conserved between human and mouse apoB. A synthetic apoB peptide spanning the 4372–4392 sequence has proved to be an effective inhibitor of Lp(a) assembly. Computer analysis of this region predicts an amphipathic alpha-helix containing two sets of paired lysine residues on opposite sides of the helix. Circular dichroism studies of the synthetic peptide have confirmed its alpha-helical nature. Our results indicate that apoB amino acids 4372–4392 play an important role in Lp(a) assembly. Additional studies are currently being performed to further characterise the structural features of this new putative apo(a) binding site.

Lipoprotein (a) as a risk factor for cardiovascular disease

Lars Berglund. *Columbia University, New York City, New York, USA*

Lipoprotein(a), [Lp(a)], has been identified as a risk factor for cardiovascular disease (CAD) in numerous but not all prospective studies. Potentially, several different features of the Lp(a) particle, such as apo(a) protein properties and the apoB/lipid core could contribute to its atherogenicity, separately or in conjunction. Curiously, mean Lp(a) levels are twice as high in Blacks compared to Whites, but studies to date have failed to establish a significant association between elevated Lp(a) levels and CAD among Blacks. The lack of understanding of this racial difference has made it difficult to conclude with full confidence that Lp(a) is a risk factor for CAD. Further, presence of small apo(a) isoform size has been associated with CAD in Whites but not in Blacks. The majority of Whites with high Lp(a) levels also possess at least one small apo(a) isoform, but for Blacks, high mean Lp(a) levels are present over a wider range of apo(a) isoforms. The high correlation between elevated levels of Lp(a) and small apo(a) isoforms in Whites makes it difficult to ascertain whether one is a confounder for the other with regards to CAD. In Blacks, the more common combination of high Lp(a) levels with larger apo(a) sizes provides opportunities to test whether Lp(a) level or apo(a) size is more predicitive of CAD. We compared Lp(a) levels, apo(a) sizes and the level of Lp(a) particles carrying small apo(a) sizes in Blacks and Whites, and found that elevated levels of Lp(a) particles carrying a small apo(a) size were significantly associated with CAD in both groups. The results provide one basis for explaining the nature of the association between Lp(a) and CAD, as well as for the previously observed difference in association between Lp(a) and CAD among Blacks and Whites. The plasma level of Lp(a) carried by small-size apo(a) may be the atherogenic subpopulation of particles that determines the degree of risk for CAD contributed by Lp(a).

LP(a) metabolism and in vivo proteolytic fragmentation

G.M. Kostner, S. Frank. *Institute of Medical Biochemistry, University of Graz, Austria*

The knowledge of specific features of the Lp(a) metabolism is still fragmentary. Early turnover studies in man revealed that individuals with high plasma Lp(a) levels exhibit a faster rate of synthesis whereas the FCR appeared to be uniform. There are currently two possibilities discussed on Lp(a) assembly: i) Apo(a) is secreted from liver and associates with LDL outside the liver cell mainly in circulating blood, and ii) Lp(a) is intracellularly assembled. These latter findings were delineated from in vivo kinetics using stable isotopes.

Concerning the catabolism of Lp(a) it appears that the liver is the major organ yet LDL-receptors may play an inferior role. There is still intensive work going on aimed at elucidating specific binding mechanisms of to the liver cell.

Another organ, which might be important in the removal of Lp(a) from circulation, is the kidney. Not only that an arterio-venous concentration difference in Lp(a) in the order of >5% was found, Lp(a) might also bind to megalin, a member of the LDL-receptor family present in kidney cells. Another point underlining the role of kidney in Lp(a) catabolism is the presence of large apo(a) fragments in the urine. Although the total apo(a) immune reactivity found in urine accounts only for 1% catabolism/day, there is the possibility that small fragments not recognized by antibodies might be also secreted.

One major question is which enzyme might be responsible for Lp(a) fragmentation and also what physiological significance might such a proteolytic cleavage have? There is little doubt that the proteases attacking Lp(a) belong to the family of metallo-proteinases of the elastase and collagenase type. Results of our ongoing studies will be presented aimed at elucidating the role of various enzymes in Lp(a) catabolism.

Sequence changes in putative enhancer regions upstream of the apolipoprotein(a) gene

L. Puckey, B. Knight. *MRC Clinical Sciences Centre, London, UK*

Objective: Plasma concentrations of the atherogenic lipoprotein(a) [Lp(a)] are almost entirely determined by sequences at or closely linked to the apolipoprotein(a) [apo(a)] gene locus. Two regions upstream of the apo(a) gene have been identified which enhance the activity of the apo(a) promoter in reporter-gene constructs in vitro, DHII, situated about 28kb, and DHIII, about 20kb upstream of the apo(a) gene. The aim of this study was to investigate whether sequence changes in these regions could influence Lp(a) concentrations.

Methods: The enhancers were amplified and sequenced from subjects chosen to cover the whole range of Lp(a) concentrations. The sequence changes were introduced into reporter-gene constructs, the resulting change in apo(a) promoter activity measured and those that had an effect were tracked through families to discover any association between the different alleles and Lp(a) levels.

Results: No base changes were found in the DHII region. In the DHIII region, 3 common base substitutions were found, an A to G change at position –1230, a C to A change at –1617 and a G to T substitution at –1712. The frequency of these sequence changes were 0.54 (A), 0.84 (C) and 0.89 (G) respectively in a Caucasian population. Changing the A to a G in reporter-gene constructs increased the activity of the downstream apo(a) promoter approximately 4-fold, while changing the C to a A and the G to a T decreased activity by 50% and 30% respectively. Family studies have shown that the G at –1230 is associated with significantly higher Lp(a) concentrations and the T at –1712 with significantly lower levels.

Conclusions: These sequence changes could provide a significant contribution to the variation of plasma Lp(a) concentrations, but are not solely responsible for determining the large range of concentrations seen in a Caucasian population.

Immunohistological localisation of Lp(a) in the human kidney

H. Dieplinger[1], I. Leiter[1], E. Trenkwalder[1], W. Salvenmoser[2], W. Horninger[3], K. Lhotta[4], P. König[4], F. Kronenberg[1]. *[1]Institute of Medical Biology and Human Genetics; [2]Institute of Zoology; [3]Department of Urology; [4]Department of Clinical Nephrology; University of Innsbruck, Austria*

Objective: Lipoprotein(a) [Lp(a)] is a genetically determined risk factor for atherosclerosis. Elevated Lp(a) concentrations have been observed also secondary to pathological conditions like end-stage renal disease (ESRD) where they significantly contribute to the high risk for atherosclerotic diseases in this patient population. Significant arteriovenous concentration differences (with lower values in the renal vein) of Lp(a) in patients with normal renal function suggest an uptake of Lp(a) by the human kidney. The precise localisation and uptake mechanisms for renal Lp(a) is unknown.

Methods: We aimed to localise Lp(a) on fixed and paraffin-embedded tissue sections obtained from resections of kidney tumor operations. Tisssue sections of patients with undetectable plasma Lp(a) concentrations served as controls.

Results: Immunostaining revealed apo(a) and apoB immunoreactivity on mesangial cells in the glomerulus. No immunoreactivity was observed in sections from Lp(a)-negative patients and in other cell types (e.g., tubulus cells) of renal tissue.

Conclusions: Mesangial cells of the human kidney are able to take up intact Lp(a) and therefore can explain the elevated plasma concentrations of Lp(a) in ESRD patients.

In vivo metabolism of apo(a) and apob-100 in human lipoprotein(a)

M.E. Frischmann[1], E. Trenkwalder[1], F. Kronenberg[1], P. König[1], H. Schweer[2], H.J. Seyberth[2], M. Soufi[2], A. Steinmetz[2], J.R. Schäfer[2], H. Dieplinger[1]. *[1]Institute of Medical Biology and Human Genetics and Department of Clinical Nephrology/Internal Medicine, University of Innsbruck, Austria; and [2]Department of Internal Medicine/ Cardiology and Children's Hospital, Philipps University of Marburg, Germany*

Objective: The atherogenic lipoprotein(a) [Lp(a)] consists of LDL and apolipoprotein(a) [apo(a)]. Detailed mechanisms of biosynthesis and catabolism are still poorly understood. Clinical studies in various patients with renal diseases suggested a possible role of the human kidney in the removal of Lp(a) from the circulation in plasma.

Methods: We studied by stable isotope methodology the in vivo turnover of Lp(a) and LDL in probands and patients with end-stage renal disease (ESRD) treated with hemodialysis. [2H3]-L-Leucine was constantly infused over 12 hours and 14 blood samples were drawn. LDL was prepared by density gradient ultracentrifugation while Lp(a) was prepared by immunoprecipitation using antibody-bound magnetic beads. The Lp(a) complex was separated by preparative SDS-PAGE under reducing conditions. Proteins were analysed by GC/MS. The level of isotope enrichment was used to calculate fractional synthesis rates (FSR). Categories 8, 9, 28.

Results: Preliminary evaluation of data shows a similar synthesis rate of apo(a) and apoB100 from Lp(a) in controls which was different from the FSR of apoB100 from LDL and a similar FSR of apo(a) in ESRD patients and controls (of the same apo(a) isoform).

Conclusions: In conclusion, first, the results are compatible with an intracellular assembly of Lp(a) from apo(a) and apoB100, and second, a role of the kidney in the catabolism of Lp(a) which would explain elevated Lp(a) plasma concentrations in ESRD.

(+)-SR-74829i/SB-270924 reduces plasma lipoprotein(a) and liver steady state apo(a) mRNA levels in the cynomolgus monkey

K. Suckling[1], T. Reape[1], A. Gee[1], K. Morasco[2], D. d'Epagnier[2], R. Coatney[2], E. Jenkins[2], E. Niesor[3], C. Bentzen[3]. *[1]SmithKline Beecham Pharmaceuticals, Harlow, UK; [2]King of Prussia, Pennsylvania, USA; and [3]Symphar, Geneva, Switzerland*

Objective: Aminophosphonates such as (+)-SR-74829i/SB-270924 (SR) signficantly reduce plasma Lp(a), apoB and LDL-cholesterol concentrations in orally treated cynomolgus monkeys. In order to investigate the mechanism by which this is achieved, steady state mRNA levels were determined in liver biopsies taken from monkeys before and after treatment with SR.

Methods: Four cynomolgus monkeys were used in the study. Before treatment with drug, plasma samples were obtained and a small liver biopsy taken. The animals were treated with SR for 2 weeks (75 mg/kg/day) and then another series of plasma and liver samples were obtained. Plasma apo(a) and apoB were measured by ELISA and liver mRNA by TaqMan quantitative PCR. The probe/primer sets selected for apo(a) were a monkey kringle IV/protease junction sequence and a monkey 5′ sequence. The same results were obtained for both. Readout from the TaqMan calibration curve was normalised to beta-actin, GAPDH and cyclophilin. All three gave the same trends.

Results: Plasma apo(a) was reduced to $49 \pm 25\%$ of pretreatment values and liver apo(a) mRNA correspondingly to $46 \pm 14\%$ of pretreatment. Liver mRNA for apoB was unchanged, but plasma apoB decreased to $69 \pm 10\%$ of pretreatment.

Conclusions: The parallel reductions in plasma Lp(a) and liver mRNA for apo(a) suggest that aminophosphonates act as the level of mRNA. The mechanism for apoB lowering appears to be different.

Hypertension, kidney disease, and atherosclerosis

Epidemiology of cardiovascular disease in chronic renal disease

Robert N. Foley. *The Patient Research Centre, Memorial Univ. of New Foundland, Canada*

The burden of cardiovascular disease in patients with chronic renal disease exceeds that of the general population, by orders of magnitude. Thus, among dialysis patients, the prevalence of coronary artery disease is approximately 40% and the prevalence of left ventricular hypertrophy is approximately 75%. Cardiovascular mortality has been estimated to be approximately 9% per year. Even after adjustment is made for the older age and higher proportion of diabetic patients that are typical of dialysis populations, the cardiovascular mortality in dialysis patients is at least 10–20 times higher than in the general population. Patients with chronic renal disease should be considered in the highest risk group for subsequent cardiovascular events.

Cardiac failure is much commoner in chronic renal disease patients than in the general population, and is an independent predictor of death in chronic renal disease. Among dialysis patients, the prevalence of cardiac failure is approximately 40% in some countries. Both coronary artery disease and left ventricular hypertrophy are risk factors for the development of cardiac failure. In practice, it is difficult to determine whether cardiac failure reflects left ventricular dysfunction or ECF volume overload. Patients who develop clinical, manifestations of cardiac failure should be evaluated for cardiovascular disease.

The high potential for reverse causation is a major barrier to use of observational studies to assess the role of "traditional", modifiable, cardiovascular risk factors like hypertension and dyslipidaemia. Factors related to chronic renal failure, such as anaemia, *the uraemic internal milieu* and abnormalities of calcium-phosphate homcostasis may also be actiological. The paucity of randomised contolled intervention trials in chronic renal failure is lamentable, and is in stark contrast contrasts to the burden of cardiovascular disease.

Inflammation as a risk factor for atherogenesis in chronic renal failure

C. Wanner, T. Metzger, K. Herfs, J. Zimmermann. *Department of Medicine, Division of Nephrology, University of Würzburg, Germany*

Objective: C-reactive protein (CRP) is a predictor of cardiovascular mortality in apparently healthy men. CRP levels in hemodialysis (HD) patients are 8–10-fold higher than in healthy controls, but the predictive value remains to be determined.

Methods: In 280 HD patients CRP was correlated with other atherogenic acute phase proteins and mortality was monitored over a two year period.

Results: CRP was found to be elevated (> 8 mg/l) in 46% of the patients in the absence of clinical apparent infection. Patients with high CRP had higher serum levels of Lp(a), higher plasma fibrinogen, and lower serum levels of HDL cholesterol, apoA-l and serum albumin than patients with normal CRP. During follow-up 72 patients had died, mostly due to cardiovascular disease (58%). Overall mortality and cardiovascular mortality were significantly higher in patients with elevated CRP and were also higher in patients with serum albumin of lower than 40 g/l. In multivariate Cox regression analysis, age and CRP were the most powerful independent predictors of both overall death and cardiovascular death.

Conclusion: In HD patients an activated acute phase response is closely related to high levels of atherogenic vascular risk factors and cardiovascular death.

Hypertension and cardiovascular disease in chronic renal failure

C.R.V. Tomson. *Southmead Hospital, Bristol, UK*

Hypertension is frequently present in patients with parenchymal renal disease even before the development of impaired excretory function, and is nearly universal in patients developing end-stage renal failure. Many patients with chronic renal failure die prematurely from cardiovascular disease — end-stage renal failure carries a risk of death comparable to many malignancies — but much of this excess mortality appears to be due to hypertensive heart failure rather than atherosclerotic myocardial infarction.

Mechanisms of hypertension in renal disease include sodium chloride retention, increased renin secretion and increased sympathetic tone, the afferent signal arising in diseased kidneys. Hypertension is poorly controlled in up to 60% of haemodialysis patients, despite aggressive drug treatment, but can be perfectly controlled, at least in selected patients, by dietary salt restriction combined with rigorous control of extracellular volume by long haemodialysis; this results, apparently paradoxically, in reduced peripheral vascular resistance. Exceptionally good survival figures have been published from one centre employing this strategy.

Observations over up to 4 years in large numbers of dialysis patients have shown that blood pressure is inversely, not directly, associated with risk of death. Very few studies have demonstrated that hypertension is a significant risk factor for death in chronic renal failure, although this can be demonstrated in the centre employing long haemodialysis with dietary salt restriction. The most tenable explanation is that the majority of dialysis patients already have significant hypertensive or ischaemic heart failure, the clinical signs of which are altered as a result of renal disease and its treatment. Treatment to alter the high cardiovascular mortality of renal patients must therefore start early in the course of renal disease.

Amelioration of lipid induced glomerulopathy by lovastatin

A.K. Walli[1], P. Fraunberger[1], E.F. Groene[2], H.J. Gröne[2], D. Seidel[1]. *[1]Department of Clinical Chemistry, Ludwig-Maximilians-University Munich; [2]Institut of Pathology, Deutsches Krebsforschungszentrum, Heidelberg, Germany*

Objective: Dyslipoproteinemia plays an important role in progression of renal disease. In contrast to rats which transport cholesterol mainly in the HDL fraction, guinea pigs like humans carry cholesterol in LDL. Rates of hepatic cholesterol synthesis and response of lipoprotein metabolism to diet and drug therapy are similar in guinea pigs to those observed in humans. The aim of the study was: 1) to characterize alterations in the lipoprotein profile, lipoprotein receptor status and HMG-CoA reductase activity in hepatic and renal tissue in the presence and absence of hypercholesterolemia and lovastatin administration; 2) to attempt to delineate hypolipidemic and direct effects of the drug on reduction of glomerular injury; and 3) to correlate biochemical data with morphological changes in the kidney of guinea pigs treated with lovastatin.

Methods: Male Dunkin Heartley guinea pigs were unilaterally nephrectomized and fed either a regular or 0.3% cholesterol enriched diet in the presence or absence of lovastatin for eight months. Lipoprotein status, LDL receptor activity and the activity of HMG-

CoA reductase were determined in liver and kidney. Quantitative analysis of glomerular and tubulointerstitial morphological changes were performed.

Results: Cholesterol feeding increased VLDL and LDL cholesterol by several folds. Administration of a high dose of lovastatin lowered plasma cholesterol by about 50% in contrast to a low dose of lovastatin. Glomerular fat content, cell number, monocyte/macrophage number, matrix increase were significantly reduced by lovastatin at both dosages.

Conclusion: Our data show that HMG-CoA reductase inhibitor Lovastatin ameliorates the lipid-induced glomerulopathy in guinea pigs possibly due to its antiproliferative and antiinflammatory effects independant of cholesterol lowering.

Sclerotic change of aorta and survival of patients with end-stage renal disease. A prospective study

T. Shoji[1], M. Emoto[1], R. Kakiya[2], K. Shinohara[1], E. Kimoto[1], A. Yamada[1], T. Tabata[2], Y. Nishizawa[1]. [1]Second Dept. of Internal Medicine, Osaka City University; [2]Division of Internal Medicine, Inoue Hospital, Osaka, Japan

Objective: Atherosclerosis is advanced and mortality rate is high in end-stage renal disease (ESRD). The purpose of this study was to examine the impact of aortic atherosclerosis on the survival of patients with ESRD.

Methods: ESRD patients on maintenance hemodialysis (n = 245) were enrolled in the study. Aortic pulse wave velocity (PWV) was measured as an index of aortic sclerosis, and their survival was followed.

Results: During the follow-up period (mean 56 months), 76 deaths (31%) were observed. Kaplan-Meier analysis indicated that diabetic patients had a higher mortality rate than nondiabetics. Also, when the subjects were divided into two groups according their initial PWV values, the high PWV group had a significantly poorer prognosis in both diabetics and nondiabetics. Cox proportional hazard model indicated that PWV was a significant factor associated with mortality in this population independent of age, gender, diabetes and serum creatinine level.

Conclusions: Aortic sclerosis as measured by PWV is an independent factor predicting the prognosis of patients with ESRD on hemodialysis.

Correlation between the carotid intimal-medial thickness and histological arteriosclerosis of radial artery in patients with chronic renal failure

H. Taniwaki[1], T. Yoshida[1], K. Sato[1], Y. Takeda[2], Y. Azuma[3], E. Ishimura[4], Y. Nishizawa[4], Y. Iida. [1]Yodogawa Christian Hospital Internal Medicine; [2]Department of Pathology; [3]Azuma clinic; and [4]2 Int. Med., Osaka City Univ., Japan

Objective: To assess the relationship between the intimal-medial thickness (IMT) of the carotid artery and the histopathological degree of arteriosclerosis of the radial artery, and to explore the factors affecting arteriosclerosis of the radial artery.

Subjects and Methods: Twenty-five patients with pre-dialysis chronic renal failure (CRF) (serum creatinine > 4.0 mg/dl; 40 to 75 years old; 12 men and 13 women) were recruited from Yodogawa Christian Hospital. The tissues from the radial artery, which were resected during the arterio-venous shunt operation, were histologically examined after H.E. staining. The IMT's of the carotid artery were measured with high-resolution B-mode ultrasonography.

Results: Out of 25 patients, arteriosclerosis was histopathologically evident in 18 patients (group 1), but not in seven patients (group 2). In group 1, three patients had intimal plaque and 6 patients had calcification in the media. The IMT's of the carotid artery of the group 1 were significantly greater than those of the group 2 (2.09 ± 1.10 vs. 0.92 ± 0.20 mm, p < 0.05). Multiple regression analysis revealed that the histolopathological degree of arteriosclerosis of the radial artery were significantly, independently affected by age and hypertension, similar to the factors affecting IMT of the carotid artery.

Conclusion: These results demonstrated that significant relationship between the carotid artery IMT and the histopathological degree of arteriosclerosis of the radial artery.

Lipoprotein-X stimulates MCP-1 expression in mesangial cells: a possible role in monocyte infiltration in familial LCAT deficiency

E.G. Lynn[1], J. Frohlich[2], K. O[1]. *[1] University of Hong Kong, Hong Kong, China; and [2] University of British Columbia, Vancouver, Canada*

Objective: Familial LCAT deficiency is a rare genetic disorder whose clinical symptoms include corneal opacities, hemolytic anemia, proteinuria and subsequent renal failure. Lipoprotein-X (Lp-X) is present in the plasma of LCAT deficient patients. Many of these patients develop glomerulosclerosis. A key event in the pathogenesis of glomerulosclerosis is the infiltration of circulating monocytes in glomeruli. Mesangial cells can express MCP-1, an important chemoattractant for monocytes. The objective of this study was to examine the effect of Lp-X on the induction of mesangial cell MCP-1 expression.

Methods: Lp-X was isolated from the plasma of a LCAT deficient patient. Mesangial cells were isolated from the kidneys of male Sprague-Dawley rats.

Results: Treatment of cells with Lp-X (50—100 nmol/ml) stimulated mesangial cell MCP-1 mRNA expression (137—220%) and MCP-1 protein secretion (233—375%). Lp-X-like liposomes (50–100 nmol/ml) also stimulated mesangial cell MCP-1 mRNA expression (124—162%) and MCP-1 protein secretion (214—317%). Lp-X-induced mesangial cell MCP-1 expression resulted in enhanced monocyte chemotaxis.

Conclusions: Lp-X may participate in the pathogenesis of glomerulosclerosis and subsequent renal failure in familial LCAT deficient patients by stimulating monocyte infiltration via a mechanism involving MCP-1. (Supported by the RGC and the ICSM).

Oxidation and atherogenesis

Isoprostanes: Indices of oxidant stress in atherosclerosis

G.A. FitzGerald. *University of Pennsylvania, Center for Experimental Therapeutics, Philadelphia, Pennsylvania, USA*

Isoprostanes are free radical catalyzed isomers of arachidonic acid. They are formed initially in situ in cell membranes from which they are cleaved, circulated and are excreted in urine. Specific assays based on mass spectrometry have been developed for a range of isoprostanes. Their urinary excretion reflects oxidant stress associated with inflammation, reperfusion after tissue ischemia, and oxidant stress in response to xenobiotics. Isoprostanes may be immunolocalized in vascular smooth muscle cells and monocyte macrophages in human atherosclerotic plaque hand are elevated in atherosclerotic vessels, circulating LDL, and in urine of humans with hypercholesterolemia. Similar biochemical abnormalities characterize a variety of mouse models of atherosclerosis. Isoprostanes also act as incidental ligands at membrane and nuclear receptors for prostanoids.

Oxidized phospholipids as ligands for macrophage scavenger receptors

D. Steinberg. *University of California, San Diego, La Jolla, California, USA*

It has generally been assumed that oxidized LDL (OxLDL) is recognized by scavenger receptors by virtue of changes in apoB, either changes its primary structure (e.g., acetylation or other masking of lysine amino groups) or changes in configuration. However, studies in this laboratory have shown that the lipid moiety of OxLDL (but not that of native LDL), when reconstituted into a microemulsion, binds in a saturable fashion to mouse peritoneal macrophages and competes for the binding of intact OxLDL. Further studies showed that liposomes containing oxidized phospholipids also completed. Unexpectedly, the reconstituted lipid and the isolated lipid-free apoB from OxLDL competed with each other. Moreover, a monoclonal antibody against oxidized phospholipids was shown to bind to both the lipid moiety and the apoprotein moiety. These findings are now shown to result from the presence of oxidized phospholipids covalently bound to apoB. Direct examination of apoB isolated from OxLDL after exhaustive extraction of lipids showed that more than 70 moles of phosphorus remained attached to the protein whereas apoB from native LDL showed almost no retained phosphorus.

Monoclonal antibodies that recognize oxidized phospholipids and oxidized LDL also react with apoptotic cell membranes (but not normal cell membrane) implying a commonality of ligand between OxLDL and apoptotic cells, probably oxidized phospholipids. These results by no means rule but the presence of additional ligands that bind to macrophage scavenger receptors. Moreover the relative importance of oxidized phospholipids as ligands may vary from one scavenger receptor to another. We have now examined the ligand-binding specificity of CD6 expressed in transfected cells. The results closely parallel those obtained with intact mouse peritoneal macrophages.

Role of LOX-1 in atherosclerosis

T. Kita. *Kyoto University Graduate School of Medicine, Geriatric Medicine, Kyoto, Japan*

One of the critical events in the pathogenesis of the early stage atherosclerotic lesions is the focal accumulation of lipid-laden foam cells derived from macrophages. In various cholesterol-fed animal models of atherosclerosis, it was found that localized attachment of circulating monocytes to arterial endothelial cells appears to precede the formation of foam cells. Recently the molecular mechanism of the formation of atherosclerosis has been elucidated. It has been suggested that monocyte recruitment into early lesions might involve, changing the endothelial adhesiveness for monocytes and lymphocytes. In vivo and in vitro studies have identified molecules, such as ICAM-1, VCAM-1 and ELAM-1, those can support the adhesion of leukocytes, monocytes and lymphocytes. Moreover oxidized LDL and lysophosphatidyl choline, (which isderived from oxidized LDL), induce the expression of these adhesion molecules. In addition, it has been demonstrated that monocyte-macrophages can ingest chemically modified LDL, such as oxidized LDL, and thereby they become foam cells. Recently we identified and characterized the novel receptor for oxidized LDL, named LOX-1. The expression of LOX-1 is found on the surface of endothelial cells smooth muscle cells and macrophages. I want focus my talk on the formation of foam cells, especially monocyte recruitmeny and significance of oxidized LDL and its receptor LOX-1, in terms of atherosclerosis.

Evidence for dissociation of lipoprotein lipid oxidation and atherosclerosis in different animals

R. Stocker[1], P. Witting[1], J. Upston[1], S. Thomas[1], A. Terentis[1], A. Lau[1], S. Leichtweis[1], X. Chafour[2], J. Burr[3], D. Liebler[3], K. Pettersson[4]. *[1] Heart Research Institute; [2] University of Sydney, Sydney, Australia; [3] University of Arizona, Tucson, USA; and [4] AstraZeneca, Mölndal, Sweden*

Oxidation of low-density lipoprotein (LDL) is now commonly thought to play a central role in atherogenesis. Indeed, oxidized lipoproteins are present in atherosclerotic lesions and in vitro oxidized LDL has many potential pro-atherogenic activities. However, direct evidence that LDL oxidation causes (rather than being a consequence of) atherosclerosis has not been forthcoming. Vitamin E a-tocopherol, TOH) is the major antioxidant associated with LDL and commonly thought to be anti-atherogenic. Surprisingly however, in human lesions relative normal concentrations of TOH coexist with small amounts of tocopherol-derived oxidation products and substantial amounts of oxidized lipids, formed largely in the presence of the vitamin. Also, overall human and animal intervention studies with vitamin E on atherosclerosis have yielded disappointing results. We discovered that the role of TOH in lipoprotein lipid oxidation is complex. As formulated by the tocopherol-mediated peroxidation (TMP) model, the vitamin requires compounds capable of eliminating the TOH-derived radical for effective protection of lipoprotein lipids. We have identified compounds that inhibit TMP in vitro. Where tested these compounds also inhibit the accumulation of the primary products of lipoprotein lipid oxidation in the vessel wall of atherosclerosis prone rabbits and mice. However, such inhibition is not always associated with a decrease in the extent of atherosclerosis. Also, probucol (an antioxidant unable to inhibit TMP) substantially attenuates atherosclerosis in the aorta of apolipoprotein E−/− mice and cholesterol-fed, ballooned rabbits without concomitant inhibition of aortic lipid oxidation. Conversely, disease can be promoted in rabbits by hypoxia without an increase in lipid oxidation. Together, our findings question whether lipoprotein lipid oxidation is a general cause of atherosclerosis.

Expression of macrophages (Mf) scavenger receptor, CD36, in cultured human aortic smooth muscle cells, in association with the expression of peroxisome proliferator activated receptor-gamma — gain of Mf-like phenotype in vitro and its implication in atherogenesis

K. Matsumoto, K. Hirano, S. Nozaki, M. Nishida, Y. Nakagawa-Toyama, M.Y. Janabi, T. Ohya, S. Yamashita, Y. Matsuzawa. *Osaka University, Osaka, Japan*

CD36 is one of the major receeptors for oxidized low density lipoproteins belonging to macrophages (Mf) scavenger receptor (SR) class B, and thought to play an important role in the foam cell formation from monocyte-Mf in the atherosclerotic lesions. Although it has been hypothesized that smooth muscle cells (SMCs) may be the other origin of foam cells in vivo, supporting data available are still very limited. In the current study, we have tested the expression of a variety of SRs including CD36 in eight lots of primary human aortic SMCs (HASMCs) explanted from eight different donors. Functional CD36 was expressed in the cultured HASMCs and the levels of expression were widely ranged between the lots. SR class A was expressed abundantly in CD36-negative (CD36 (–)) lots. Other Mf markers such as CD32 and CD68 were expressed in all lots tested. These data suggest that the cultured HASMCs gained Mf-like phenotype. To know the mechanism for the above phenotypic change, we have tested the expression of a nuclear receptor, peroxisome proliferator activated receptor-g (PPARg) in those cells. This nuclear receptor was abundantly expressed in CD36-positive (CD36 (+)) lots, whereas c-fms was expressed abundantly in CD36 (–)/SR-A (+) lots. The synthetic ligand of PPARg, troglitazone, up-regulated the expression of CD36 only in CD36 (+) lots. These observations demonstrate that cultured HASMCs can gain Mf-like phenotype, and that expression of CD36 may be associated with that of PPARg in these cell types. The present study may support the possibility that HASMCs is one of the origins of foam cells in vivo.

Monocyte chemoattractant protein-1 promotes macrophage oxidation of low density lipoprotein

Rajendra K. Tangirala[1], Domenico Pratico[1], Uwe J.F. Tietge[1], Oswald Quehenberger[2], Garret A. FitzGerald[1], Daniel J. Rader[1]. *[1]Dept. of Medicine, University of Pennsylvania, Philadelphia, Pennsylvania; and [2]UC San Diego, California, USA*

Objective: To investigate the atherogenic role of MCP-1/CCR2 interaction beyond monocyte recruitment and to test the hypothesis that MCP-1 promotes oxidation of LDL and generation of oxidative stress by macrophages.

    Methods: CCR2 expression in normal and atherosclerotic aortas of apolipoprotein E-deficient (apoE$^{-/-}$) mice and its modulation by native LDL in mouse peritoneal macrophages was evaluated by RT-PCR. Macrophages were incubated with LDL in the presence of increasing concentrations of MCP-1 (0–100 ng/ml). The effect of MCP-1 on the oxidation of LDL was assessed by two independent measures: analysis of thiobarbituric acid reactive substances (TBARS) and gas chromatography-mass spectrometric (GC-MS) determination of isoprostane F2α-VI, (iPFα-VI), a sensitive marker of lipid peroxidation and oxidative stress. In vivo studies to examine the effect of MCP-1 inhibition on aortic oxidative stress were performed in 6-month old apo $E^{-/-}$ mice divided into three groups: one group sacrificed at baseline and the second and third were injected intravenously with a neutralizing anti-MCP-1 monoclonal antibody and a control isotype-matched IgG, respectively. After 2 weekly injections with respective antibodies, the mice were sacrificed at day-14 and the aortas prepared were analyzed for iPF2 a-VI levels by GC-MS.

Results: CCR2 mRNA was abundantly expressed in established aortic atherosclerotic lesions but absent from arteries lacking grossly-visible atherosclerotic lesions in apoE$^{-/-}$ mice. Both resident and adherent peritoneal macrophages expressed CCR2 and the expression was markedly augmented by native LDL. MCP-1 induced a dose-dependent increase in macrophage oxidation of LDL assessed by analysis of TBARS and iPFα-VI generation. Futhermore, intravenous injection of neutralizing anti-MCP-1 monoclonal antibody significantly reduced oxidative stress in the artery wall by 40% compared with baseline and control IgG injection in apoE$^{-/-}$ mice. The aortic iPFα-VI levels of baseline and control antibody-injected mice were not significantly different.

Conclusions: These results provide first evidence that MCP-1 promotes oxidation of LDL by macrophages and generation of aortic oxidative stress. Thus, MCP-1/CCR2 interactions could play atherogenic role(s) beyond monocyte recruitment and potentially contribute to the inflammatory nature and progression of atherosclerotic lesions.

Sites of action of Protein Pinase C (PKC) and Phosphatidylinositol 3-Kinase (Pl3K) are distinctin oxidized low-density lipoprotein-induced macrophage proliferation

S. Horiuchi, M. Sakai, A. Miyazaki. *Kumamoto Univ Sch Med., Kumamoto, Japan*

Background and Objective: Oxidized low density lipoprotein (Ox-LDL) can induce macrophage proliferation in vitro. To explore the mechanisms involved in this process, we reported that activation of protein kinase C (PKC) is involved in its signaling pathway (ATVB 17;3013:1997) and that expression of granulocyte/macrophage colony-stimulating factor (GM-CSF) and its subsequent release in the culture medium are important (JBC 273;28305:1998). However, a recent study from other laboratory showed the involvement of phosphatidylinositol 3-kinase (Pl3K) in this process (JBC 273;4915:1998). In the present study, we compared the contribution of PKC and Pl3K to Ox-LDL-induced macrophage proliferation.

Results: Ox-LDL-induced macrophage proliferation was inhibited by 90% by a PKC inhibitor, calphostin C, and 50% by a Pl3K inhibitor, wortmannin. Ox-LDL-induced expression of GM-CSF and its subsequent release were inhibited by calphostin C but not by wortmannin, whereas recombinant GM-CSF-induced macrophage proliferation was inhibited by wortmannin by 50% but not by calphostin C. Ox-LDL activated Pl3K at two time points (10 minutes and 4 hours), and the activation at the second but not first point was significantly inhibited by calphostin C and anti-GM-CSF antibody.

Conclusions: The present results suggest that PKC plays a role upstream in the signaling pathway to GM-CSF induction, whereas Pl3K is involved, at least in part, downstream in the signaling pathway after GM-CSF induction.

Genetics of lipoprotein metabolism

The relative role of invariant and context dependent genetic effects in predicting cardiovascular disease

C. Sing[1], K. Zerba[1], M. Nelson[3], S. Lussier-Cacan[4], S. Kardia[2]. *[1]Dept. of Human Genetics; [2]Dept. of Epidemiology, University of Michigan, Ann Arbor, Michigan; [3]Esperion Therapuetics, Ann Arbor, Michigan, USA; and [4]IRCM, Montreal, Quebec, Canada*

No gene has been established as having invariant context independent effects on the risk of cardiovascular disease (CVD). Most geneticists agree that the causation of phenotypic variability is a consequence of non-linear, dynamic interactions between genes, proteins, cellular organelles, cells, tissues and organ systems as well as the interactions between each of these classes of agents. Furthermore, it is widely acknowledged that these interactions are influenced by interactions with exposures to environments external to the individual that are indexed by time and ecological space. So why does medical science continue to seek to identify and characterize independent invariant Cartesian effects of candidate agents using study designs and analytical models that assume no interactions? Disciplinary hubris, lack of mathematical skills, narrowness of intellectual interest, intellectual property considerations and inadequate training in biology have been suggested as reasons for the inconsistency. We review here genetic studies that test the assumptions of biological and statistical independence of predictors of CVD risk. These studies document that the influence of genotypic variation in candidate genes on risk of CVD are not independent of background genotype, age, body size, gender, alcohol consumption, smoking and other measures of context. Such studies clearly establish that the full utilization of genomic information can only be expected if the forgotten role of context is reinstated in the search for the genetic predictors, and an etiological understanding, of CVD. The cost to medicine and public health of ignoring context in the search through the immense resource of genetic data now available for meaningful information will be great. Awareness of the complexity of the problem in the academic and industrial communities is a necessary first step to avoiding this cost. (Supported by NIH grants HL39107, HL51021 and HL54457).

ABCA7, A novel ABC transporter potentially involved in Macrophage Lipid Metabolism

W.E. Kaminski, J. Klucken, G. Schmitz. *Institute for Clinical Chemistry and Laboratory Medicine, University of Regensburg, 93042 Regensburg, Germany*

Objective: Identification of macrophage cholesterol-responsive genes

Methods: Human lipid-laden macrophages were screened for the expression of ATP binding cassette (ABC) transporters. ABC transporters translocate a variety of substances, ranging from ions to small peptides, across cell membranes.

Results: We recently demonstrated that the ABC transporter ABCA1 is a key regulator of HDL metabolism [1–3], which is mutated in Tangier disease, a syndrome associated with premature atherosclerosis. Here we report the cloning of a novel member of the A subfamily of full-size ABC transporters, tentatively termed ABCA7, from human macrophages. The ABCA7 cDNA predicts a polypeptide, consisting of 12 transmembrane domains and two ATP binding cassettes, that exhibits significant homology with ABCA1. The identification of alternative mRNA splice variants suggests the existence of potential ABCA7 isoforms. Unlike ABCA1, which is expressed in a multitude of tissues, ABCA7 mRNA expression was detected predominantly in myelo-lymphatic tissues.

Conclusions: Our finding that ABCA7 is regulated by cholesterol import and export in human macrophages suggests that this ABC transporter may be involved in macrophage lipid metabolism.

References

1. Bodzioch et al., Nat Gen 1999; 22:347—435
2. Klucken et al., Proc Natl Acad Sci USA 2000
3. Orso et al., Nat Gen 2000

A cholesterol-lowering gene maps to chromosome 13Q

H. Knoblauch[1], B. Müller-Myhsok[2], A. Busjahn[1], L. Ben Avi[3], H. Schuster[1], F.C. Luft[1], E. Leftersdorf[3]. *[1]Franz Volhard Clinic and Max Delbrück Center for Molecular Medicine; [2]Bernhard Nocht Institute for Tropical Medicine, Hamburg, Germany; [3]The Center for Research, Prevention, and Treatment of Atherosclerosis; Department of Medicine, Hadassah University Hospital, Jerusalem, Israel*

Objective: To map a putative Cholesterol-lowering gene in a large Arab family.

Methods: We studied an Arab family with familial hypercholesterolemia (FH) in which certain relatives with a mutated LDL receptor gene have normal or minimally elevated LDL levels. Certain homozygous FH individuals have LDL levels similar to heterozygous FH persons. Furthermore, part of the non-FH family members display lower than normal LDL levels. We performed a genome wide search and used parametric as well as non-parametric linkage analysis.

Results: We identified a locus on the long arm of chromosome 13 defined by markers D13S156 and D13S158 linked to the LDL-cholesterol lowering phenotype by means of an affected sibpair analysis and parametric linkage analysis. We extended our study and performed a multipoint quantitative-trait (QTL) linkage analysis and verified this locus as a QTL for LDL levels within this family. To test the relevance of this QTL in an independent normal population we then performed an IBD linkage analysis on healthy young DZ twins from the German population with markers at the 13q locus. We found strong evidence for linkage at this locus with LDL ($p < 0.0002$), HDL ($p < 0.004$), total cholesterol ($p < 0.0002$), and body mass index ($p < 0.0001$).

Conclusions: These data provide further support for the existence of a new gene influencing lipid concentrations in man.

A genome-wide scan for low HDL-cholesterol in genetically isolated Finnish families with premature coronary heart disease

H. Lilja[1], A. Soro[2], P. Pajukanta[1], K. Ylitalo[2], Ilpo Nuotio[3], Jorma Viikad[3], M-R. Taskinen[2], L. Peltonen[1]. *[1]Department of Human Genetics, University of California, Los Angeles, USA; [2]Department of Medicine, University of Helsinki; and [3]Department of Medicine, University of Turku, Finland*

Background: Low HDL-C is one of the most important risk factors for CHD. At least 50% of the variation in the HDL levels is seems to be genetically. determined. Identification of major genes affecting this trait would provide basis for the characterization of the molecular pathogenesis of CHD.

Objective: To use a genome-wide scan to identify major loci for low HDL-C using families with multiple affecteds collected from the genetically isolated population of Finland.

Methods: 25 well documented Finnish pedigrees with premature CHD and isolated low HDL-C. Inclusion criteria for the probands were: Age of 30–60 years, angiographically or clinically verified CHD and HDL-C level below the: age and sex specific 10 th population percentile. The genome scan was performed using 388 informative multiallelic markers with average marker to marker interval of 7.5 cM (modified Weber set 9.0). A total of 176 individuals, including 83 affected family members, were genotyped and both parametric and non-parametric linkage and affected sib pair methods were adapted for statistical analyses.

Results and Conclusions: A total of seven chromosomal regions were identified to reveal a pairwise LOD score > 1.0, one of them being the region of the ATP-binding cassette transporter 1 gene on chromosome 9. We are currently performing fine mapping of these chromosomal regions with markers providing an average intermarker interval of 2 cM to obtain conclusive evidence for the involvement of some of these loci in the genetic predisposition to low HDL-C.

Fine mapping of the human familial combined hyperlipidemia locus on chromosome 1q21-q23 using conserved synteny to the mouse locus on chromosome 3

P. Pajukanta, J. Bodnar, Michael Chu, Qunong Xiao, A.J. Lusis, L. Peltonen. *Dept of Human Genetics, UCLA, Los Angeles, California, USA*

Objective: Familial combined hyperlipidemia (FCHL) is a complex disorder predisposing to coronary heart disease. To identify the first human FCHL gene mapped to chromosome 1q21–q23, we restricted the syntenic mouse region on chromosome 3 and defined the borders of the syntenically conserved region between human and mouse.

Methods and Results: The interval containing the mouse gene *Hyplip1*, the potential mouse homolog for the 1q21–q23 FCHL gene, was originally about 3.5 cM. Recombinations observed in F2 animals from a large interspecific intercross between strain HcB-19/*Dem*, carrying the *Hyplip1* mutation, and strain *Mus musculus castaneus* helped us to restrict the critical interval between markers *D3Mit157* and *D3Mit76*, a distance of 1.8 cM. Importantly, this localization confirms the regional synteny to chromosome 1q21–q23 where the first human FCHL locus was mapped in Finnish families. We also constructed a physical contig of bacterial artificial chromosomes (BACs) across the most probable *Hyplip1* region surrounding *D3Mit101* which shows the highest evidence of linkage. By sequencing the ends of these mouse BACs, we identified three known genes and five new mouse genes. We are currently identifying single nucleotide polymorphisms (SNPs) in the human homologues of these genes and in genes nearby on chromosome 1q21–q23 to monitor for linkage disequilibrium in Finnish FCHL families.

Conclusions: The mouse *Hyplip1* gene is restricted to a region syntenic to human chromosome 1q21-q23. Further studies are warranted to identify the gene resulting in FCHL.

Prevention of CVD

Global mandate in CVD prevention: from molecules to markets

A.D. Mbewu. *Medical Research Council, Cape Town, South Africa*

A major component of the process of globalisation sweeping across the planet is the consolidation of the pharmaceutical industry with widening "knowledge gap" between them rich and poor countries. This is accompanied by a resurgence of small biotechnology companies whose explosive growth parallels that of startups in the telecommunications and information technology sectors.

To ameliorate (and even exploit) this commercial trend of globalisation, research agencies, donors and industry itself are forming global alliances to ensure that, not only are drugs and vaccines developed for the diseases that affect developing countries, but that these agents when they reach market are affordable for these countries.

Particular challenges for these initiatives lie in the realm of public health law, particularly international trade law as pertains to the World Trade Organisation and the TRIPS agreements.

Global alliances for cardiovascular prevention provide leadership and coordination of efforts in for example health advocacy (such as the Tobacco Free Initiative); and research and development (such as the this Cardiovascular Health Initiative in Developing Countries initiative). There is little doubt that the world will become an increasingly unpredictable and exciting place to live in new millenium; with unimagineable possibilities for mankind to transform his body, his mind and his environment.

Conventional risk factors: evolving concepts of risk and expanding strategies for prevention

B. Ncal, S. MacMahon. *Institute for International Health, Sydney, New South Wales, Australia*

The importance of the conventional risk factors for cardiovascular disease is widely underestimated. The principal reasons for this are twofold. First, random and systematic errors in the measurement of risk factors such as cholesterol, blood pressure and smoking result in substantial underestimates of the strengths of the associations. And second, the arbitrary division of risk factor levels into normal and abnormal levels (when many associations are actually continuous) fails to take account of the effects of risk factors in the large proportion of most populations. The conventional risk factors are therefore likely to have stronger effects on risk in a much larger proportion of the population than is typically recognised. As a consequence of this, many at-risk individuals may well have been denied potentially lifesaving preventive interventions. Preventive strategies that recognise the true strengths of the associations between risk factors and disease and interventions that are based upon an individual's absolute disease risk (rather than a single risk factor level) may prove to be more effective and efficient. Identification of the most cost-effective means for disease prevention is particularly important for low-income countries since they suffer most of the burden of cardiovascular disease. In such countries, resources for the prevention of cardiovascular disease are scarce and the selective implementation of the most efficient strategies will be essential. New studies to determine the best mechanisms for the implementation of established low-cost interventions, within the constraints imposed by the limited resources available in low-income countries, are required.

High apolipoprotein (apo) B and low apoA-i improve the prediction of fatal myocardial infarction at all levels of cholesterol and triglycerides — mortality data from the amoris (apolipoprotein-related mortality risk) study

G. Walldius[1], I. Jungner[2], I. Holme[3], A. Aastveit[4], W. Kolar[2], E. Steiner[2]. [1]King Gustaf V Research Institute, Stockholm and AstraZeneca; [2]CALAB Research, Stockholm, Sweden; [3]Institute for Medical Statistics, Ulleval Sykehus, Oslo; and [4]Agricultural University, As, Norway

Objective: To evaluate the importance of apoB (reflecting atherogenic particles LDL, VLDL and IDL) and apoA-I (anti-atherogenic particles) in predicting fatal acute myocardial infarction (AMI).

Methods: In 98,722 males and 76,831 females (< 20 to > 80 years old) examined 1985–1996 at health controls total cholesterol (TC), total triglycerides (TG), apoB and apoA-I (automated im. turb. method, fresh serum, acc. to WHO-IFCC) were measured. After a mean follow-up of 67 months 864 males and 359 females died in AMI.

Results: A high apoB and a low apoA-I were stronger risk factors than TC in both males and females below and over 70 yrs (age standardized, univariate analysis). Similarly TG was a strong risk factor both in males and even stronger in females. When adjusting AMI risk for age, TC and TG there still remained a highly significant and graded increase in risk ratios of 3–9 times for those with highest apoB and lowest apoA-I levels as compared to those with lowest apoB and highest apoA-I values. The ratio apoB/apoA-I summarizes the additional risk over and above that of TC and TG at all lipid levels. Similar findigs were obtained for both males and females irrespective of age.

Conclusions: By measuring both apoB and apoA-I, which are easily standardized, automated and insensitive to dietary variation, the predictivity of AMI is considerably increased. These measurements may help to select out those at highest/lowest risk at all lipid levels and may therefore be useful in clinical practice when deciding upon lipid lowering therapy.

Relations of lipoprotein subclass levels and ldl size to reduction in coronary atherosclerosis in the PLAC I trial

R. Rosenson[1], I. Shalaurova[2], J. Otvos[3]. [1]Rush-Presbyterian-St. Luke's Medical Center, Chicago, Illinois; [2]LipoMed, Inc., Raleigh, North Carolina; and [3]North Carolina State University, Raleigh, North Carolina, USA

Objective: To evaluate the influence of pravastatin therapy mon coronary atherosclerosis in subjects who have predominantly large LDL (pattern A, LDL size > 20.6 nm) or small LDL (pattern B, LDL size < 20.5 nm).

Methods: Frozen plasma samples were analyzed from a subset of participants in the PLAC I trial at baseline and after 6 months treatment with pravastatin (n = 119) or placebo (n = 104). Lipids, lipoprotein subclasses, and mean LDL and HDL particle size were measured by NMR spectroscopy. The primary angiographic endpoint was change in minimum lumen diameter (MLD).

Results: In the placebo group, subjects classified as pattern B at baseline had MLD that decreased more than pattern A (0.09 vs. 0.04 mm/y, p = 0.05). As compared to placebo, pravastatin limited atherosclerosis progression in the entire treatment group (0.02 vs. 0.06 mm/y; p = 0.003), and this response was greater for pattern B (0.02 vs. 0.09 mm/y; p = 0.008) as compared to pattern A subjects (0.01 vs. 0.04 mm/y; p = 0.11). For the whole group, progression was correlated positively with on-trial levels of intermediate-size VLDL (p = 0.01), total cholesterol (p = 0.009), LDL cholesterol (p = 0.003), LDL particles (p = 0.0004), small LDL (p = 0.003) and small HDL (p = 0.01). A negative associations was observed for HDL size (p = 0.03).

Conclusions: (1) LDL pattern B subjects have more coronary atherosclerosis progression than pattern A subjects; (2) pravastatin reduces progression rates in both pattern A and B subjects, but more in pattern B; (3) LDL and HDL particle size and subclass levels are important predictors of coronary atherosclerosis progression.

Moderate physical exercise prevents carbohydrate-induced hypertriglyceridaemia and accumulation of postprandial chylomicron remnants

C. Koutsari[1], F. Karpe[2], S.M. Humphreys[2], A.E. Hardman[1]. *[1]Human Muscle Metabolism Group, Loughborough University; and [2]Oxford Lipid Metabolism Group, University of Oxford, UK*

Background: Low-fat, high-carbohydrate (CHO) diets are associated with elevation of fasting and postprandial plasma triglyceride (TG) concentrations as well as accumulation of atherogenic small dense LDL.

Objectives: To investigate (i) whether moderate physical exercise can prevent the high CHO diet-induced increase in postprandial lipaemia and (ii) the underlying mechanisms by studying the effect on postprandial apo B-48 and B-100 concentrations in the triglyceride-rich lipoproteins (TRL).

Methods: Eight healthy, normolipidaemic, postmenopausal women aged 60 ± 4 years underwent oral fat-tolerance tests in a random order 1) after 3 days on a diet with 35%, 50% and 15% of energy (E) derived from CHO, fat and protein, respectively, 2) after 3 days on a high-CHO diet (70 E%, 15 E% and 15 E%, respectively) and 3) after 3 days on the same high-CHO diet and daily 60 minute sessions of brisk walking. ApoB-48 and B-100 concentrations were measured in the fasting and postprandial TRL fraction by quantitative SDS-PAGE.

Results: The increase in plasma TG concentration (fasting +59% and postprandial +36%, both p<0.01) induced by the high-CHO diet compared with the high fat diet was significantly attenuated by exercise. In the fasting state there was a marked accumulation of TRLs containing apo B-100 (+296%, p<0.01) after consuming the high-CHO diet without exercise compared with the high fat diet. This effect was normalised by exercise. The high-CHO diet induced a significant accumulation of postprandial TRLs containing apo B-48 compared with the high fat diet (+111%, p<0.05), which was completely normalised by the exercise.

Conclusions: Elevation of postprandial lipaemia due to high-CHO diets may be explained by expansion of the fasting VLDL pool. This in turn could increase the competition of these particles with chylomicrons postprandialty. The CHO-induced increase in chylomicron remnants was entirely prevented by moderate exercise.

Comparison of a mediterranean (med) diet to low fat (lf) diet on lipids in patients (pts) with coronary heart disease (chd)

D. Colquhoun[1], P. Glasziou[2], P. Horsley[3], S. Somerset[3], B. Gallagher[1], J. Weyers[1].
[1]Core Research Group; [2]University of Queensland; [3]Griffith University, for OLIVE Group, Brisbane, Australia

Objective: To compare LF to Med diet effects on lipids and major lipoproteins in pts with CHD on statin therapy.

Method: 68 patients with CHD documented by coronary angiography were randomised to LF (20–25% energy (E) from fat and 8–10% saturated) or Med (35–40% E from fat and > 50% of fat being monounsaturated). Lipids were measured prior to lipid lowering drug therapy, at randomisation ($\times 2$) and 3 mths ($\times 2$).

Results: At randomisation and 3 months 86% patients LF and 80% patients Med were on statins. Similarly, 80% LF and 85% Med pts were taking aspirin.

	Pre Statin (LF & Med)	LF (n = 34)		Med (n = 34)	
		Week 0	3 months	Week 0	3 months
Cholesterol	6.59	4.48	4.44	4.43	4.34
Triglycides	2.81	1.59	1.63	1.48	1.38
HDL-C	1.18	1.11	1.17	1.17	1.2
LDL-C	3.92	2.61	2.51	2.58	2.46

Conclusion: A Med diet is as efficacious for lipid management as a LF diet in pts with CHD on statin therapy. Current dietary recommendations for CHD could consider a Med diet as a treatment and preventative dietary option. This would extend choice for pts and possibly enhance adherence.

Intracellular lipid metabolism

Multiple roles of cholesterol in hedgehog signaling

Philip A. Beachy. *Johns Hopkins University/Howard Hughes Medical Institute Baltimore, Maryland, USA*

The cellular responses elicited by the Hedgehog (Hh) family of secreted signaling proteins play an important role in the growth and patterning of multicellular embryos, from insects to man. The loss or attenuation of Hh signaling can lead to severe birth defects, such as cyclopia, limb deformities, and absence of the axial skeleton. Inappropriate activation of Hh signaling pathways in contrast is associated with neoplastic growth, as in basal cell carcinoma, one of the most common forms of human cancer.

The role of cholesterol in the Hedgehog signaling pathway first became apparent several years ago upon the discovery that, in the presence of cholesterol, the C-terminal domain of Hedgehog executes an autoproteolytic cleavage reaction. This reaction results in attachment of cholesterol to the N-terminal fragment, the fragment active in signaling. This covalent cholesterol-peptide product adheres to the signaling cell so as to localize the signal and produce spatially patterned responses in tissues such as the spinal cord, where differentiation into distinct neuronal types is exquisitely sensitive to the level of Hh pathway activation.

In addition to its role in Hedgehog biogenesis, pharmacologic and genetic studies suggest that cholesterol has a distinct role in cellular response to the Hedgehog signal. Treatment of laboratory animals with synthetic compounds that interfere with cholesterol biosynthesis and/or transport causes cyclopia and other birth defects that are reminiscent of severe holoprosencephaly in humans. In addition, cyclopamine and related steroidal alkaloids from plants have long been known to cause cyclopia. Finally, several genetic perturbations of cholesterol transport and synthesis are associated with various birth defects including an abnormally high incidence of holoprosencephaly. In our studies of these perturbations of cholesterol homeostasis, we have demonstrated that both natural and synthetic teratogens produce birth defects by inhibiting Hedgehog protein signaling, acting at the level of cells' ability to respond to the Hedgehog signal. Although the precise mechanism by which these compounds block cellular response to the Hedgehog signal is not resolved, we are utilizing cultured cell studies to identify the cellular targets of these compounds and to understand how Hedgehog signaling is affected.

Apolipoprotein A-I stimulates transport of intracellular cholesterol to cell surface caveolae

Dmitri Sviridov, Noel Fidge, Christopher Fielding. *Baker Medical Research Institute, Melbourne, Australia; and Cardiovascular Research Institute, University of California, San Francisco, USA*

The effect of lipid-free human plasma apolipoprotein A-I (apoA-I) on the transport of newly synthesized cholesterol to cell-surface caveolae in human skin fibroblasts was studied. Changes in transport of newly synthesized cholesterol were assessed after labeling cells with [14C]acetate at 15C, warming cells to allow transfer of cholesterol, followed by selective oxidation of cholesterol in caveolae prior to their partial purification. ApoA-I, but not bovine serum albumin added in an equimolar concentration, enhanced transport of cholesterol to the caveolae up to 5-fold in a dose- and time-dependent manner. Stimulation of cholesterol trafficking was independent of cholesterol efflux. Transport of cholesterol to the cell surface in general was not affected by apoA-I.

Methyl-beta-cyclodextrin, added at a concentration promoting cholesterol efflux to the same extent as apoA-I, also stimulated cholesterol trafficking, but was 3 times less effective than apoA-I. Progesterone inhibited transport of newly synthesized cholesterol to the caveolae. Treatment of cells with apoA-I stimulated the expression of caveolin, increasing the amount of caveolin mRNA by about 40% and the amount of caveolin protein by about 60%. We conclude that apoA-I induces transport of intracellular cholesterol to cell surface caveolae, possibly in part through stimulation of caveolin expression.

Biosynthesis of lipoproteins

H.N. Ginsberg[1], J-S. Liang[1], M. Pan[1], D. Mitchell[2], M. Zhou[1], R. Pariyarath[2], E.A. Fisher[2]. [1]Columbia University, New York; [2]Mt. Sinai School of Medicine, New York City, New York, USA

Apolipoprotein B (apoB) lipoproteins carry the bulk of triglyceride (TG) and cholesteryl esters (CE) in plasma, and have atherogenic potential. ApoB is essential for the assembly and secretion of apoB lipoproteins, and the biosynthesis of these lipoproteins in hepatocytes has been extensively examined during the past 20 years. It is clear from these studies that apoB is a very unusual secretory protein in that it has very hydrophobic sequences that seem to interact with the translocation (T) channel (C) of the endoplasmic reticulum (ER) so that T is can be very slow or even stop, leaving nascent apoB in a bitopic orientation in the TC and exposing domains of apoB to the cytosol. Cytosolic apoB interacts with heat shock protein-70, facilitating ubiquitination and proteasomal degradation of the protein. The proteasomal degradation occurs co- or post-translationally while apoB is still in the TC and associated with Sec61. In the presence of adequate TG or CE, the T of nascent apoB is more efficient and less proteasomal degradation occurs. The effects of core lipids on T depends on the presence of microsomal triglyceride transfer protein (MTP). The resulting partially lipidated apoB lipoprotein can later accumulate additional lipid by MTP independent pathways. This may occur by fusion of the partially lipidated apoB lipoprotein with a lipid droplet already in the ER.

Intracellular lipidation of ApoB

S.-O. Olofsson, L. Asp, P. Stillemark, K. Lindberg, C. Claesson, M. Rutberg, D. Marchesan, J. Borén. Dept. Medical Biochemistry University of Göteborg, Sweden

ApoB acquires lipids in at least two steps during the formation of VLDL. The first step occurs cotranslationally and is terminated shortly after the completion of the molecule. The product is a partially lipidated VLDL-precursor. This VLDL precursor acquires the major amount of lipids in the second step, forming VLDL. The assembled VLDL is first observed in a non-Rough ER compartment suggesting that the second step occur outside Rough ER. VLDL particles isolated from the microsomal lumen contains a network of chaperons (BiP, PDI, GRP 94, Calreticulin and CaBP2), indicating an ongoing protein folding process also when the VLDL-precursor is converted to VLDL. Investigation of the relation between the length of apoB and the efficiency of the second step demonstrated that this efficiency increased dramatically when apoB reached the length of apoB 48, indicating that the last portion of apoB-48 contains sequences of importance for the second step. The second step can be inhibited by Brefeldin A. A similar inhibition was also observed when a GDP restrictive mutant of ARF1 (T31N) was transiently over-expressed in McA RH 7777 cells, indicating that ARF 1 is involved in the regulation of the second step. A cell free system carrying out the second step was developed and used to follow the signal from ARF1 to the VLDL assembly. Brefeldin A inhibited the VLDL assembly also in the cell free system. Moreover such an inhibition was also observed when a synthetic polypeptide corresponding to the N-terminal 17 aa of ARF was included in the incubation. Together these results strengthen the conclusion that ARF1 regulated the VLDL assembly. Using the cell free system, we could demonstrate that an ARF1 dependent activation of Phospholipase D and the subsequent formation of phosphatidic acid were essential for the VLDL assembly.

Insulin, PI 3-Kinase and apolipoprotein B biogenesis

J. Sparks, A. Wagner, T. Phung, C. Sparks. *University of Rochester, Rochester, New York, USA*

Insulin action inhibits the secretion of very low density lipoprotein (VLDL) by liver through a mechanism that favors the degradation of freshly synthesized apo B. A direct action of post-receptor signaling molecules on an "apo B-specific" process is implicated because of the selectivity of the insulin effect for apo B.

Our recent findings indicate that the insulin effect on apo B requires the activation of phosphatidylinositide 3-kinase (PI 3-K). A role for PI 3-K in effects on apo B is further strengthened by the following new findings. 1) p85, the regulatory subunit of PI 3-K, cross-links to apo B in situ using a cell permeant, cross-linking agent, indicating that apo B is within 12 A of PI 3-K. 2) Incubation of hepatocytes with IL-4, but not EGF, mimics insulin effects supporting that an insulin receptor substrate is a likely intermediate in signal transduction. 3) The S6-kinase inhibitor, rapamycin is unable to block insulin-mediated effects on apo B secretion suggesting effects are not related to transcriptional events. 4) Label incorporation studies support that apo B degradation is accompanied by inhibition of B100 synthesis. The inhibition of B100 translation occurs even when cotranslational degradation is inhibited by pre-incubation of hepatocytes with lactacysin, a specific proteasomal inhibitor.

The significance of insulin-mediated suppression of hepatic apo B secretion is that the process most likely reduces hepatic VLDL secretion during the time interval that intestinal triglyceride-rich lipoproteins are being secreted. The inhibition thereby minimizes competition of VLDL and chylomicrons for catabolic pathways modulating post-prandial hypertriglyceridemia.

Internalization of apolipoprotein e by hepatocytes via the ldl receptor is coupled to retroendocytosis

P.C.N. Rensen[1], M.C. Jong[2], L.C. van Vark[2], H. van der Boom[2], W.L. Hendriks[2], T.J.C. van Berkel[1], E.A.L. Biessen[1], L.M. Havekes[2]. *[1]Div. Biopharmaceutics, LACDR, Leiden University; and [2]TNO-Prevention and Health, Gaubius Laboratory, Leiden, The Netherlands*

ApoE plays a key role in the LDLr-mediated uptake of triglyceride (TG)-rich lipoproteins and emulsions by the liver, but the intracellular pathway of apoE following particle internalization is poorly defined. In the present study, we investigated whether retroendocytosis is a unique feature of apoE as compared to apoB by studying the intracellular fate of VLDL-sized apoE-containing emulsions and LDL after LDLr-mediated uptake. Incubation of HepG2 cells with [^{3}H]cholesteryl oleate (CO)-labeled particles at 37°C led to rapid hydrolysis of [^{3}H]CO within 30 min for both LDL and emulsions. In contrast, emulsion-derived ^{125}I-apoE was more resistant to degradation (onset $\geqslant$ 120 min) than LDL-derived ^{125}IapoB $\leqslant$ 30 min). Incubation at 18°C, which allows endodomal uptake but prevents lysosomal degradation, followed by a heparin wash and subsequent incubation at 37°C resulted in a time-dependent release of intact apoE from the cells, as shown by nonreducing SDS-PAGE. The apoE release was accelerated by the presence of HDL (26% of internalised apoE at 4 h). Retroendocytosis of intact particles could be excluded since little intact [^{3}H]CO was released ($<$ 3%). In contrast, the degradation of LDL was complete with virtually no secretion of intact apoB into the medium. The intracellular stability of apoE was also demonstrated after hepatic uptake in C57BI/6 mice. Intravenous injection of ^{125}I-apoE and [^{3}H]CO-labeled emulsions resulted in efficient LDLr-mediated uptake of both components by the liver (45—50% after 20 min). At 1 h after injection, only 15—20% of the hepatic ^{125}I-apoE was degraded whereas 75% of the [^{3}H]CO was hydrolysed. From these date we conclude that following LDLr-mediated internalization by liver cells, apoE can escape lysosomal degradation and can be secreted intactly. This sequence of events may allow apoE to participate in intracellular lipid trafficking and VLDL assembly.

Proliferation and differentiation of smooth muscle cells

Coronary smooth muscle differentiation from proepicardial cells

M. Majesky, T. Landerholm, J. Lu, X.-R. Dong, P.-T. Ku. *Baylor College of Medicine, Houston, Texas, USA*

Lineage maps in vertebrate embryos indicate that the vascular system is a mosaic structure made up of different types of smooth muscle cells (SMCs) that arise from independent embryonic origins. Guided by these lineage maps, we isolated committed progenitors for coronary SMCs from the proepicardial organ (PEO) of HH17 quail embryos and studied their differentiation in vitro. We found that the default pathway for PEO differentiation was cytokeratin-positive epicardial cells. By contrast, exposure to endothelial-derived factors (PDGF-BB, TGF-β1, desert hedgehog) produced epicardial to mesenchymal transformation (EMT) and stepwise differentiation to coronary SMCs. SMC differentiation was strictly dependent on intact rhoA/p160-rho kinase (p160ROCK) signaling and required transcriptionally active serum response factor (SRF). To test the role of rhoA-p160ROCK signaling in coronary wall formation in vivo, we prepared chick-quail chimeric embryos by grafting gene-modified quail PEOs into the pericardial coelom of HH17 host chick embryos. Hearts and coronary vessels were examined 10d later. Chick hearts that received vehicle-treated quail PEOs were indistinguishable from native hearts. By contrast, chick hearts that received quail PEOs pretreated with inhibitors of rhoA-p160ROCK signaling had few, if any, coronary SMCs and exhibited a hypoplastic myocardial wall. QCPN-positive quail nuclei were largely absent from the subepicardial and myocardial layers of chick hearts that received rhoA-p160ROCK-inhibited quail PEOs, indicating a failure of epicardial cells to complete EMT at the surface of the heart. These finding suggest that formation of coronary SMCs from proepicardial cells in vivo requires signaling via rhoA-p160ROCK, and that epicardial-derived cells are required in multiple ways for normal heart development.

Role of diverse plaque smooth muscle cells in atherosclerotic progression

L.D. Adams, S.M. Schwartz. *Dept. of Pathology, University of Washington, Seattle, Washington, USA*

Langerhans suggested that a special set of smooth muscle cells (SMC) contribute to the atherosclerotic plaque. PCR methods show that the smooth muscle cells of the fibrous cap of the atherosclerotic plaque are clonal. These clones probably arise early since focal intimal thickening (FIT) predicts the distribution of lesions in adults. Origins of the cells are unclear, possibly including blood borne cells or a unique intimal lineage.

A large number of genes have been identified as "marking" intimal cells by differential expression vs. medial smooth muscle. Most of these genes, however, are the reflection of activation — either by the inflamed state of the atherosclerotic plaque or by the processes involved in forming a neointima after injury.

To study this in a more systematic way, we have used array display to define genes that mark both the normal intima and the fibrous cap. Approximately 27,000 genes were studied. A subset of about 180 shows overexpression in the intima vs. the media while only two genes were overexpressed in the media over the intima. Surprisingly this set suggests an increase, rather than a decrease in intimal cell differentiation, including expression of one gene that is arterial specific. A further subset of about 78 genes mark the fibrous cap from the intima. Again these are largely ESTs, suggesting that unique transcripts may define the clone that forms the atherosclerotic plaque.

The role of vascular smooth muscle cells in the development and progression of atherosclerosis

P.L. Weissberg. *Department of Medicine, University of Cambridge, UK*

Vascular smooth muscle cells (VSMC) exhibit remarkable phenotypic plasticity, making them capable of considerable functional diversity. Studies of VSMC gene expression during development have identified an early intrauterine commitment to VSMC-specific gene expression. During early post-natal vascular growth VSMCs express both contractile and matrix proteins and in the mature adult they express predominantly contractile proteins. Following vascular injury, and in response to the development of an atherosclerotic plaque, VSMCs re-express a similar pattern of gene expression to that seen in early post-natal growth, consistent with a reparative role. Indeed, the change from contractile to "repair" phenotype, far from being detrimental, as was once thought, is essential for the synthesis and maintenance of the fibrous cap. However, VSMCs in the fibrous cap appear to undergo further phenotypic changes in that they become senescent and inherently susceptibility to apoptosis. Since clinical outcome in atherosclerosis is determined by the dynamic balance between the destructive influence of inflammatory cells and the reparative capacity of intimal VSMCs, it is likely that by understanding the molecular regulation of VSMC gene expression it may be possible to manipulate VSMC phenotype to promote and maintain plaque stability.

Fibronectin activates the p42/44 map kinase cascade and facilitates cell cycle entry of smooth muscle cells in primary culture

J. Roy, M. Kazi, J. Thyberg, U. Hedin. *Division of Vascular Surgery, Karolinska Hospital, Stockholm, Sweden*

Objectives: Rat arterial injury is accompanied by an accumulation of fibronectin (FN) around smooth muscle cells (SMCs). In order to elucidate the role of FN in SMC activation, we studied the effect of FN on the expression of Cyclin D1, Cyclin A, p27^{KIP1}, and Rb protein and on the activation of the p42/44 mitogen-activated protein kinase (MAPK) cascade.

Methods: SMCs were enzymatically isolated from rat aortas, seeded on FN and cultured under serum-free conditions for up to 6 days. Some of the cultures were stimulated with serum for 24 h. After regular time intervals, samples were prepared for immunoblotting and immunocytochemistry.

Results: There was a gradual increase in Cyclin D1 and p27^{KIP1} expression during the 6-day period of culture. However, the expression of Cyclin A and hyperphosphorylation of the Rb protein required serum stimulation. We also detected phosphorylated ERK1 and ERK2 throughout the culture period.

Conclusions: FN facilitates the cell cycle entry of quiescent SMCs into the G1 phase of the cell cycle, but further progression into the S-phase is mitogen-dependent. Furthermore, there was a distinct pattern of sustained MAPK phosphorylation that differs significantly from growth factor induced MAPK activation. Our results suggest that FN plays a permissive role for the action of growth factors on SMC proliferation after arterial injury.

Rho-associated kinase regulates migration and proliferation of vascular smooth muscle cells both in vitro and in vivo

N. Sawada[1], H. Itoh[1], K. Ueyama[2], J. Yamashita[1], T.-H. Chun[1], M. Inoue[1], K. Masatsugu[1], T. Saito[1], S. Sakaguchi[1], M. Sone[1], M. Komeda[2], K. Nakao[1]. *Depts. of [1]Cardiovascular Surgery and [2]Medicine and Clinical Science, Kyoto University Grad. Sch. of Med., Kyoto, Japan*

Objective: Rho-associated kinase (ROCK), a putative effector of small GTPase Rho, has been shown to mediate the calcium sensitization of vascular smooth muscle cells (VSMCs) and play a key role in the pathogenesis of hypertension. However its role in vascular remodeling has remained unknown.

Methods: We examined the effect of a newly-developed specific ROCK inhibitor, Y-27632 (0–10 µM), on migration and proliferation of cultured human aortic SMCs in vitro and on neointimal formation of balloon-injured rat carotid arteries in vivo (Wistar rats, 14–16 weeks).

Results: [1] Y-27632 dose-dependently suppressed PDGF-BB- and LPA-induced VSMC migration. Both Y-27632 treatment and overexpression of dominant negative ROCK inhibited PDGF-BB, LPA and serum-induced DNA synthesis of VSMCs. In Y-27632-treated VSMCs, mitogen-induced tyrosine phosphorylation of FAK and paxillin was blocked. Serum-induced deprivation of CDKI cip1 and kip1 was attenuated by Y-27632. [2] Systemic administration of Y-27632 (35–70 mg/kg/day) via osmotic pumps started three days prior to injury and decreased systolic blood pressure by 20 mmHg. Fourteen days post-injury, in Y-27632-administered rats, neointimal formation was dramatically reduced to 22% of the control rats (Intima/media ratio; 0.20 ± 0.08, Y-27632-treated rats vs. 0.90 ± 0.16, vehicle). ROCK activation in injured vessels was detected by the elevated phosphorylation of myosin phosphatase and myosin light chain.

Conclusion: Activation of ROCK underlies the pathogenesis of both hypertension and proliferative vascular disorders. Rho/ROCK blockade can be a common therapeutic strategy for hypertension and atherosclerosis.

Cell density determines apoptosis and cell cycle arrest in vascular smooth muscle cells in association with p21WAF1/CIP1

J. Ako, M. Yoshizumi, M. Akishita, S. Kim, M. Hashimoto, K. Iijima, N. Sudoh, Y.Q. Liang, T. Watanabe, Y. Ohike, K. Toba, Y. Ouchi. *Department of Geriatric Medicine, Graduate School of Medicine, The University of Tokyo, Tokyo, Japan*

There is a controversy about the fate of vascular smooth muscle cells (VSMC) treated with antioxidants, cell cycle arrest or apoptosis. We hypothesized that cell density affects the effect of antioxidants on VSMC.

Methods: Rat aortic smooth muscle cell s (RASMC) were cultured in DMEM with 10% FBS. RASMC were plated at two different concentrations, high cell density (HCD; 50,000/cm^2), and low cell density (LCD; 10,000/cm^2). Pyrrolidinedithiocarbamate (PDTC) was added to exponentially growing RASMC. Apoptotic change was examined using Hoechst 33258 under fluorescent microscopy. DNA synthesis was measured with [3H] thymidine incorporation.

Results: Incubation with 0.1 mM PDTC for 24 h induced apoptosis in RASMC in LCD confirmed by fluorescent staining with Hoechst 33258. In contrast, RASMC in HCD did not undergo apoptosis. The DNA synthesis decreased in a dose-dependent manner in both groups after 24-h incubation with PDTC (2.4% of control in LCD, 14.6% in HCD: 0.01 mM PDTC, 0.6% in LCD, 2.8% in HCD: 0.1 mM). In HCD, the down-regulation of DNA synthesis was reversible after the removal of PDTC. However, DNA synthesis did not resume in LCD due to induction of apoptosis. The expression of cyclin D1 and cyclin A did not change significantly in either LCD or HCD. A potent cdk inhibitor, p21WAF1/CIP1, was expressed as early as 8 h after the treatment of PDTC only in HCD. p21 WAF1/CIP1 was not expressed in LCD after PDTC treatment.

Conclusion: Cell density may be a key regulator of PDTC-induced apoptosis in VSMC, and the expression of p21WAF1/CIP1 is associated with PDTC-induced cell cycle arrest.

The heparan sulfate chains on perlecan affects smooth muscle cell adhesion and spreading when co-coated with fibronectin

K. Lundmark[1], P.K. Tran[1], U. Hedin[1], A.W. Clowes[2], T.N. Wight[2]. *[1]Divsion of Vascular Surgery, Karolinska Hospital, Stockholm, Sweden; and [2]University of Washington School of Medicine, Seattle, USA*

Objective: We work on the notion that composition of the basement membrane may play a key role in regulating smooth muscle cell (SMC) functions. In this study we have focused on how the heparan sulfate proteoglycan perlecan modifies the effect of fibronectin on cell-adhesion and morphology.

Methods: Matrices were prepared by co-coating fibronectin (FN) or laminin (LN) with either heparin (Hep), perlecan (PN), choindroitin sulfate (CS) or hyaluronan (HA). SMC were allowed to adhere to the substrate for 3 h before fixation, staining and quantification in an ELISA reader. SMC were also stained for actin and examined under light and interference reflection microscope.

Results: SMC adhesion to FN (10 µg/ml) was reduced in a dose-dependent manner by both PN and Hep. PN (2 µg/ml) and Hep (1 µg/ml) reduced adhesion by 70–90%. The presence of either PN or Hep also inhibited cell-spreading, stress fiber formation and development of focal contacts. Heparinase treatment of PN abolished these effects. PN and Hep did not inhibit SMC adhesion to LN (10 µg/ml). Other glycosaminoglycans such as CS and HA had no effects on adhesion and morphology of SMC plated on a FN- or LN-containing matrix.

Conclusion: Both the heparan sulfate chains of perlecan and heparin reduce cell-adhesion and spreading when co-coated with fibronectin.

Lipoprotein receptors

Complex genetic functions of the LDL receptor gene family

Joachim Herz. *Department of Molecular Genetics, UT Southwestern, Dallas, Texas, USA*

The low density lipoprotein (LDL) gene family represents a class of multifunctional cell surface receptors that is involved in the cellular uptake of biologically diverse ligands. Five members of this gene family are currently known, that control distinct physiological processes. For instance, the LDL receptor and the LDL receptor-related protein (LRP) work in concert to mediate the removal of cholesterol and triglyceride-containing lipoproteins by the liver and LRP also participates in the homeostasis of proteases and protease inhibitors. All members of the family are abundantly expressed in the brain where they bind ApoE, an integral component of several lipoproteins. Genetic association studies indicate that ApoE has important roles in neurodegenerative processes but the underlying mechanisms are presently not understood. We have recently described a molecular pathway by which neuronal ApoE receptors transmit signals across the plasma membrane, leading to the activation of intracellular signaling cascades. Signaling through this pathway may be altered in neurodegenerative disorders like Alzheimer disease. Similar signaling events may take place in other tissues, for instance the vascular wall, where the expression of lipoprotein receptors is highly regulated during atherogenesis.

Structure and function of the class B type I scavenger receptor, SR-BI, an HDL and LDL receptor which mediates selective lipid uptake

Monty Krieger. *Dept. of Biology, Massachusetts Institute of Technology, Massachusetts, USA*

The class B type I scavenger receptor, SR-BI, is a physiologically relevant, high affinity cell surface HDL receptor which mediates selective lipid uptake. It also binds LDL with high affinity. The mechanism of selective lipid uptake is fundamentally different from that of classic receptor-mediated uptake via coated pits and vesicles (e.g., the LDL receptor pathway) in that it involves efficient transfer of the lipids, but not the outer shell proteins, from HDL to cells. In mice, SR-BI (mSR-BI) plays a key role in determining the levels of plasma HDL cholesterol and in mediating the selective delivery of HDL-cholesterol to steroidogenic tissues and the liver. The structure, ligand binding properties and physiologic functions of SR-BI will be discussed.

Roles of ApoE receptors and their family

Tokuo Yamamoto. *Tohoku University Gene Research Center, Sendai, Japan*

ApoE plays a key role in the transportation and metabolism of plasma cholesterol and triacylglycerol. It is recognized by several receptors including the LDL receptor, LDL receptor related proteins, VLDL receptor (VLDLR), and apoE receptor 2 (apoER2). VLDLR and apoER2 consist of five common functional domains that resemble LDLR. Although they are structurally closely related, their expressions are completely different: VLDLR mRNA is abundant in heart and skeletal muscle, and apoER2 mRNA predominates in brain, but they are almost absent in the liver. In chicken, VLDLR is expressed almost exclusively in oocytes and mediates the uptake of yolk precursors, VLDL and vitellogenin. Chicken mutants lacking VLDLR are sterile and exhibit severe hyperlipidemia, demonstrating that VLDLR is crucial in nonmammalian vertebrate oogenesis. In contrast to nonmammalian vertebrates, mice lacking VLDLR exhibit modest decreases in body weight, body mass index and adipose tissue mass, while their plasma cholesterol levels, triacylglycerol levels, and lipoprotein profiles are not altered. Furthermore, knockout mice lacking both VLDLR and LDLR exhibit a modest hypercholesterolemia, whereas apoE knockout mice exhibit a profound hypercholesterolemia. These data suggests the presence of several apoE receptors. To identify these, we characterized several cDNAs containing the ligand-binding region. Our recent characterization on apoE receptors and their family proteins will be presented.

Intracellular trafficking — consequence of receptor mediated uptake of lipoproteins

U. Beisiegel, J. Heeren. *Medical Clinic, UKE, Hamburg, Germany*

Objective: To study the intracellular pathway of chylomicron remnant (CR) constituents after endocytosis by lipoprotein receptors, most probably by the LDL receptor-related protein (LRP).

Methods: Human chylomicrons were isolated from Apo C-II deficient patients and hydrolyzed in vitro by lipoprotein lipase (LpL) to obtain CR. The CR were labeled with iodine and used for biochemical studies (binding, uptake, degradation and recycling) in human hepatoma cells and human fibroblasts with and without LDL receptor (LDLR). In addition native CR and CR labeled with DiI (fluorescent phospholipid analogue) were incubated on the same cells for immunofluorescence analysis.

Results: The biochemical studies showed that apo E and apo C were not degraded, in contrast to LDL-apo B. The labeled apoproteins remained in the cell and apo E was detected within peripheral endosomal compartments. In the presence of HDL, as an extracellular acceptor, the radioactivity was re-secreted into the medium and labeled apo E was associated with HDL. The DiI-label, in contrast, was found in the lysosomal compartment. This intracellular pathway which leads to lipoprotein disassembly occurred in both LDLR positive and negative cells, suggesting that LRP is a candidate receptor for CR recycling.

Conclusions: The uptake of human CR, possibly via LRP, leads to the intracellular disassembly of the particles. The surface constituents, mainly apo E, are recycled when HDL is present as an extracellular acceptor.

TGF-β_1 increases the expression of lectine-like oxidized LDL receptor-1 (LOX-1)

M. Minami, N. Kume, H. Kataoka, M. Morimoto, T. Kita. *Department of Geriatric Medicine, Kyoto University, Kyoto, Japan*

Objective: LOX-1 is a novel membrane receptor for atherogenic oxidized LDL, which can be expressed by vascular endothelial cells and macrophages. We have examined whether TGF-β_1, which inhibits the expression of class A scavenger receptors in macrophages and plays crucial roles in vascular diseases including atherosclerosis, can induce expression of LOX- 1.

Methods: 1. Cultured bovine aortic endothelial (BAEC) or smooth muscle (BASMC) cells were treated with recombinant human TGF-β_1 (0.1—10 ng/ml), then immunoblot analyses and Northern blot analyses were performed. 2. After pretreatment with or without actinomycin D (2.5—5 µg/ml) for 30 min, BAEC or BASMC were treated with 1 ng/ml of TGF-β_1, then Northern blot analyses were performed. 3. Murine peritoneal macrophages were cultured overnight and treated with TGF-β_1 (0.1—10 ng/ml), and then Northern blot analyses were performed.

Results: 1. Immunoblot and Northern blot analyses showed that treatment with TGF-β_1 increased the expression of LOX-1 protein and mRNA in both BAEC and BASMC. Treatment with 1 ng/ml of TGF-β_1 for 8 h resulted in 4.2-fold and 2.8-fold increases in the amounts of LOX-1 protein in BAEC and BASMC, respectively. 2. Pretreatment with actinomycin D completely abolished LOX-1 mRNA induction elicited by TGF-β_1, suggesting that TGF-β_1 may stimulate transcription of the LOX-1 gene. 3. TGF-β_1 also induced LOX-1 expression in murine peritoneal macrophages in a dose- and time-dependent fashion; treatment with 10 ng/ml of TGF-β.1 for 4 hours resulted in a 4.7-fold increase in the amount of LOX-1 mRNA.

Conclusions: TGF-β_1 can highly induce LOX-1 expression in vascular endothelial cells, smooth muscle cells and macrophages. TGF-β_1 appears one of the key regulators that can modulate the expression of scavenger receptors.

Very-low-density lipoprotein receptor deficient mice are protected against diet-induced obesity and insulin resistance

J.R. Goudriaan[1], M.C. Jong[1], V.E.H. Dahlmans[1], P.J. Tacken[2], L.M. Havekes[1].
[1]Gaubius Lab; and [2]Leiden Univ Med Centre, Leiden, Netherlands

Objective: To investigate whether very-low-density lipoprotein receptor deficient (VLDLR−/−) mice develop a clear phenotype when fed a high-fat diet.

Methods: Homozygous knockout male mice that lack the VLDL receptor and wild-type littermates were fed a high-fat diet (HF; 46% of the calories are provided by corn oil) for a period of 17 weeks. Their body weight, food intake, plasma insulin, lipid, and ketone levels, glucose tolerance, intestinal fat absorption and the fatty acid composition of liver, heart, muscle and fat tissues were measured.

Results: After 17 weeks on the HF diet, VLDLR−/− mice showed a slight increase in their body weight (from 25.3 ± 2.3 g to 29.7 ± 4.8 g), whereas wild-type littermates became obese (from 28.7 ± 1.6 g to 44.1 ± 5.7 g). No differences were observed with respect to food intake. Furthermore, after 17 weeks of HF feeding, VLDLR−/− mice exhibited significant lower plasma insulin levels as compared to wild-type mice (1.3 ± 0.8 vs. 4.6 ± 2.5 ng/ml) and were able to clear an intraperitoneal injected glucose bolus more rapidly than wild-type mice. These results clearly indicate that VLDLR−/− mice are protected against HF diet-induced insulin resistance. There were no significant differences found between VLDLR−/− mice and their controls with respect to plasma lipids, fatty acid oxidation (ketone bodies), intestinal fat absorption or fatty acid tissue-composition.

Conclusion: In contrast to their wild-type littermates, VLDLR−/− mice do not become obese, nor insulin resistant after 17 weeks of high-fat feeding. These findings are indicative for a fundamental role of the VLDL receptor in the entry of fat-derived calories into tissues.

Evidence for the role of megalin in renal resorption of transthyretin

M.M. Sousa[1,2], A.G. Norden[3], C. Jacobsen[4], P.J. Verroust[5], S.K. Moestrup[4], M.J. Saraiva[1,2]. [1]Amyloid Unit, Instituto de Biologia Molecular e Celular; [2]Instituto de Ciências Biomédicas Abel Salazar, University of Porto, Portugal; [3]Department of Chemical Pathology, Chase Farm Hospitals Trust, Middlesex, UK; [4]Department of Medical Biochemistry, University of Aarrhus, Denmark; [5]Institut National de la Santé et de la Recherche Medicale, U489, Hopital Tenon, Paris, France

Megalin is expressed on the luminal surface of various epithelia including the renal proximal tubules. In the kidney it plays an important role in tubular uptake of macromolecules filtered through the glomerulus. By two-dimensional gel electrophoresis followed by mass spectrometry analysis we identified transthyretin (TTR) as an abundant protein in the urine of patients with renal tubule failure. TTR is a plasma protein that functions as a transporter of thyroxine and retinol. It was recently shown that by binding RBP, megalin has an essential role in transepithelial transport of retinol. It is possible that in vivo, megalin might also be responsible for the tubular resorption of TTR. To investigate this hypothesis we performed different TTR binding assays by surface plasmon ressonance (SPR) analysis and by using immortalized rat yolk sac cells with high expression levels of megalin. Binding of purified TTR, free as well as in complex with thyroxine or retinol, to immobilized megalin was shown by the SPR analysis. Radiolabeled TTR was rapidly taken up by cultured cells and the uptake was partially inhibited by a polyclonal megalin antibody and by the receptor-associated protein (RAP), a chaperone-like protein inhibiting ligand binding to megalin and other LDLr family receptors. The present data indicate that TTR represents a novel megalin ligand of potential importance in the transepithelial transport of retinol and thyroxine.

Monogenic hyperlipidemia

Familial hypercholesterolemia: factors affecting phenotypic expression

Joep C. Defesche, Pernette de Sauvage Nolting, John J.P. Kastelein. *Department of Vascular Medicine, Academic Medical Centre, Amsterdam, The Netherlands*

Aim: To assess the contribution of genetic variants in several genes to the phenotypic expression of Familial Hypercholesterolemia (FH).

Method: Genetic analysis by conventional PCR in a well-defined and well-documented cohort of patients with FH.

Results: Specific mutations in the low-density lipoprotein receptor (LDL-R) gene were associated with mildly elevated LDL-cholesterol levels (below P95), while other mutations predominantly led to severely elevated levels. Mutations in the lipoprotein lipase (LPL) gene further deteriorated lipoprotein levels and significantly increased the risk for cardiovascular disease (CVD) in FH patients. The D-variant in the gene for the angiotensine converting enzyme (ACE) was more frequent in FH patients with CAD, while the ID-genotype was associated with higher blood pressure. The TT-genotype of the microsomal triglyceride transfer protein (MTP) gene was associated with significantly lower LDL-cholesterol levels. Genetic variation in the genes coding for the cholesterylester transfer protein (CETP) and apolipoprotein E (apoE) was associated with variation in LDL-levels, with the Taq1B2- and apoE2-variants resulting in higher LDL-cholesterol levels. In patients with the apoE2-variant the frequency of cardiovascular disease was higher. A functional mutation (C677T) in the methylene-tetrahydrofolate reductase (MTHFR) gene was not associated with elevated homocysteine levels nor with CVD risk.

Conclusion: The phenotype of FH in terms of levels of LDL-cholesterol and CVD risk is determined by LDL-R mutation type and genetic variation in the genes coding for LPL, ACE, MTP, CETP and apoE.

The underlying gene in Tangier disease

S. Rust. *Institut für Arterioskleroseforschung, Münster, Germany*

Objective: One of the major features in homozygous Tangier disease is an almost complete deficiency of normal high density lipoprotein (HDL). Heterozygous relatives show half normal HDL values. As low HDL is a strong predictor of ischaemic heart disease and myocardial infarction, we aimed on identification and analysis of the gene underlying Tangier disease.

Methods: For chromosomal localization of Tangier disease a modified linkage analysis procedure was developed, the so-called traffic light scheme. Candidate genes were mapped to contigs of the resulting candidate region and sequenced in Tangier patients. The established contigs were furthermore exploited for analysis of the genomic structure of the final candidate gene.

Results: We identified the ABCA1 (also called ABC1) gene on chromosome 9q31 to be the Tangier disease gene. Sequencing revealed numerous mutations in ABCA1 in Tangier patients, some of them obviously destroying the function of the gene. The complete mRNA encoded by 50 exons and the promoter region were characterised.

Conclusions: The ABCA1 has an essential influence on HDL in Tangier patients and their heterozygous relatives and the codominant fashion of inheritance regarding this trait indicates a clear gene dosage effect. Thus, ABCA1 is a very promising target for an intervention that aims on improving so-called reverse cholesterol transport by increasing HDL. Our data provide the basis for developing such a strategy that is aimed on upregulation of ABCA1.

Phenotypic expression and pathophysiology of genetic cholesteryl ester transfer protein deficiency

K. Hirano. *Osaka University, Osaka, Japan*

Genetic deficiency of cholesteryl ester transfer protein (CETP), which was found in 1985 in Japan, is characterized by the marked elevation of HDL-cholesterol. We found various different mutations in the CETP gene, responsible for the majority of CETP-deficient patients. Their lipoprotein profiles were characterized by the presence of small polydisperse LDL as well as markedly large and cholesterol-rich HDL. These abnormal lipoproteins had such atherogenic biological property that the former had reduced affinity for LDL receptor and that the latter did not have ability to mediate cholesterol efflux. We found a unique area (Omagari, Japan) where a CETP gene mutation accumulates. In this area, prevalence of marked HALP was 10 times higher than in other areas of Japan and there was a U-shaped relationship between HDL-cholesterol levels and ischemic ECG changes. The quantification of carotid and aortic atherosclerosis determined by ultrasoundgraphy showed the significantly increased atherosclerotic area in the CETP-deficient patients, comparing with normolipidemic control subjects. Combined reduction of CETP and hepatic triglyceride lipase worsened the susceptibility for atherosclerosis in the patients. Recently, we have found the expression of CETP in both cultured human macrophages (Mf) and foam cells in the atherosclerotic lesions. Cholesterol efflux from Mf obtained from CETP deficiency was markedly reduced, whereas overexpression of CETP increased HDL-mediated cholesterol efflux from the cells. These findings indicate that CETP facilitates cholesterol efflux from the cells as well as transfer of CE between lipoproteins, suggesting that this molecule plays crucial roles in multiple steps of the reverse cholesterol transport (RCT). In conclusion, the genetic deficiency of CETP is expressed as an atherogenic phenotype resulted from the above impairments of RCT, even though those patients have very high plasma HDL-cholesterol levels.

Non-apoB related familial hypobetalipoproteinemia: Genetic and metabolic studies

Gustav Schonfeld, Rosalind Neuman, Bo Yuan, Bruce Patterson, Nizar Elias, Zhouji Chen. *Washington University-St. Louis, USA*

Virtually all of the well-characterized cases of FHBL are due to defects in the apoB gene on chromosome 2, specifying unnatural truncations or null alleles. In heterozygotes, both the normal apoB100 and the truncated apoBs circulate in plasma in greatly reduced concentrations. Metabolic studies in heterozygous humans indicate that low rates of production VLDLapoB are responsible. In some cases high fractional rates of catabolism of VLDLapoB also contibute. The limited low production of apoB100 is accompanied by reduced production rates of triglycerides. The latter may account for the reported cases of fatty liver in FHBL. Animal and cell culture studies confirm the human results, and further demonstrate that while the liver removes most of ciculating apoB100, renal proximal tubular cells remove most of the apoB truncations, mediated by the megalin receptor. However, the genetics of the vast majority of cases of FHBL remain unexplained. We report a FHBL kindred in which linkage to apoB, apoE, and MTP have been ruled out. Rather, we have identified a heretofore undetected candidate locus at 3p21.1-22. We used genome screening, followed by two-point and multi-point linkage calculations, using dichotomous or quantitative traits and a variety of parametric and non-parametric programs (e.g. GENEHUNTER, SOLAR, LOKI). In the affected members of this family, VLDLapoB100 production is reduced and LDLapoB100 (not VLDLapoB) fractional catabolic rates are increased. Thus, the genetic and metabolic bases of FHBL in this family differ from those in the apoB-linked families, demonstrating the heterogeneity of FHBL.

Investigation of a novel defect in patients with familial hypercholesterolaemia (FH): identification of a protein that binds to the cytoplasmic tail of the low density lipoprotein (LDL) receptor

J. Burden, E. Eden, X-M. Sun, A. Soutar. *Lipoprotein Group, MRC Clinical Sciences Centre, Hammersmith Hospital, London, UK*

Objective: To identify proteins involved in the internalisation of the LDL-receptor via clathrin-coated pits that might be defective in a novel form of familial hypercholesterolaemia in which LDL-receptor internalisation has been shown to be defective (Norman et al. J Clin Invest 1999;104:616–628).

Methods: The inducible Lex A-based yeast two hybrid system (Clontech) was used to screen a human liver cDNA library fused to a prey protein with a bait comprising the cytoplasmic tail of the human LDL receptor. Positive clones were re-tested, and the inserts amplified by PCR and identified by sequencing and database searching.

Results: Out of 35 positives, 16 different clones were probable false positives, six were identical to human pigment epithelium derived factor, and 13 were identical to a known cDNA for a hypothetical protein (Nomura et al. DNA Res 1994;1:223–229), which is predicted to have domains that suggest a possible role in receptor organisation. Mammalian cells transfected with this cDNA in pcDNA4/HISMAX (Invitrogen) expressed a soluble His-tagged protein of expected size. Mutations in the LDL receptor cytoplasmic tail known to influence internalisation reduced binding of the novel protein in the yeast two hybrid system. Northern analysis and cDNA sequencing show that the mRNA is normal in the patient's cells; this was confirmed by linkage analysis in the family.

Conclusion: A novel protein of previously unknown function has been identified that binds to the cytoplasmic tail of the LDL receptor. Preliminary evidence suggests that it may play some part in internalisation, but that it is not the defective gene in our patients with unusual phenotypic FH.

A novel molecular basis for genetic cholesteryl ester transfer protein (CETP) deficiency — G to A mutation in consensus ETS binding site at the promoter region of CETP gene

M. Nagano[1], M. Ito[1], Y. Sagehashi[1], H. Hattori[1], T. Egashira[1], K. Hirano[2], S. Yamashita[2], T. Maruyama[2], N. Nakajima[3], Y. Matsuzawa[2]. *[1]BML, Inc., Saitama; [2]Osaka University, Osaka; [3]Nakajima Clinic, Akita, Japan*

Genetic CETP deficiency is not associated with longevity, but rather pro-atherogenic, showing that this molecule plays a crucial role in reverse cholesterol transport, the major protective system against atherosclerosis. We heve reported various mutations at the coding region as well as exon/intron boundary in the CETP gene. In the present study, we have identified a novel mutation located at the promoter region.

Plasma concentrations of CETP were measured by the sandwich ELISA using two monoclonal antibodies specific for human CETP. 117 hyperalphalipoproteinemic (HALP) Japanese patients with low CETP levels were subjected. The entire coding region and all intron/exon boundaries as well as 186 bp promoter regions were sequenced. Activities of 165 bp wild type and mutated promoter regions were measured by the luciferase reporter gene assay in HepG2 cells.

Proband was an 18-year-old female with HALP. We have found a novel G to A substitution at nucleotide (nt) –69 in the promoter region of CETP gene, corresponding to the second nt of consensus ETS binding sequence (CGGAA) located just upstream of putative TATA box. Out of 117 subjects, four (3.4%) were revealed to be heterozygous. The allelic frequency was 0.0171 in patients with HALP. Family study suggested that this mutation had a dominant effect on plasma HDL-cholesterol levels. Luciferase reporter gene assay demonstrated that the mutated promoter appeared to lose transcriptional activity in HepG2 cells (5% of wild type).

The present results show a novel molecular mechanism for genetic CETP deficiency.

Overproduction of apoE in patients with type III hyperlipoproteinemia and in patients with other forms of hypertriglyceridemia

R. Batal, M. Tremblay, P.H.R. Barrett, H. Jacques, A. Fredenrich, O. Mamer, J. Davignon, J.S. Cohn. *Clinical Research Institute of Montreal, Quebec, Canada*

Objective: Recent studies in transgenic mice have shown that overexpression of human apoE results in hypertriglyceridemia (HTG) and increased secretion of VLDL-TG by the liver. The aim of the present study was to investigate the role of apoE overproduction in the etiology of human HTG.

Methods: The plasma kinetics of total, VLDL and HDL apoE were investigated in normolipidemic (NL) subjects (n = 5), HTG patients (pts., TG > 2.3 mmol/l, n = 5) and in pts. (n = 2) with type III (TypIII) hyperlipoproteinemia. Each subject, after an overnight fast, underwent a primed constant (12 h) infusion of stable-isotope labelled [D3]-leucine, and apoE kinetics were determined by multicompartmental analysis of apo. enrichment curves.

Results: HTG and TypIII pts. had reduced rates of VLDL apoB catabolism and no evidence of VLDL apoB overproduction. Elevated total plasma and VLDL apoE concs. in TypIII pts. (10- and 40-fold, respectively) were associated with reduced apoE catabolism, but also sig. elevated rates of apoE production. Similarly, HTG pts. (with 2- and 6-fold higher total and VLDL apoE levels) had significantly elevated apoE production rates — plasma apoE transport rates (TRs, mean ± SEM): (NL) 2.94 ± 0.78, (HTG) 5.80 ± 0.59 (p < 0.05), and (TypIII) 11.80 mg. kg-1.d-1; VLDL apoE TRs: (NL) 1.59 ± 0.18, (HTG) 4.52 ± 0.61 (p < 0.01), and (TypIII) 11.95 mg. kg-1.d-1. In fasted NL subjects, one-half of newly-synthesized apoE was found in VLDL and one-half was in HDL. In TypIII and HTG pts., more than 80% off newly-synthesized apoE was found in VLDL.

Conclusion: These results demonstrate that patients with TypIII HLP or HTG, having reduced rates of VLDL apoB-100 catabolism, are characterized by overproduction of plasma and VLDL apoE.

Management of cardiovascular risk in women

Coronary risk factors for atherosclerosis in women (CORA) a case-control study

B. Zyriax[2], H. Boeing[1], R. Fischer[2], P. Nielsen[2], E. Windler[2]. [1]*Universitäts-Krankenhaus Eppendorf, Hamburg;* [2]*Deutsches Institut für Ernährungsforschung, Bergholz-Rehbrücke, Germany*

Design: Population based case-control study. 200 women aged 30–80 years with incidental CHD and at least 200 population based controls free of CHD.

Objective: To define environmental (nutriton, lifestyle, anthropometry, hormones) and genetic risk factors predisposing particulary women for CHD.

Results: Preliminary results of the first 100 cases indicate that a waist-to-hip ratio of > 0.8 is a strong predictor for CHD risk at any age, while BMI is less powerful. This is in line with the findings that diabetes, elevated fasting C-peptide and low HDL are several fold more frequent in CHD patients. Also, hypertension is more frequent in cases, while elevated LDL is less predictive. Cases do smoke more often, but especially at older age of > 60 years.

Conclusions: These preliminary data point to the metabolic syndrome as the principle risk factor for CHD in women at any age. Interestingly smoking is more characteristic of older women with CHD. The results underline the importance of developing effective interventions and implementing general measures like hormone replacement therapy.

The effects of hormone replacement therapy on plasma homocysteine and C-reactive protein levels

A. Yildirir, F. Aybar, L. Tokgözöğlu, H. Yarali, G. Kabakçi, O. Bükülmez, İ. Sinici, İ. Ünsal, T. Gürgan, A. Oto. *Hacettepe University Faculty of Medicine, Ankara, Turkey*

Objective: To evaluate the effects of hormone replacement therapy (HRT) on plasma C reactive protein (CRP) and homocysteine levels.

Methods: Forty-six postmenopausal women (age 48 ± 5, range 40–60) were prospectively evaluated for the effects 6 months of HRT on lipid parameters, CRP and homocysteine levels. HRT regimens were continuos 0.625 mg/day conjugated equine estrogen (CEE) + 2.5 mg/day medroxyprogesterone acetate (MPA) or 0.625 mg/day CEE alone depending on the hysterectomy status.

	CEE (n = 16)		CEE + MPA (n = 30)	
	Pre	Post	Pre	Post
CRP (mg/dl)	0.66 ± 0.48	$0.81 \pm 0.35^*$	0.77 ± 0.64	0.88 ± 0.80
Homocysteine (μmol/l)	10.7 ± 4.9	$8.8 \pm 3.0^*$	12.0 ± 5.8	$9.1 \pm 3.2^{**}$
Cholesterol (mg/dl)	217 ± 41	224 ± 46	217 ± 42	215 ± 39
LDL (mg/dl)	132 ± 37	123 ± 34	125 ± 30	116 ± 26
HDL (mg/dl)	52 ± 7	$64 \pm 13^{**}$	60 ± 12	55 ± 12
Triglyceride (mg/dl)	121 ± 34	150 ± 82	137 ± 69	$188 \pm 88^{**}$

$^*p < 0.05$; $^{**}p < 0.01$. Compared to pretreatment value. Paired sample t-test.

Results: Estrogen alone significantly increased CRP levels, but the combination therapy did not have significant effect on CRP. However, the decrease in homocysteine levels was maintained with both regimens. The HDL increasing effect of estrogen was blunted by the addition of progesterone which also increased the triglycerides.

Conclusions: Plasma homocysteine levels were significantly reduced by both estrogen and the combined regimen. However, the increase in CRP levels due to estrogen was blunted by the addition of progesterone.

Hormone replacement therapy (HRT) reduces expression of cell adhesion molecules in healthy postmenopausal women

B. Gužič Salobir[1], I. Keber[1], I. Seljeflot[2], H. Arnesen[2], L. Vrabič[3]. [1]*University Clinical Center, Ljubljana;* [3]*Novo Nordisk A/S, Ljubljana, Slovenia; and* [2]*Ullevaal University Hospital, Oslo, Norway*

Objective: HRT may reduce the risk for atherosclerosis. One of the mechanisms could be the improvement of endothelial dysfunction as evaluated by circulation cell adhesion molecules (CAM), which are markers of dysfunctional endothelium. As the effect of norethisterone acetate (NETA) combined with estradiol has not been studied yet, we investigated the effect of this combination on the soluble CAM in healthy postmenopausal women.

Methods: Sixty-one healthy postmenopausal women (mean age 55 years) were randomly assigned to oral continuous combined HRT (estradiol 2 mg and NETA 1 mg/d) or placebo. The levels of estradiol and soluble forms of vascular cell adhesion molecule-1 (VCAM-1), intercellular cell adhesion molecule-1 (ICAM-1), E-selectin and P-selectin were determined before and after 3 and 6 month of therapy.

Results: Fifty-two women completed the study. According to the increases in estradiol levels we identified 22 women who responded adequately to HRT (R). The control group (C) consisted of 27 women with no change in estradiol. We found a significant decrease in ICAM-1 in R group compared to C group (278 vs. 289 before, 239 vs. 295 after 3 month and 226 vs. 301 ng/ml after 6 month of HRT; $p < 0.01$ for both). There was also a significant decrease in E-selectin (49.9 vs. 49.7 at the beginning, 37.1 vs. 50.8 after 3 months and 34.7 vs. 51.7 after 6 months for R and C group, respectively, $p < 0.01$ for both). The changes in VCAM-1 and P-selectin were smaller and nonsignificant.

Conclusions: Combined HRT of estradiol and NETA reduced the levels of some soluble CAM after 3 and 6 months in healthy postmenopausal women. These findings could indicate a less activated state of the endothelium with consequent reduced risk for atherosclerotic disease.

Index of authors